"An unusual—and unusually profound—self-help manual that teaches the application of ancient meditative techniques to modern living. . . . Kabat-Zinn here details the lessons of the course—from how to undertake a breathing-attentive 'sitting' meditation to how to apply insights gained to the obvious stresses of physical and emotional pain, as well as the more subtle stresses of work, other people, time pressure, etc.—the 'poignant enormity of our life experience.' "

—*Kirkus Reviews*

"In personable, enlightening prose, Kabat-Zinn first explains how to develop a meditation schedule, and in later chapters pragmatically applies his plan to the main sources of stress. An impressive middle section clearly marshals scientific and anecdotal evidence relating state of mind to state of health. And while emphasizing meditation's healing potential, Kabat-Zinn makes no sweeping claims, suggesting that the discipline serve not as a means but as an end."

—*Publishers Weekly*

Comments from graduates of the program:

"My bouts with severe pain remind me to practice what I learned in the stress clinic. And it still works!"

—Gladys McGauley, age 88

"The program saved my life."

—Gregg Hathaway, Leominster firefighter

"Meditation has become the fifteenth club in my golf bag."

—Bill Morrow, retired businessman

"Ten years after my initial experience with the Stress Reduction and Relaxation Program, which I attended after being diagnosed with cancer, I continue to practice, expanding my universe, enhancing wellness, balancing my emotions, and quickening my spirit. It is a powerful journey."

—Marie Sullivan, therapist

What referring physicians and other health professionals say about the clinic:

"I have found the stress reduction program invaluable in helping to manage stress and anxiety problems in my patients. Not only do the patients benefit from the program in the short term, they learn techniques to help them face future stressful situations more confidently. The nearly unanimous opinion of patients completing the program is that they feel they again can take charge of their own lives."

—Mary R. Hawthorne, M.D.
General Internal Medicine
Worcester, Massachusetts

"Dr. Jon Kabat-Zinn's meditative approach to stress reduction is the answer for the majority of our patients who present with stress-related symptoms or illnesses. This self-regulating modality helps people improve their coping skills in their work life. It is a necessary pressure relief valve in this era of increased productivity and expectations from employers."

—Thomas H. Winters, M.D.
Director, Medsite Occupational Health Center
Quincy, Massachusetts
Former Director, Primary Care
Clinic, U Mass Medical Center

"The usefulness of Dr. Kabat-Zinn's stress reduction program cannot be overestimated. I have had many patients for whom this program was the most important part of their therapeutic regimen."

—Joseph Alpert, M.D.
Director of Cardiovascular Medicine
U Mass Medical School

"I know the stress clinic works. It has helped my patients with chronic low back pain and neck pain many times over the past ten years plus."

—John J. Monahan, M.D.
Department of Orthopedics
U Mass Medical School

"I have sent innumerable patients to the Stress Reduction and Relaxation Program over the years and most have found it quite useful. It has allowed me to minimize the use of medications for many conditions, including hypertension, anxiety, arrhythmia, etc. I have utilized many of Dr. Kabat-Zinn's techniques in my practice of medicine as well as in dealing with my own hectic lifestyle."

—Bruce E. Gould, M.D.
Chief of Community Medicine
Mount Sinai Hospital
Hartford, Connecticut
Former Director, Primary Care
Clinic, U Mass Medical School

"The divisions between body, mind and spirit are not absolute, and the higher reaches of human consciousness can heal the lower. This book shows how this can be done. If you think harnessing the mind and spirit are complicated and painful, read this book and be surprised. It is a paragon of simplicity—full of gentle, caring instructions on reaching our highest potential. This book is not an experience in reading, but healing. It reflects great insight by someone who has been there."

—Larry Dossey, M.D.
Author of *Space, Time and Medicine*
and *Recovering the Soul*

"Based upon sound scientific research, his extensive clinical experience (at the University of Massachusetts Medical School), and practical instructions for the development of a personal stress management program, Dr. Jon Kabat-Zinn has distilled his tested program into an effective, emotionally moving, and compelling new book. Each person can draw upon Dr. Kabat-Zinn's extensive experience to develop their own unique approach to achieving an optimal state of mental, physical, spiritual, and environmental health."

—Kenneth R. Pelletier, Ph.D.
Author of *Mind as Healer, Mind as Slayer*
Associate Clinical Professor
of Medicine and Psychiatry
School of Medicine,
University of California, San Francisco

"*Full Catastrophe Living* represents a true breakthrough in the area of behavioral medicine and self-control. My recommendation for readers seeking relief from stress is to read *Full Catastrophe Living*. If you are looking for the best available book on this topic, this is it!"

—G. Alan Marlatt, Ph.D.
Professor of Psychology
Director of the Addictive Behaviors
Research Center
University of Washington

"Despite the spectacular advances in medical sciences in the 20th century, our patients continue to struggle with stress, pain and illness. Jon Kabat-Zinn has added the critical ingredient to our therapeutic armamentarium, self-control. His stress reduction program at the University of Massachusetts Medical Center has helped thousands of patients. His book, *Full Catastrophe Living*, will help people throughout the world to conquer stress, pain and illness."

—James E. Dalen, M.D., M.P.H.
Dean, College of Medicine
University of Arizona Health Sciences Center

FULL CATASTROPHE LIVING

Using the Wisdom
of Your Body and
Mind to Face Stress,
Pain, and Illness

**FIFTEENTH
ANNIVERSARY EDITION**

THE PROGRAM OF THE
STRESS REDUCTION CLINIC AT THE
UNIVERSITY OF MASSACHUSETTS
MEDICAL CENTER

Jon Kabat-Zinn, Ph.D.

DELTA TRADE PAPERBACKS

FULL CATASTROPHE LIVING
A Delta Book

PUBLISHING HISTORY
Delacorte Press hardcover edition published 1990
Delta trade paperback edition / July 1991
Delta trade paperback reissue / January 2005

Published by
Bantam Dell
A Division of Random House, Inc.
New York, New York

Library of Congress Catalog Card Number: 89-027829

ISBN 0-385-30312-2

Manufactured in the United States of America
Published simultaneously in Canada

BVG 35 34 33 32 31

for
Myla, Will, Naushon, and Serena

for
Sally and Elvin

and for the people in the stress clinic—past,
present, and future—who come to face
the full catastrophe and grow

This book describes the program of the Stress Reduction Clinic at the University of Massachusetts Medical Center. The content does not necessarily reflect the position or policy of the University of Massachusetts Medical Center, and no official institutional endorsement of the content should be inferred.

The recommendations made in this book are generic and are not meant to replace formal medical or psychiatric treatment. Individuals with medical problems should consult with their physicians about the appropriateness of following the program and discuss appropriate modifications relevant to their unique circumstances and condition.

CONTENTS

I
The Practice of Mindfulness: Paying Attention

‖ V
‖ The Way of Awareness

PREFACE

This very readable and practical book will be helpful in many ways. I believe many people will profit from it. Reading it, you will see that meditation is something that deals with our daily life. The book can be described as a door opening both on the dharma (from the side of the world) and on the world (from the side of the dharma). When the dharma is really taking care of the problems of life, it is true dharma. And this is what I appreciate most about the book. I thank the author for having written it.

THICH NHAT HANH
Plum Village, France
October 1989

FOREWORD

I still remember walking into a big conference room at the University of Massachusetts Medical School in the winter of 1981. There were about thirty people, young and old, sitting in a circle. The energy was expectant, electric, as the group gathered for the sixth in their series of eight stress reduction and relaxation sessions with Dr. Jon Kabat-Zinn. Faces that bore the telltale signs of chronic pain and stress—furrowed brows, clenched jaws, worried eyes—were beginning to soften and change. I remember one man in particular, a gentleman in his fifties, whose face was shining with the kind of wonder and curiosity that is so endearing in children. This man's delighted enthusiasm drew me right in. Although I had come to this session with a colleague, Dr. Ilan Kutz, as an "observer," I was eager to become a participant in the morning's events.

Before long we were all meditating, becoming progressively more aware of the exquisite interplay of subtle energies that create feelings of tension, pain, pleasure, and myriad other physical and emotional sensations. With consummate skill Jon led us out of the mind's tendency to hold on to the past and future and into the moment. We were invited to witness the ever-changing flow of our inner experience rather than to be carried away with the currents of our minds. As the observers and experiencers of life rather than its victims, we began to sense a radical power in this seemingly simple practice called mindfulness.

When we opened our eyes I was fully relaxed and absolutely amazed that forty-five minutes had passed! Although I had been meditating for over a decade, twenty minutes of meditation at home in the mornings often seemed like a long time. Yet, this room full of novice meditators—many of them chronic pain patients who had trouble sitting still to begin with—had committed to forty-five minutes a day of home practice. And in just a few weeks' time, many people were reporting remarkably positive changes in their relationship to their bodies and minds as well as to other people.

As the group began to ask questions and share experiences from their week of practice, Jon responded with a delightful no-nonsense blend of science, wisdom rooted in his own long practice of meditation, and refreshing common sense. It was clear that the group's commitment to practicing the meditation exercises was a reflection of Jon's own commitment. Here was a man with clarity and purpose who exuded a kind of confident strength that invited people to make an all-out effort in their own behalf. I thought to myself, "This guy doesn't pussyfoot around." As you read this book and experience the gentle strength in its pages, you will most likely come to the same conclusion. Jon asks of his reader the same radical commitment to self-awareness and self-acceptance that he asks of the people who come to the clinic. What makes him so effective as a teacher is that he asks no less of himself.

Ilan Kutz and I had first met Dr. Kabat-Zinn through our mutual interest in mind/body medicine and meditation practice. At the time, Dr. Kutz and I were both on the staff of the Division of Behavioral Medicine at Boston's Beth Israel Hospital under the direction of Dr. Herbert Benson, where we were conducting research and engaged in clinical practice. Dr. Kabat-Zinn had come to give a seminar about his results using mindfulness meditation training with groups of medical patients; he invited us to visit his clinic and share his experiences and resources in order to help us launch a similar effort. His program became both the inspiration and the model for the mind/body clinic that we established soon after at the Beth Israel.

Drawing from ancient traditions of self-inquiry and healing, Jon teaches meditation and hatha yoga as part of a comprehensive whole that is too often lost by focusing on just the physiological or even the psychological effects of the practices. Jon is really a teacher of wholeness—a spiritual concept whose wisdom has recently been harvested in medical and psychological studies that speak persuasively to the healing power of connectedness that Jon discusses in Part Two of this book. Which of us, in our heart of hearts, is unaware that those moments when we feel deeply connected to another person, to nature, or to the quiet stillness in our own being are deeply healing? To those of us willing to quest for wholeness, this book will be of enormous value. And as Jon so ably reminds us, the quest need not be lengthy. Wholeness is as close as the next breath—as the next moment we are willing to be fully aware of.

Jon's teaching of mindfulness remains true to the roots of the venerable tradition that spawned it some 2,500 years ago. Then, as now, people faced the suffering associated with sickness, old age, poverty, death, and the inevitability of change whose insistent tendrils seek out the edifices we have so carefully wrought and return them once again to dust. Then, as now, people sought help in living what Jon calls the "full catastrophe" of life. Mindfulness is more than a meditation practice that can have profound medical and psychological benefits; it is also a way of life that reveals the gentle and loving wholeness that lies at the heart of our being, even in times of great pain and suffering. The success of his program comes in part from its unique synthesis of East and West—of meditation and yoga with science and mainstream medicine—and in part out of Jon's gift for making the meditation and the science exciting and clearly relevant to our health and the quality of our lives. I am glad that Jon has now written an in-depth book about his clinic. It provides us with profoundly healing principles and practices that couldn't be more timely or more needed in today's stressful world.

JOAN BORYSENKO, PH.D.
president of Mind/Body Health Sciences, Inc.,
author of *Minding the Body, Mending the Mind*
and *Guilt Is the Teacher, Love Is the Lesson*

ACKNOWLEDGMENTS

Many people contributed directly and indirectly to this book. Without the faith and support of Tom Winters, M.D., Hugh Fulmer, M.D., and John Monahan, M.D., the stress clinic would never have existed. James E. Dalen, M.D., Chief of Medicine at UMMC until 1988 and now dean of the University of Arizona College of Medicine, was an early and staunch supporter. Judith K. Ockene, Ph.D., director of the Division of Preventive and Behavioral Medicine at the University of Massachusetts Medical School, has given continuing support and encouragement over the years and throughout the writing of this book, for which I am deeply grateful. Her endless warmth of heart and her generosity are all too rare for people in leadership positions. Dr. Ockene believes not only in the importance of encouraging her colleagues to exercise imagination, intuition, and creativity in their own work—she actually makes the psychic space available for them to do so.

I would also like to thank the more than five hundred physicians at the University of Massachusetts Medical Center and in the greater New England community who have referred their patients to the stress reduction clinic over the past ten years. Their faith in the clinic and, above all, in their patients' abilities to grow, change, and, ultimately, to influence the course of their own health as a complement to their medical treatment sets an essential tone for our efforts to help their patients to mobilize their own inner resources for healing.

A number of people read this book in part or in its entirety at various stages of the writing and gave me wise editing advice, helpful criticism, and practical suggestions. Their candid views helped me to probe more deeply and ask myself what I really wanted to convey. Myla Kabat-Zinn contributed enormously through her sensitivity to excesses and to lapses in clarity and by her keen sense of what works on the printed page and what doesn't. Saki Santorelli, M.A., the associate director of the clinic, provided many helpful suggestions and much encouragement. Since we have shared this work daily over the past seven years, Saki was able to indicate where I was accurately portraying the spirit of the clinic and where I was introducing distortions or leaving out key points. Sarah Doering, David Breakstone, and Canan Avunduk, M.D., also read and critiqued the whole manuscript at various stages and offered key suggestions, insights, and editorial advice that greatly improved the final work.

Larry Rosenberg, Phil Hunt, John Miller, M.D., Jean Kristeller, Ph.D., Linda Peterson, M.D., Ann Massion, M.D., Judith K. Ockene, Ph.D., James Hebert, Ph.D., Joel Weinberger, Ph.D., Eric Kolvig, Ph.D., Tony Schwartz, and Alan Shapiro read and critiqued portions of the book or individual chapters and offered important insights and suggestions. At an earlier stage, Frank Urbanowski, Ray Montgomery, and Daniel Goleman were extremely helpful in advising me about the book proposal and in their enthusiasm for the project.

My editor, Bob Miller, believed there was a book here from the moment he first read about mindfulness and the stress clinic. With clarity, great skill, and a keen editorial perspective, he shepherded the book through to completion and made the process a pleasure and an adventure. His kindness and gentleness and his willingness to let me participate in decision-making at all levels are profoundly appreciated.

I also thank my formal and informal teachers for being who they are and for the many gifts they have bestowed on me. Some I have known only through their writings or at a distance. Many I count as my closest friends. Above all, I acknowledge my live-in teachers—Myla, my soulmate, and my children, Will, Naushon, and Serena—who mirror the teaching of moment-to-moment awareness back to me each day in their love and the luminosity of their being and continually challenge me to be my best, that is, my most relaxed and mindful self. For too long they patiently and generously made room in their lives for me to work on this project, enduring endless book talk and long periods when my attention was not all there for them.

I also acknowledge my gratitude to my very first teachers, my parents, Sally and Elvin Kabat. They gave me and continue to give me far more than they know or that I can express in words. We have been blessed with a mostly joy-filled unfolding of mutual love and caring in our years together. With my brothers Geoffrey and David and their families, we continue to explore what it means to be a family and to share and marvel in the complex and sometimes difficult bonds of the past and present. On the other side of the family, my in-laws, Roslyn and Howard Zinn, have also long been teachers and friends and I have benefited greatly from their loving support and encouragement. I am also deeply grateful to my dharma brother, Larry Rosenberg, for his friendship and love and for his many gentle teachings during our shared adventures in meditation and in living over the past twenty-five years.

I am greatly indebted to many other teachers as well: to the late Alfred Satterthwaite of Haverford College, who taught me a love of writing; to Salvador Luria, Victor Weiskopf, and Huston Smith of MIT days and beyond, who taught me a love of science and the importance of taking responsibility for its social, philosophical, and spiritual implications; to Philip Kapleau, for *The Three Pillars of Zen* and for coming to MIT to conduct meditation retreats among the scientists, where he influenced at least one; to John Lauder, a genius of a yoga teacher, for his wonderfully understated classes in the basement of the church in Harvard Square more than twenty years ago; to Ram Dass and the Lama Foundation for the mysterious cardboard box filled with wonderful things to explore, including *Be Here Now*, which someone gave to me one day in the desert in New Mexico; to Swami Chinmayananda for his marvelous energy and example and his love for the Bhagavad Gita; to J. Krishnamurti for his uncompromising integrity and insistence on the need to chart one's own spiritual course and not someone else's; to Suzuki Roshi for his beginner's mind and his cow pasture; to Zen Master Seung Sahn, who, as Stephen Mitchel says in the dedication to his book of sacred poems, *The Enlightened Heart*, also taught me everything I don't know; to Quan Ja Nim, who taught the mind sword path; to Thich Nhat Hanh for his gentleness of being, for his unwavering and total commitment to healing the deep psychic wounds of the Vietnam War and those we incur simply in being alive, for the title of Chapter 8, which comes from *The Miracle of Mindfulness*, and for his gentle teachings of mindfulness and peacefulness; to Corrado Pensa for the clarity of his view of meditation practice; to Jack Kornfield (who first gave me raisins to eat mindfully, much as the old man gave Jack the three magic beans that grew to be a beanstalk), Joseph Goldstein, Sharon Salzberg, Christopher Titmus, and Christina Feldman (from whom I first learned the value of differentiating between reacting and responding), teachers at the Insight Meditation Society, all of whom have given me periodic refuge and much guidance over the past fifteen years and set a shining example in their deep commitment to the practice and in the generosity of their own hearts; to Ken Pelletier for his trailblazing efforts in bringing together the domains of science, medicine, and meditation; to Roger Walsh for his brilliant articulation of the new paradigm in the behavioral sciences and his equally brilliant efforts in voicing the urgency of our ecological dilemma and our need to transcend our precocious intelligence for the sake of planetary survival; to Ken Wilbur for the jewel of *No Boundary* and his vast wisdom and penetrating intellect; to Dan Brown, for his efforts to bring together science and meditation and for advising me on how to begin outcome studies in the clinic; to Robert Bly, poet/shaman/wild man extraordinaire, for his vision and example of what it means and takes to be a man in these times and whose love and kindness have touched me deeply; to Dean Ornish for his belief in the reversibility of coronary disease through life-style change and his single-minded efforts to demonstrate scientifically that this was so; and to Joan Borysenko for her staunch willingness to grow no matter what, to face and transcend pain if that is what it takes, and for the keenness of her intellect and the kindness and purity of her heart.

I also acknowledge the support and warm collegiality of a number of people, past and present, at the University of Massachusetts Medical Center: Michael Weiss, M.P.A., JoAnn Scott, Leigh Emery, R.N., M.S., Sylvia Spencer, Karen Pye, John Agasian, Bill Stickley, Ph.D., Sarah Jane Williams, John Nespoli, Keith Waterbrook, Joseph Alpert, M.D., Robert Burney, M.D., Leslie Lipworth, M.D., William Sellers, M.D., Ira Ockene, M.D., James Rippe, M.D., Jim Michaels, R.P.T., Thomas Edwards, M.D., Debbie Hannah, R.N., Nilima Patwardhen, M.D., H. Brownell Wheeler, M.D., John Paraskos, M.D., Jeffrey Bernhard, M.D., Richard Irwin, M.D., Cindy French, M.R.N., Fred Curley, M.D., Steven Baker, Ph.D., Elizabeth Kabachenski, L.P.N., Carolyn Appel, L.P.N., Joan Goyette, L.P.N., Thea Ashkenaze, Doreen Kupstas, and Pat Walsh. All have contributed to the work of the stress clinic over the years in important ways. I am also indebted to Beth Maynard for her fine artwork for the book, to Annie Skillings for her tireless and good-natured help with data analysis for our many research studies, and to a generous anonymous donor for major funding to support our research efforts in the clinic.

I wish to express deep gratitude and respect for my past and present colleagues in the stress clinic: Peggy Roggenbuck-Gillespie, Larry Rosenberg, and Trudy Goodman, who taught in the program in the early years; Brian Tucker, the clinic's first secretary; Norma Rosiello, the heart, soul, and voice of the clinic, who came as a pain patient and, when she finished the program, occasionally took time off from her work as a hairdresser to help out in the office, and has now been working full-time in the clinic for more than six years, in the course of which she learned to type, do word processing, and anticipate the immediate future like a wizard; Kathy Brady, who also came first as a patient, started volunteering in the office, and made a job for herself, putting her kind heart and her thoughtfulness and organizational skills to work for the benefit of patients and staff alike; Saki Santorelli, M.A., my close friend and colleague, who selflessly took more work upon himself so that I might have time to write, and whose compassion and concern for patients and staff alike is immeasurable, matched only by his skill as a teacher; Elana Rosenbaum, L.I.C.S.W., whose heart is immense and completely available for her patients; and Kacey Carmichael, B.A., who loves the work and brings her whole being to it. Each has given me great support and shared his or her wisdom and caring with me as I devoted myself to this project. I am continually grateful for the way we manage to work together as a family, meditating before meetings and allowing our work to be above all an expression of meditation in action.

And finally I thank all the people in the stress clinic who shared their stories with us and consented to let them appear in this book. They did so expressing a virtually unanimous hope that their personal experiences with the meditation practice might help inspire others who suffer from similar problems to find peace and relief in their lives.

FULL CATASTROPHE
LIVING

INTRODUCTION TO THE
═══15TH ANNIVERSARY EDITION═══

It is now fifteen years since this book was published, and I am grateful to Dell and Random House for reissuing it in this new format. My hopes and intentions in writing it in the first place haven't changed in the intervening years. They have only grown stronger. Being about intimacy with the present moment, the practice of mindfulness is not bound by time. For this reason alone, its applicability to the human condition and to the rich potential of our minds and bodies for facing stress, pain, and illness with the deep wisdom that we are capable of as human beings is not likely to diminish with the passage of time.

Nevertheless, harking back to 1990, when this book first appeared, the world has changed hugely, unthinkably, in the years since, perhaps more than it has ever changed before in such a brief interval. Just think of laptops, cell phones, the Internet, the impact of the digital revolution on just about everything, and the speed-up of the pace of life and our 24/7 lifestyles, to say nothing of the huge social, economic, and political changes that have occurred globally during this period. The speed at which things are changing nowadays is not likely to slow, and its effects will be increasingly felt and will be increasingly unavoidable. You could say that the revolution in science and technology and its effects on the way we live our lives has hardly gotten started. Certainly the stress of adjusting to it on top of everything else will only mount in the coming decades.

My original objective in writing this book was that it might serve as an effective counterbalance to all the ways we get pulled out of ourselves and wind up losing sight of what is most important. We are apt to get so caught up in the urgency of everything we have to do, and so caught up in our heads and in what we *think* is important, that it is easy to fall into a state of chronic tension and anxiety that continually drives our lives on automatic pilot. This stress is only compounded when we are faced with a serious medical condition, with chronic pain or a chronic disease.

The way of being described here, which emerges naturally

out of the cultivation and practice of mindfulness, can serve as a doorway into a profound way of knowing ourselves better and for mobilizing the inner resources we all have, no matter what our situation and our condition, for learning, for growing, for healing, and for transformation across the life span, starting from where we find ourselves, no matter where or how that is.

Given the changes we have experienced in the past fifteen years and those we will undoubtedly find ourselves facing in the future, mindfulness is now more relevant than ever as an effective and dependable counterbalance to insure and strengthen our health and well-being, and perhaps our very sanity.

For while we are now blessed with "24/7 connectivity" so we can be in touch with anybody anywhere at any time, we may be finding, ironically enough, that it is more difficult than ever to actually be in touch with ourselves. What is more, we may feel that we have less time in which to do it, although each of us still gets the same twenty-four hours a day as everybody else. It's just that we fill up those hours with so much doing, we scarcely have time for being anymore, or even for "catching our breath."

The first chapter of this book is called *You Have Only Moments to Live*. It is still true, and it will continue to be true, for all of us. Yet so much of the time, we are out of touch with the richness of the present moment, and the fact that inhabiting this moment, our only moment, with greater awareness shapes the moment that follows, and if we can sustain it, actually shapes the future and the quality of our lives and relationships in ways we often simply do not appreciate. The only way we have of influencing the future is to own the present, however we find it. Then we just might find ways to live the life that is actually ours to live.

Another aim in writing this book was to make mindfulness and meditation understandable and commonsensical for regular people, all of us really, because all of us, having minds and bodies, suffer inevitably from one aspect or another of the human condition. We are all subject to old age, illness, and death. The real question, and the real adventure, is how do we *live* our lives while we have the chance? And how do we work with what comes our way in ways that are healing, that nourish us deeply, and that make use of the full spectrum of our experiences, the good, the bad, and the ugly, Zorba's full catastrophe? Can we experience joy and satisfaction as well as suffering? What about being at home in our own skin within the maelstrom? What about tasting ease of well-being, and even genuine happiness? Thousands of people have found the path described here to be helpful in dealing with their own version of the full catastrophe, medical or otherwise. Many have personally communicated with me to say that the practice of mindfulness "saved my life" or "gave me back to myself."

I never tire of hearing this, and I never take it for granted. To me, it is a confirmation of how much we humans are miraculous beings, and how creative and imaginative we are when we nurture what is deepest and best in ourselves with kindness, self-compassion, and patience. Clearly, we are all in this together. Mindfulness is not merely a good idea or a nice philosophy. It is something we need to embody moment by moment for ourselves, if it is to have any value for us at all. And that requires practice on the part of all of us who care.

◆

A great deal has happened on so many fronts since this book first appeared. For one, the Stress Reduction Clinic described here, now under the direction of my long-time colleague and friend, Dr. Saki Santorelli, continues to thrive, thanks in large measure to his remarkable leadership through a very difficult time in medicine. In September 2004, the clinic celebrated its twenty-fifth year in continual operation. Over 16,000 medical patients have completed its eight-week program. The present teachers and staff of the clinic are unsurpassed in their devotion to articulating the practice of mindfulness effectively, in the quality of the work they do, and in the profound effects they have on the people who take the program in helping them to know themselves better and grow more fully into themselves to whatever degree might be possible. And my colleagues and I have deep gratitude for all the past MBSR instructors and staff who contributed to the successes of the CFM over the years.

In the past fifteen years, the work described in this book has spread to hospitals, medical centers, and clinics around the world, in part thanks to its having been featured in the Public Television Special, *Healing and the Mind, with Bill Moyers* in 1993, as well as in many other television programs and articles in the media. That work is now known as *mindfulness-based stress reduction,* or MBSR. Since 1995, the Stress Reduction Clinic has been nested within the Center for Mindfulness in Medicine, Health Care, and Society (CFM) at UMass. The CFM offers MBSR programs in schools and businesses in addition to our work with medical patients, and a series of programs for training interested health professionals. The CFM also houses our ongoing research program.

From 1992 to 1999, we ran a free MBSR clinic in the inner city in Worcester, with free onsite mindful childcare, free transportation, and in which classes were taught in Spanish as well as in English. This clinic and the hundreds of people it served demonstrated the universality of MBSR and its adaptability to multicultural settings. We also conducted a four-year program for inmates and staff of the Massachusetts Department of Corrections, and demonstrated an ability to reach large numbers of inmates with MBSR and reduce measures of hostility and stress. One of our colleagues trained both the Chicago Bulls and then the Los Angeles Lakers in mindfulness during some of their champion seasons. You can find out more about the CFM and the Stress Reduction Clinic, its professional training opportunities, and where MBSR programs that we know about are located around the world by visiting the CFM's website at *www.umassmed.edu/cfm.*

Much has happened in medicine in the past fifteen years. For one, mind/body approaches to healing have become far more accepted and widespread than they were in 1990. Research exploring MBSR in particular has blossomed, and there are now over one hundred scientific papers on aspects of the clinical applications of mindfulness, and the number is growing rapidly.

The study I describe in Chapter 13 on the effect of meditation on people with the skin disease psoriasis undergoing ultraviolet light treatments was replicated and the results published in 1998. In that study, we found that the meditators healed at approximately four times the rate of the non-meditating control group.[1]

In another study, in collaboration with Dr. Richard

---

[1] Kabat-Zinn, J., Wheeler, E., Light, T., Skillings, A., Scharf, M., Cropley, T.G., Hosmer, and Bernhard, J. Influence of a mindfulness-based stress reduction intervention on rates of skin clearing in patients with moderate to severe psoriasis undergoing phototherapy (UVB) and photochemotherapy (PUVA). *Psychosomatic Medicine* (1998) 60:625-632.

Davidson and his colleagues at the University of Wisconsin, that looked at the effects of MBSR delivered in a corporate setting during working hours with healthy but stressed employees rather than with medical patients, we found that over the eight weeks of the program, the electrical activity in certain areas of the brain that are known to be involved in the expression of emotions (within the prefrontal cerebral cortex) shifted in the MBSR participants in a direction that suggested that the meditators were handling emotions such as anxiety and frustration more effectively, in ways that we now think of as emotionally more intelligent, than the control subjects, who were not taking the program but were going into the lab to go through all the testing. We also found that when we gave all the people in the study a flu shot, the meditation group mounted a significantly stronger antibody response in their immune system than did the controls, and showed a significant linear relationship between the amount of brain shift in a positive direction and the amount of antibody production. No such relationship was found in the control group.[2] More research with mindfulness along these and other lines is currently underway, and a great deal more is in the planning stages.

The fields of mind/body and integrative medicine have come into their own since the writing of this book. Integrative Medicine is the umbrella term we now use to cover mind/body healing approaches as well as all other scientifically supported therapeutic modalities in what is sometimes referred to as complementary and alternative medicine (CAM). There is now an Academic Consortium on Integrative Medicine, which has representatives of twenty-two medical schools in the U.S. and Canada, and the number is rapidly growing. There is a general agreement among practitioners of integrative medicine that mindfulness itself forms the "container" for this discipline. Without mindfulness and the nonjudgmental "presencing" it encourages and nurtures in health-care practitioners, the sacred dimension of the practitioner-patient relationship is all too easily eroded or lost, and the profound potential of each human being for learning, growing, healing, and personal transforma-

---

[2] Davidson, R.J., Kabat-Zinn, J., Schumacher, J. Rosenkranz, M.S., Muller, D., Santorelli, S.F., Urbanowski, F., Harrington, A., Bonus, K., and Sheridan, J.F. Alterations in brain and immune function produced by mindfulness meditation, *Psychosomatic Medicine* (2003) 65:564-570.

tion across the life span either ignored or unwittingly actively thwarted.

◆

Much has happened in the world itself since 1990. Some of the places where we wept for the world in those days are named here at various points in the text: South Africa, Cambodia, El Salvador, Northern Ireland, Chile, Nicaragua, Bolivia, Ethiopia, the Philippines, Beirut, Jerusalem. In 2005, there is no longer a Soviet Union, or an East Germany, a Yugoslavia, or a Czechoslovakia. There are now many more independent countries in Europe and Asia. Yet the global suffering continues in the places originally cited, as well as others with names like Rwanda, Bosnia, Herzegovina, Kosovo, East Timor, places and names that have already come and gone from the news. The date September 11, 2001, along with Afghanistan, Iraq, Darfur, Chechnya, Beslan, Gaza, and the West Bank could be added to the list and we all would instantly nod our heads in recognition of the magnitude of what has been unfolding in the interim. What we have called here "world stress" has only grown over the intervening years, and while the salient names that dominate our news and foreign policy have changed and will continue to change, the themes are depressingly familiar, and the weeping goes on even in the face of all the beauty and good that has also been unfolding during that time. The world itself is weeping and begs for us to bring an entirely different level of attention and resolve to its suffering, based on our inherent beauty, goodness, and creative imagination as human beings. Perhaps mindfulness can play a significant role in the healing not only of ourselves but also of our world in ways little and big, and yet to be imagined.

◆

More and more, mindfulness meditation has made its way into the mainstream of society during the past fifteen plus years. More and more people are adopting this simple route toward greater sanity and well-being for themselves. Mindfulness meditation is becoming increasingly a natural part of the American landscape, and it is in that atmosphere and spirit that I welcome you to this edition of *Full Catastrophe Living*.

The text of the book has not changed, aside from the addition of this new Introduction, an updated reading list in the Appendix, and a broader offering of my guided meditation tapes and CDs to support, enhance, and deepen your personal practice of mindfulness meditation. These are now available by direct order on the Internet, as described on the last page of the book.

May your mindfulness practice grow and flower and nourish your life and work from moment to moment and from day to day.

JON KABAT-ZINN
September 21, 2004

INTRODUCTION

Stress, Pain, and Illness: Facing the Full Catastrophe

This book is an invitation to the reader to embark upon a journey of self-development, self-discovery, learning, and healing. It is based on ten years of clinical experience with over four thousand people who have begun this lifelong journey via their participation in an eight-week course known as the Stress Reduction and Relaxation Program (SR&RP) at the University of Massachusetts Medical Center. The SR&RP—or stress clinic, as it is often called—is a new kind of clinic in a new branch of medicine known as behavioral medicine, which believes that mental and emotional factors, the ways in which we think and behave, can have a significant effect, for better or worse, on our physical health and on our capacity to recover from illness and injury.

The people who embark on this journey in the stress clinic do so in an effort to regain control of their health and to attain at least some peace of mind. They come referred by their doctors for a wide range of medical problems ranging from headaches, high blood pressure, and back pain to heart disease, cancer, and AIDS. They are young and old and in-between. What they learn in the stress clinic is the *how* of taking care of themselves, not as a replacement for their medical treatment but as a vitally important complement to it.

Over the years numerous people have made inquiries about how they can learn what our patients learn in this eight-week course, which amounts to an intensive self-directed training program in the art of conscious living. This book is a response to those inquiries. It is meant to be a practical guide for anyone, well or ill, who seeks to transcend his or her limitations and move toward greater levels of health and well-being.

1

The SR&RP is based on rigorous and systematic training in mindfulness, a form of meditation originally developed in the Buddhist traditions of Asia. Simply put, mindfulness is moment-to-moment awareness. It is cultivated by purposefully paying attention to things we ordinarily never give a moment's thought to. It is a systematic approach to developing new kinds of control and wisdom in our lives, based on our inner capacities for relaxation, paying attention, awareness, and insight.

The stress clinic is not a rescue service in which people are passive recipients of support and therapeutic advice. Rather it is a vehicle for active learning, in which people can build on the strengths that they already have and come to do something for themselves to improve their own health and well-being.

In this learning process we assume from the start that as long as you are breathing, there is more right with you than there is wrong, no matter how ill or how hopeless you may feel. But if you hope to mobilize your inner capacities for growth and for healing and to take charge in your life on a new level, a certain kind of effort and energy on your part will be required. The way we put it is that it can be stressful to take the Stress Reduction Program.

I sometimes explain this by saying that there are times when you have to light one fire to put out another. There are no drugs that will make you immune to stress or to pain or that will by themselves magically solve your life's problems or promote healing. It will take conscious effort on your part to move in a direction of healing and inner peace. This means learning to work with the very stress and pain that is causing you to suffer.

The stress in our lives is now so great and so insidious that more and more people are making the deliberate decision to understand it better and to bring it under personal control. They realize the futility of waiting for someone else to make things better for them. Such a personal commitment is all the more important if you are suffering from a chronic illness or disability that imposes additional stress in your life on top of the usual pressures of living.

The problem of stress does not admit to simpleminded solutions or quick fixes. At root, stress is a natural part of living from which there is no more escape than from the human condition itself. Yet some people try to avoid stress by walling themselves off from life experience; others attempt to anesthetize themselves one way or another to escape it. Of course, it is only sensible to avoid undergoing unnecessary pain and hardship. Certainly we all need to distance ourselves from our troubles now and again. But if escape and avoidance become our habitual ways of dealing with our problems, the problems just multiply. They don't magically go away. What does go away, or get covered over when we tune out our problems or run away from them, is our power to grow and to change and to heal. When it comes right down to it, facing our problems is usually the only way to get past them.

There is an art to facing difficulties in ways that lead to effective solutions and to inner peace and harmony. When we are able to mobilize our inner resources to face our problems artfully, we find we are usually able to orient ourselves in such a way that we can use the pressure of the problem itself to propel us through it, just as a sailor can position a sail to make the best use of the pressure of the wind to propel the boat. You can't sail straight into the wind, and if you only know how to sail with the wind at your back, you will only go where the wind blows you. But if you know how to use the wind's energy and are patient, you can sometimes get where you want to go. You can still be in control.

If you hope to make use of the force of your own problems to propel you in this way, you will have to be tuned in, just as the sailor is tuned in to the feel of the boat, the water, the wind, and his or her course. You will have to learn how to handle yourself under all kinds of stressful conditions, not just when the weather is sunny and the wind blowing exactly the way you want it to.

We all accept that no one controls the weather. Good sailors learn to read it carefully and respect its power. They will avoid storms if possible, but when caught in one, they know when to take down the sails, batten down the hatches, drop anchor, and ride things out, controlling what is controllable and letting go of the rest. Training, practice, and a lot of firsthand experience in all sorts of weather are required to develop such skills so that they work for you when you need them. Developing skill in facing and effectively handling the various "weather conditions" in your life is what we mean by the art of conscious living.

The issue of control is central to coping with problems and with stress. There are many forces at work in the world that are totally beyond our control and others that we sometimes think are beyond our control but really aren't. To a great extent, our ability to influence our circumstances depends on how we see things. Our beliefs about ourselves and about our own capabilities as well as how we see the world and the forces at play in it all affect what we will find possible. How we see things affects how much energy we have for doing things and our choices about where to channel what energy we do have.

For instance, at those times when you are feeling overwhelmed by the pressures in your life and you see your own efforts as ineffectual, in all likelihood you will wind up feeling depressed and helpless. Nothing will seem controllable or even worth trying to control. On the other hand, at those times when you are seeing the world as threatening but only potentially overwhelming, then feelings of insecurity rather than depression may predominate, causing you to worry incessantly about all the things you think threaten or might threaten your sense of control. These could be real or imagined; it hardly matters in terms of the stress you will feel and the effect it will have on your life.

Feeling threatened can easily lead to feelings of anger and hostility and from there to outright aggressive behavior, driven by deep instincts to protect your position and maintain your sense of things being under control. When things do feel "under control," we might feel content for a moment. But when they go out of control again, or even *seem* to be getting out of control, our deepest insecurities can erupt. At such times we might even act in ways that are self-destructive and hurtful to others. And we will feel anything but content.

If you have a chronic illness or a disability that prevents you from doing what you used to be able to do, whole areas of control may go up in smoke. And if your condition causes you physical pain that has not responded well to medical treatment, the distress you might be feeling can be compounded by emotional turmoil caused by knowing that your condition seems to be beyond even your doctor's control.

What is more, our worries about control are hardly limited to our major life problems. Some of our biggest stresses actually come from our reactions to the smallest, most insignificant events when they threaten our sense of control in one way or another, from the car breaking down just when you have someplace important to go, to your children not listening to you for the tenth time in as many minutes, to the lines being "too long" at the supermarket checkout or at the bank.

It is not easy to find a word or phrase that really captures the broad range of experiences in life that cause us distress and pain and that promote in us an underlying sense of fear, insecurity, and loss of control. If we were to make a list, it would certainly include our own vulnerability and mortality. It might also include our collective capacity for cruelty and violence, as well as the colossal levels of ignorance and greed, delusion and deception, that seem to drive us and the world much of the time. What could we possibly call the sum total of our vulnerabilities and inadequacies, our limitations and weaknesses as people, the illnesses and injuries and disabilities we may have to live with, the personal defeats and failures we have felt or fear in the future, the injustices and exploitations we suffer or fear, the losses of people we love and of our own bodies sooner or later? It would have to be a metaphor that would not be maudlin, something that would also convey the understanding that it is not a disaster to be alive just because we feel fear and we suffer; it would have to convey the understanding that there is joy as well as suffering, hope as well as despair, calm as well as agitation, love as well as hatred, health as well as illness.

In groping to describe that aspect of the human condition that the patients in the stress clinic and, in fact, most of us, at one time or another, need to come to terms with and in some way transcend, I keep coming back to one line from the movie of Nikos Kazantzakis's novel *Zorba the Greek*. Zorba's young companion turns to him at a certain point and inquires, "Zorba, have you ever been married?" to which Zorba replies (paraphasing somewhat) "Am I not a man? Of course I've been married. Wife, house, kids, everything . . . *the full catastrophe!*"

It was not meant to be a lament, nor does it mean that being married or having children is a catastrophe. Zorba's response embodies a supreme appreciation for the richness of life and the inevitability of all its dilemmas, sorrows, tragedies, and ironies. His way is to "dance" in the gale of the full catastrophe, to celebrate life, to laugh with it and at himself, even in the face of personal failure and defeat. In doing so, he is never weighed down for long, never ultimately defeated either by the world or by his own considerable folly.

Anybody who knows the book can imagine that living with Zorba must in itself have been quite the "full catastrophe" for his wife and children. As is so often the case, the public hero that others admire can leave quite a trail of private hurt in his wake. Yet ever since I first heard it, I have felt that the phrase "the full catastrophe" captures something positive about the human spirit's ability to come to grips with what is most difficult in life and to find within it room to grow in strength and wisdom. For me, facing the full catastrophe means finding and coming to terms with what is most human in ourselves. There is not one person on the planet who does not have his or her own version of the full catastrophe.

Catastrophe here does not mean disaster. Rather it means the poignant enormity of our life experience. It includes crises and disaster but also all the little things that go wrong and that add up. The phrase reminds us that life is always in flux, that everything we think is permanent is actually only temporary and constantly changing. This includes our ideas, our opinions, our relationships, our jobs, our possessions, our creations, our bodies, everything.

In this book we will be learning and practicing the art of embracing the full catastrophe. We will be doing this so that rather than destroying us or robbing us of our power and our hope, the storms of life will strengthen us as they teach us about living, growing, and healing in a world of flux and change and sometimes great pain. This art will involve learning to see ourselves and the world in new ways, learning to work in new ways with our bodies and our thoughts and feelings and perceptions, and learning to laugh at things a little more, including ourselves, as we practice finding and maintaining our balance as best we can.

In our era the full catastrophe is very much in evidence on all fronts. A brief reading of any morning newspaper will drive home the impression of an unending stream of human suffering and misery in the world, much of it inflicted by one human being or group of human beings on another. If you listen with an attentive ear to what you hear on radio or television news programs, you will find yourself assaulted daily by a steady barrage of terrible and heartbreaking images of human violence and misery, reported in the matter-of-fact tones of broadcast journalism, as if the suffering and death of people in South Africa, Cambodia, El Salvador, Northern Ireland, Chile, Nicaragua, Bolivia, Ethiopia, the Philippines, in Beirut or Jerusalem or Paris or Beijing or Boston were just part of the prevailing climatic conditions that follow in the same matter-of-fact tones, without so much as a nod to the incomprehensible juxtaposition of the two.

Even if we don't read or listen to or watch the news, we are never far from the full catastrophe of living. The pressures we feel at work and at home, the problems we run into and the frustrations we feel, the balancing and juggling that is required to keep our heads above water in this fast-paced world are all part of it. We might extend Zorba's list to include not only wife or husband, house and children, but also work, paying the bills, parents, lovers, in-laws, death, loss, poverty, illness, injury, injustice, anger, guilt, fear, dishonesty, confusion, and on and on. The list of stressful situations in our lives and of our reactions to them is very long. It is also constantly changing as new and unexpected events demanding some form of response continue to surface.

No one who works in a hospital can be unmoved by the infinite variations of the full catastrophe that are encountered every day. Each person who comes to the stress clinic has his or her own unique version, just as do all the people who work in the hospital. Although people are referred to the stress clinic with specific medical problems including heart disease, cancer, lung disease, hypertension, headaches, chronic-pain problems, seizures, sleep disorders, panic attacks, stress-related digestive problems, skin problems, voice problems, and many more, the diagnostic labels they come with mask more about them as people than they reveal. The full catastrophe lies within the complex web of their past and present experiences and relationships, their hopes and their fears, and their views of what is happening to them. Every person, without exception, has a unique story that gives meaning and coherence to that person's perception of his or her life, as well as of his illness and his pain and what he or she believes is possible.

Often these stories are heartbreaking. Not infrequently our patients come feeling that not only their bodies but their very lives are out of control. They feel overwhelmed by fears and worries, often caused or compounded by painful family relationships. We hear stories of physical and emotional suffering, of frustration with the medical system; poignant stories of people overwhelmed by feelings of anger or guilt, deeply lacking in self-confidence and self-esteem from having been beaten down by circumstances, often since childhood. And many times we see people who were or are literally beaten down through physical and psychological abuse.

Many of the people who come to the stress clinic have not seen much improvement in their physical condition despite years of medical treatment. Many do not even know where to look for help anymore and come to the clinic as a last resort, often skeptical about it but willing to do anything to get some relief.

Yet by the time they have been in the program for a few weeks, the majority of these people are taking major steps toward transforming their relationship to their bodies and minds and to their problems. From week to week, there is a noticeable difference in their faces and their bodies. By the end of eight weeks, when the program comes to an end, their smiles and more relaxed bodies are evident to even the most casual observer.

Although they were originally referred to the clinic to learn how to relax and to cope better with their stress, it is apparent that they have learned a lot more than that. They often leave with fewer and less severe physical symptoms and with greater self-confidence, optimism, and assertiveness. They are more patient with and more accepting of themselves and their limitations and disabilities. They are more confident about their ability to handle physical and emotional pain, as well as the other forces in their lives. They are also less anxious, less depressed, and less angry. They feel more in control, even in very stressful situations that previously would have sent them spinning out of control. In a word, they are handling "the full catastrophe" of their lives, the entire range of life experience, including impending death in some cases, much more skillfully.

One man who came into the program recently had had a heart attack that had forced him to retire from his work. For forty years he had owned a large business and lived right next door to it. For forty years, as he described it, he worked every day, never taking a vacation. He loved his work. He was sent to stress reduction by his cardiologist following cardiac catheterization (a procedure for diagnosing coronary artery disease), angioplasty (a procedure for expanding the coronary artery at the point of narrowing), and participation in a cardiac rehabilitation program. As I walked by him in the waiting room, I saw a look of utter despair and bewilderment on his face. He seemed on the verge of tears. He was waiting for my colleague, Saki Santorelli, to see him, but his sadness was so apparent that I sat down and talked with him then and there. He said, half to me and half to the air, that he no longer wanted to live, that he didn't know what he was doing in Stress Reduction . . . his life was over, there was no more meaning in it, he had no joy in anything, not even his wife and children, and no desire to do anything anymore.

After eight weeks of involvement in the stress clinic this man had an unmistakable sparkle in his eyes. When I met with him following the course, he told me that work had consumed his entire life without his realizing what he had been missing and that it had damn near killed him in the process. He went on to say that he had never told his children he loved them when they were growing up but was going to get started now while he still had the time. He was hopeful and enthusiastic about his life and was able for the first time to think about selling his business. He also gave me a big hug when he left, probably the first he had ever given another man.

This man still had the same degree of heart disease that he had had when he started, but at that time he saw himself as a sick man. He was a depressed cardiac patient. In eight weeks he had become healthier and happier. He was enthusiastic about living, even though he still had heart disease and plenty of problems in his life. In his own mind he went from seeing himself as a heart patient to seeing himself as a whole person again.

What happened in between to bring about such a transformation? We can't say with certainty. Many different factors were involved. But he did take the stress reduction program during that time and he took it seriously. It crossed my mind that he would probably drop out after the first week because, on top of everything else, he had to travel fifty miles to come to the hospital and when a person is depressed, that is hard to do. But he stayed and did the work we required of him, even though at the beginning he had no idea of how it could help him.

Another man, in his early seventies, came to the clinic with severe pain in his feet. He came to the first class in a wheelchair. His wife came with him to each class and sat outside the room for the two hours. That first day he told the class that the pain was so bad he just wanted to cut off his feet. He didn't see what meditating could possibly do for him, but things were so bad that he was willing to give anything a try. Everybody felt incredibly sorry for him.

Something about that first class must have touched him because this man showed a remarkable determination to work with his pain in the weeks that followed. He came to the second class on crutches rather than in the wheelchair. After that he used only a cane. The transition from wheelchair to crutches to cane spoke volumes to us all as we watched him from week to week. He said at the end that the pain hadn't changed much but that his attitude toward his pain had changed a lot. He said it just seemed more bearable after he started meditating and that by the end of the program his feet were less of a problem. When the program was over, his wife confirmed that he was much happier and more active.

A young physician's story comes to mind as another example of embracing the full catastrophe. She was sent to the program for high blood pressure and extreme anxiety. She was going through a difficult period in her life, which she described as full of anger and depression and self-destructive tendencies. She had come from another part of the country to finish her residency training. She was feeling isolated and burned out. Her doctor had urged her to give stress reduction a try, saying, "What can it hurt?" But she was scornful and dubious of a program that didn't actually "do something *to* you." And the fact that it involved meditation just made it worse. She didn't show up for the first class on the day she was scheduled, but Kathy Brady, one of the clinic secretaries, who had been through the program herself as a patient years before, had called her to find out why and was so nice to her and sounded so concerned on the phone, she told me later, that she sheepishly showed up for another class the next evening.

As part of her job this young doctor had to fly in the medical-center helicopter on a regular basis to the scene of accidents and bring back severely injured patients. She hated the helicopter. It terrified her, and she always got nauseous flying in it. But by the end of eight weeks in the stress clinic, she was able to fly in the helicopter without getting nauseous. She still hated it with a passion, but she was able to tolerate it and get her job done. Her blood pressure came down to the point where she took herself off her medication to see if it would stay down (doctors can get away with this), and it did. By this point she was in the last few months of her residency training and was exhausted a good deal of the time. On top of that, she continued to be emotionally hypersensitive and reactive. But now she was much more aware of her fluctuating states of body and mind. She decided to repeat the entire course because she felt she was just getting into it when it ended. She did, and has continued to keep up her meditation practice over the years since then.

Her experience in the stress clinic also led this doctor to a newfound respect for patients in general and for her own patients in particular. During the program she was among medical patients every week in class, not in her usual role as "the doctor" but as just another person with her own problems. She did the same things they were doing in the course week by week. She listened to them talking about their experiences with the meditation, and she watched them change over the weeks. She said she was astonished to see how much some people had suffered and what they were able to do for themselves with a little encouragement and training. She also came to respect the value of meditation as her view that people could only be helped by doing something *to* them yielded to what she was seeing. In fact she came to see that she was no different from the other people in the class and that what she could do, they could do, and what they could do, she could also do.

Transformations similar to the ones these three people experienced occur frequently in the stress clinic. They are usually major turning points in the lives of our patients because they expand the range of what they thought was possible for them.

Usually people leave the clinic thanking *us* for their improvement. But actually the progress they make is entirely due to their own efforts. What they are really thanking us for is the opportunity to get in touch with their own inner strength and resources and also for believing in them and not giving up on them and for giving them the tools for making such transformations possible.

We take pleasure in pointing out to them that to get through the program, they had to not give up on themselves. They had to be willing to face the full catastrophe of their own lives, in both pleasant and unpleasant circumstances, when things were going the way they wanted and when they were not, when they felt things were under control and when they didn't, and to use these very experiences and their own thoughts and feelings as the raw materials for healing themselves. When they began, it was with thoughts that the program could or might or probably wouldn't *do* something *for* them. But what they found was that they could do something very important for themselves that no one else could possibly do for them.

In the above examples each person took up the challenge we extended to them to live life as if each moment was important, as if each moment counted and could be worked with, even if it was a moment of pain, sadness, despair, or fear. This "work" involves above all the regular, disciplined practice of moment-to-moment awareness or *mindfulness*, the complete "owning" of each moment of your experience, good, bad, or ugly. This is the essence of full catastrophe living.

All of us have the capacity to be mindful. All it involves is cultivating our ability to pay attention in the present moment. Cultivating mindfulness plays a central role in the changes that the people who come to the stress clinic experience. One way to think of this process of transformation is to think of mindfulness as a lens, taking the scattered and reactive energies of your mind and focusing them into a coherent source of energy for living, for problem solving, and for healing.

We routinely and unknowingly waste enormous amounts of energy in reacting automatically and unconsciously to the outside world and to our own inner experiences. Cultivating mindfulness means learning to tap and focus our own wasted energies. In doing so, we learn to calm down enough to enter and dwell in states of deep relaxation. This nourishes and restores body and mind. At the same time it makes it easier for us to *see* with greater clarity the way we actually live and therefore how to make changes to enhance our health and the quality of our life. In addition it helps us to channel our energy more effectively in stressful situations, or when we are feeling threatened or helpless. This energy comes from inside us and is therefore always within our reach and potential control.

Cultivating mindfulness can lead to the discovery of deep realms of relaxation, calmness, and insight within yourself. It is as if you were to come upon a new territory, previously unknown to you or only vaguely suspected, which contains a veritable wellspring of positive energy for self-understanding and healing. Moreover it is easy to get to this territory. The path to it in any moment lies no farther than your own body and mind and your own breathing. And this territory is always accessible. It is always here, independent of your problems. Whether you are facing heart disease or cancer or pain or just a very stressful life, its energies can be of great value to you.

The systematic cultivation of mindfulness has been called the heart of Buddhist meditation. It has flourished over the past 2,500 years in both monastic and secular settings in many Asian countries. In recent years the practice of this kind of meditation has become widespread in the world. This has been due in part to the Chinese invasion of Tibet and the continual war in Southeast Asia, both of which made exiles of many Buddhist monks and teachers; in part to young Westerners who went to Asia to learn and practice meditation in monasteries and then became teachers in the West; and in part to Zen masters and other meditation teachers who have come to the West to visit and teach, drawn by the remarkable interest in this country in meditative practices.

Although at this time mindfulness meditation is most commonly taught and practiced within the context of Buddhism, its essence is universal. Mindfulness is basically just a particular way of paying attention. It is a way of looking deeply into oneself in the spirit of self-inquiry and self-understanding. For this reason it can be learned and practiced, as we do in the stress clinic, without appealing to Oriental culture or Buddhist authority to enrich it or authenticate it. Mindfulness stands on its own as a powerful vehicle for self-understanding and healing. In fact one of its major strengths is that it is not dependent on any belief system or ideology, so that its benefits are therefore accessible for anyone to test for himself or herself. Yet it is no accident that mindfulness comes out of Buddhism, which has as its overriding concerns the relief of suffering and the dispelling of illusions.

◆

This book is designed to give the reader full access to the training program our patients undergo in the stress clinic. Above all, it is a manual for helping you to develop your own personal meditation practice and for learning how to use mindfulness to promote improved health and healing in your own life. The section entitled "The Practice of Mindfulness" (Part I) describes what takes place in the stress reduction program and the experiences of people who have taken it. It will guide you through the major techniques we use in the clinic and gives explicit and easily followed directions for how to practice them and how to integrate mindfulness into daily-life activities. It also provides a detailed eight-week practice schedule so that, if you choose, you can follow the exact program our patients undergo while you are reading other sections of the book. This is the way we recommend you proceed.

The section entitled "The Paradigm" (Part II) provides a simple but revealing look at some of the latest research findings in behavioral medicine as background for understanding how the practice of mindfulness is related to physical and mental health. This section develops an overall "philosophy of health" based on the notions of "wholeness" and "connectedness" and on what science and medicine are learning about the relationship of the mind to health and the process of healing.

The section called simply "Stress" (Part III) discusses what stress is and how our awareness and understanding of it can help us to handle it more appropriately. It includes a model for understanding the value of bringing moment-to-moment awareness to stressful situations in order to cope more effectively with them.

Part IV "The Applications," provides detailed information and guidance for utilizing mindfulness in a wide range of specific areas that cause people significant stress, including medical symptoms, physical and emotional pain, anxiety and panic, time pressures, relationships, work, food, and events in the outside world.

The last section, "The Way of Awareness," (Part V) will give you practical suggestions for maintaining momentum in the meditation practice once you understand the basics and have begun practicing, as well as for using mindfulness effectively in all aspects of your life. It also contains information about how to find groups of people to practice with, hospitals and community-based institutions that have programs nurturing meditative awareness, and a reading list to support continued practice and growth.

The serious reader who wishes to put mindfulness to work to change his or her life may wish to order the mindfulness practice tapes that our patients use when practicing the formal meditation techniques described in this book. There is an order form to do so in the back of the book. Some people find it easier, when embarking for the first time on a daily meditation practice, just to plug in a tape and let it guide them rather than to follow instructions from a book, however clear and detailed they may be. If you feel this way, the tapes may help you to get launched in this process more effectively. They can increase your chances of giving the formal meditation techniques a fair try. Then, once you understand what is involved, you can practice on your own without the tapes, as many of our patients do.

However, whether you use the tapes or not, anybody who is interested in achieving the kind of results seen in the stress clinic should understand that our patients make a strong commitment to practice the formal techniques as described in this book on a daily basis for a period of at least eight weeks. They are required to practice with the tapes for forty-five minutes per day, six days per week, over the eight weeks. From follow-up studies we know that most continue to practice on their own long after the eight weeks are over. For many, mindfulness rapidly becomes a way of being.

As you embark on your own journey of self-development and discovery of your inner resources for healing and for working with the full catastrophe, all you need to remember is to suspend judgment for the time being and to commit yourself to practicing the techniques described in this book in a disciplined way, observing for yourself what is happening as you go along. What you will be learning will be coming primarily from inside you, from your own experience as your life unfolds from moment to moment rather than from some external authority or teacher or belief system. Our philosophy is that you are the world expert on your life, your body, and your mind, or at least you are in the best position to become that expert if you observe carefully. Part of the adventure of meditation is to use yourself as a laboratory to find out who you are and what you are capable of doing. As Yogi Berra once said, "You can observe a lot by just watching."

I

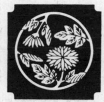

THE PRACTICE OF
MINDFULNESS:
PAYING
ATTENTION

1

You Have Only Moments to Live

—

"Oh, I've had my moments, and if I had to do it over again, I'd have more of them. In fact, I'd try to have nothing else. Just moments, one after another, instead of living so many years ahead of each day."

—Nadine Stair, eighty-five years old, Louisville, Kentucky

As I look around at the thirty or so people in this new class in the stress clinic, I marvel at what we are coming to engage in together. I assume they all must be wondering to some extent what the hell they are doing here in this room full of total strangers this morning. I see Edward's bright and kind face and ponder what he must be carrying around daily. He is a thirty-four-year-old insurance executive with AIDS. I see Peter, a forty-seven-year-old businessman who had a heart attack eighteen months ago and is here to learn how to take it easy so that he doesn't have another one. Next to Peter is Beverly, bright, cheerful, and talkative; sitting next to her is her husband. At forty-two Beverly's life changed radically when she had a cerebral aneurysm that burst, leaving her uncertain about how much she is her real self. Then, there is Marge, forty-four years old, referred from the pain clinic. She had been an oncology nurse until she injured her back and both knees several years ago trying to prevent a patient from falling. Now she is in so much pain that she can't work and walks only with great effort, using a cane. She has already had surgery on one knee and now, on top of everything else, faces surgery for a mass in her abdomen. The doctors won't know for sure what it is until they operate. Her injury knocked her for a loop from which she has yet to recover. She feels wound up like a spring and has been exploding at the littlest things.

17

Next to Marge is Arthur, fifty-six, a policeman who suffers from severe migraine headaches and frequent panic attacks, and sitting next to him is Margaret, seventy-five, a retired schoolteacher who is having trouble sleeping. A French-Canadian truck driver named Phil is on the other side of her. Phil was also referred here by the pain clinic. He injured himself lifting a dock pallet and is out on disability from chronic low-back pain. He will not be able to drive a truck anymore and needs to learn how to handle this pain better and figure out what other type of work he will be able to do to support his family, which includes four small children.

Next to Phil is Roger, a thirty-year-old carpenter who injured his back at work and is also in pain. According to his wife, he has been abusing pain medications for several years. She is enrolled in another class. She makes no bones about Roger's being the major source of her stress. She is so fed up with him that she is certain they are going to get divorced. I wonder as I look over at him where his life will carry him and whether he will be able to do what is necessary to get his life on an even keel.

Hector sits facing me across the room. He wrestled professionally for years in Puerto Rico and has come here today because he has a hard time controlling his temper and is feeling the consequences of it in the form of violent outbursts and chest pains. His large frame is an imposing presence in the room.

Their doctors have sent them all here for stress reduction, and we have invited them to come together one morning a week at the medical center for the next eight weeks in this class. *For what, really?* I find myself asking as I look around the room. They don't know it as well as I do yet, but the level of collective suffering in the room this morning is immense. It is truly a gathering of people suffering not only physically but emotionally as well from the full catastrophe of their lives.

In a moment of wonder before the class gets under way, I marvel at our *chutzpah* in inviting all these people to embark on this journey. I find myself thinking *What can we possibly do for the people gathered here this morning and for the hundred and twenty others who are beginning the stress reduction program in different classes this week, young people and older people, single, married or divorced, people who are working, others who are retired or on disability, people on Medicare and people who are well off? How much could we influence the course of even one person's life? What can we possibly do for all these people together in eight short weeks?*

The interesting thing about this work is that we don't really do anything for them. If we tried, I think we would fail miserably. Instead we invite them to do something radically new for themselves, namely to experiment with living intentionally from moment to moment. When I was talking to a reporter, she said, "Oh, you mean to live for the moment." I said "No, it isn't that. That has a hedonistic ring to it. I mean to live *in* the moment."

The work that goes on in the stress clinic is deceptively simple, so much so that it is difficult to grasp what it is really about unless you become involved in it personally. We start with where people are in their lives right now, no matter where that is. We are willing to work with them if they are ready and willing to work *with* and *on* themselves. And we never give up on anyone, even if they get discouraged or have setbacks or are "failing" in their own eyes. We see each moment as a new beginning, a new opportunity to start over, to tune in, to reconnect.

In some ways our job is hardly more than giving people permission to live their moments fully and completely and providing them with some tools for going about it systematically. We introduce them to ways that they can use to listen to their own bodies and minds and to begin trusting their own experience more. What we really offer people is a sense that there is a way of being, a way of looking at problems, a way of coming to terms with the full catastrophe that can make life more joyful and rich than it otherwise might be, and a sense also of being somehow more in control. We call this way of being *the way of awareness* or *the way of mindfulness*. The people gathered here this morning are about to encounter this new way of being and seeing as they embark on this journey in the stress clinic. We will have occasion to meet them again and others as well along the way as we now embark upon our own exploration of mindfulness and healing.

◆

If you were to look in on one of our classes at the hospital, the chances are you would find us with our eyes closed, sitting quietly or lying motionless on the floor. This can go on for anywhere from ten minutes to forty-five minutes at a stretch.

To the outside observer it might look strange, if not a little crazy. It looks like nothing is going on. And in a way nothing is. But it is a very rich and complex nothing. These people you would be looking in on are not just passing time daydreaming or sleeping. You cannot see what they are doing, but they are working hard. They are practicing *non-doing*. They are actively tuning in to each moment in an effort to remain awake and aware from one moment to the next. They are practicing mindfulness.

Another way to say it is that they are "practicing being." For once, they are purposefully stopping all the doing in their lives and relaxing into the present without trying to fill it up with anything. They are purposefully allowing body and mind to come to rest in the moment, no matter what is "on" their mind or how their body feels. They are tuning in to the basic experiences of living. They are simply allowing themselves to be in the moment with things exactly as they are, without trying to change anything.

In order to be admitted to the stress clinic in the first place, each person had to agree to make a major personal commitment to spend some time every day practicing this "just being." The basic idea is to create an island of being in the sea of constant doing in which our lives are usually immersed, a time in which we allow all the "doing" to stop.

Learning how to stop all your doing and shift over to a "being" mode, learning how to make time for yourself, how to slow down and nurture calmness and self-acceptance in yourself, learning to observe what your own mind is up to from moment to moment, how to watch your thoughts and how to let go of them without getting so caught up and driven by them, how to make room for new ways of seeing old problems and for perceiving the interconnectedness of things, these are some of the lessons of mindfulness. This kind of learning involves settling into moments of being and cultivating awareness.

The more systematically and regularly you practice, the more the power of mindfulness will grow and the more it will work for you. This book is meant to serve as a map, a guide to you in this process, just as the weekly classes are a guide to the people who come to the stress clinic at the urging of their doctors.

As you know, a map is not the territory it portrays. In the same way you should not mistake reading this book for the actual journey. That journey you have to live yourself, by cultivating mindfulness in your own life.

If you think about it for a moment, how could it be otherwise? Who could possibly do this kind of work for you? Your doctor? Your relatives or your friends? No matter how much other people want to help you and can help you in your efforts to move toward greater levels of health and well-being, the basic effort still has to come from you. After all, no one is living your life for you and no one's care for you could or should replace the care you can give to yourself.

In this regard, cultivating mindfulness is not unlike the process of eating. It would be absurd to propose that someone else eat for you. And when you go to a restaurant, you don't eat the menu, mistaking it for the meal, nor are you nourished by listening to the waiter describe the food. You have to actually eat the food for it to nourish you. In the same way you have to actually *practice* mindfulness in order to reap its benefits and come to understand why it is so valuable.

Even if you send away for our tapes to support your efforts in practicing, you will still have to use them. Tapes sit on shelves and gather dust very nicely. Nor is there any magic in them. Just listening to them from time to time will not help you much, although it can be relaxing. To benefit deeply from this work, you will have to *do* the tapes, as we say to our patients, not just listen to them. If there is magic anywhere, it is in you, not in any tape or technique.

Until recently the very word *meditation* tended to evoke raised eyebrows and thoughts about mysticism and hocus-pocus in many people. In part, that was because people did not understand that meditation is really about paying attention. This is now more widely known. And since paying attention is something that everybody does, at least occasionally, meditation is not as foreign or irrelevant to our life experience as we might once have thought.

However, when we start paying attention a little more closely to the way our own mind actually works, as we do when we meditate, we are likely to find that much of the time our mind is more in the past or the future than it is in the present. Consequently in any moment we may be only partially aware of what is actually occurring in the present. We can miss many of the moments we have to live because we are not fully here for them. This is true not just while we are meditating. Unawareness can dominate the mind in any moment and consequently, it can affect everything we do. We may find that much of the time we are really on "automatic pilot," functioning mechanically, without being fully aware of what we are doing or experiencing. It's as if we are not really at home a lot of the time or, put another way, only half awake.

You might verify for yourself whether this description applies to your own mind the next time you are driving a car. It is a very common experience to drive someplace and have little or no awareness of what you saw along the way. You may have been on automatic pilot for much of the drive, not really fully there but there enough, one would hope, to drive safely and uneventfully.

Even if you deliberately try to concentrate on a particular task, whether it's driving or something else, you might find it difficult to be in the present for very long. Ordinarily our attention is easily distracted. The mind tends to wander. It drifts into thought and reverie.

Our thoughts are so overpowering, particularly in times of crisis or emotional upheaval, that they easily cloud our awareness of the present. Even in relatively relaxed moments they can carry our senses along with them whenever they take off, as when driving we find ourselves looking intently at something we have passed in the car long after we should have brought our attention back to the road in front of us. For that moment we were not actually driving. The car was on autopilot. The thinking mind was "captured" by a sense impression, a sight, a sound, something that attracted its attention, and was literally pulled away. It was back with the cow or the tow truck, or whatever it was that caught our attention. As a consequence, at that moment, and for however long our attention was captured, we were literally "lost" in our thoughts and unaware of other sense impressions.

Is it not true that the same thing happens most of the time, whatever you are doing? Try observing how easily your own awareness is carried away from the present moment by your thoughts, no matter where you find yourself, no matter what the circumstances. Notice how much of the time during the day you find yourself thinking about the past or about the future. You may be shocked at the result.

You can experience this pull of the thinking mind for yourself right now if you perform the following experiment: Close your eyes, sit so that your back is straight but not stiff, and become aware of your breathing. Don't try to control your breathing. Just let it happen and be aware of it, feeling how it feels, witnessing it as it flows in and out. Try being with your breath in this way for three minutes.

If, at some point, you think that it is foolish or boring to just sit here and watch your breath go in and out, note to yourself that this is just a thought, a judgment that your mind is creating. Then simply let go of it and bring your attention back to your breathing. If the feeling is very strong, try the following additional experiment, which we sometimes suggest to our patients who feel similarly bored with watching their breathing: Take the thumb and first finger of either hand, clamp them tightly over your nose, keep your mouth closed, and notice how long it takes before your breathing becomes very interesting to you!

When you have completed three minutes of watching your breath go in and out, reflect on how you felt during this time and how much or how little your mind wandered away from your breathing. What do you think would have happened if you had continued for five or ten minutes, or for half an hour, or an hour?

For most of us, our minds tend to wander a lot and to jump quite rapidly from one thing to another. This makes it difficult to keep our attention focused on our breathing for any length of time unless we train ourselves to stabilize and calm our own mind. This little three-minute experiment can give you a taste of what meditation is. It is the process of observing body and mind intentionally, of letting your experiences unfold from moment to moment and accepting them *as they are*. It does not involve rejecting your thoughts nor trying to clamp down on them or suppress them, nor trying to control anything at all other than the focus and direction of your attention.

Yet it would be incorrect to think of meditation as a passive process. It takes a good deal of energy and effort to regulate your attention and to remain genuinely calm and nonreactive. But, paradoxically, mindfulness does not involve trying to get anywhere or feel anything special. Rather it involves allowing yourself to be where you already are, to become more familiar with your own actual experience moment by moment. So if you didn't feel particularly relaxed in these three minutes or the thought of doing it for half an hour is inconceivable to you, you don't need to worry. The relaxation comes by itself with continued practice. The point of this three-minute exercise was simply to try to pay attention to your breathing and to note what actually happened when you did.

If you start paying attention to where your mind is from moment to moment throughout the day, chances are you will find that considerable amounts of your time and energy are expended in clinging to memories, being absorbed in reverie, and regretting things that have already happened and are over. And you will probably find that as much or more energy is expended in anticipating, planning, worrying, and fantasizing about the future and what you want to happen or don't want to happen.

Because of this inner busyness, which is going on almost all the time, we are liable either to miss a lot of the texture of our life experience or to discount its value and meaning. For example, let's say you are not too preoccupied to look at a sunset and are struck by the play of light and color among the clouds and in the sky. For that moment you are just there with it, taking it in, really seeing it. Then thinking comes in and perhaps you find yourself saying something to a companion, either about the sunset and how beautiful it is or about something else that it reminded you of. In speaking, you disturb the direct experiencing of that moment. You have been drawn away from the sun and sky and the light. You have been captured by your own thought and by your impulse to voice it. Your comment breaks the silence. Or even if you don't say anything, the thought or memory that came up had already carried you away from the real sunset in that moment. So now you are really enjoying the sunset in your head rather than the sunset that is actually happening. You may be *thinking* you are enjoying the sunset itself, but actually you are only experiencing it through the veil of your own embellishments with past sunsets and other memories and ideas that it triggered in you. All this may happen completely below the level of your conscious awareness. What is more, this entire episode might last only a moment or so. It will fade rapidly as one thing leads to the next.

Much of the time you may get away with being only partially conscious like this. At least it seems that way. But what you are missing is more important than you realize. If you are only partially conscious over a period of years, if you habitually run through your moments without being fully in them, you may miss some of the most precious experiences of your life, such as connecting with the people you love, or with sunsets or the crisp morning air.

Why? Because you were "too busy" and your mind too encumbered with what you *thought* was important in that moment to take the time to stop, to listen, to notice things. Perhaps you were going too fast to slow down, too fast to know the importance of making eye contact, of touching, of being in your body. When we are functioning in this mode, we may eat without really tasting, see without really seeing, hear without really hearing, touch without really feeling, and talk without really knowing what we are saying. And of course, in the case of driving, if your mind or somebody else's happens to check out at the "wrong" moment, the immediate consequences can be dramatic and very unfortunate.

So the value of cultivating mindfulness is not just a matter of getting more out of sunsets. When unawareness dominates the mind, all our decisions and actions are affected by it. Unawareness can keep us from being in touch with our own body, its signals and messages. This in turn can create many physical problems for us, problems we don't even know we are generating ourselves. And living in a chronic state of unawareness can cause us to miss much of what is most beautiful and meaningful in our lives. What is more, as in the driving example or in the case of alcohol and drug abuse or habits such as workaholism, our tendency toward unawareness may also be lethal, either rapidly or slowly.

♦

When you begin paying attention to what your mind is doing, you will probably find that there is a great deal of mental and emotional activity going on beneath the surface. These incessant thoughts and feelings can drain a lot of your energy. They can be obstacles to experiencing even brief moments of stillness and contentment.

When the mind is dominated by dissatisfaction and unawareness, which is much more often than most of us are willing to admit, it is difficult to feel calm or relaxed. Instead, we are likely to feel fragmented and driven. We will think this *and* that, we want this *and* that. Often the *this* and the *that* are in conflict. This mind state can severely affect our ability to do anything or even to see situations clearly. In such moments we may not know *what* we are thinking, feeling, or doing. What is worse, we probably won't know that we don't know. We may think we know what we are thinking and feeling and doing and what is happening. But it is an incomplete knowing at best. In reality we are being driven by our likes and dislikes, totally unaware of the tyranny of our own thoughts and the self-destructive behaviors they often result in.

Socrates was famous in Athens for saying, "Know thyself." It is said that one of his students said to him: "Socrates, you go around saying "Know thyself," but do you know yourself?" Socrates was said to have replied, "No, but I understand something about this not knowing."

As you embark upon your own practice of mindfulness meditation, you will come to know something for yourself about your own not knowing. It is not that mindfulness is the "answer" to all life's problems. Rather it is that all life's problems can be seen more clearly through the lens of a clear mind. Just being aware of the mind that thinks it knows all the time is a major step toward learning how to see through your opinions and perceive things as they actually are.

◆

One very important domain of our lives and experience that we tend to miss, ignore, abuse, or lose control of as a result of being in the automatic-pilot mode is our own body. We may be barely in touch with our body, unaware of how it is feeling most of the time. As a consequence we can be insensitive to how our body is being affected by the environment, by our actions, and even by our own thoughts and emotions. If we are unaware of these connections, we might easily feel that our body is out of control and we will have no idea why. As you will see in Chapter 21, physical symptoms are messages the body is giving us that allow us to know how it is doing and what its needs are. When we are more in touch with our body as a result of paying attention to it systematically, we will be far more attuned to what it is telling us and better equipped to respond appropriately. Learning to listen to your own body is vital to improving your health and the quality of your life.

Even something as simple as relaxation can be frustratingly elusive if you are unaware of your body. The stress of daily living often produces tension that tends to localize in particular muscle groups, such as the shoulders, the jaw, and the forehead. In order to release this tension, you first have to know it is there. You have to feel it. Then you have to know how to shut off the automatic pilot and how to take over the controls of your own body and mind. As we will see farther on, this involves zeroing in on your body with a focused mind, experiencing the sensations coming from within the muscles themselves, and sending them messages to let the tension dissolve and release. This is something that can be done at the time the tension is accumulating if you are mindful enough to sense it. There is no need to wait until it has built to the point that your body feels like a two-by-four. If you let it go that long, the tension will have become so ingrained that you will have probably forgotten what it felt like to be relaxed, and you may have little hope of ever feeling relaxed again.

One man who came to the stress clinic ten years ago with back pain put the dilemma in a nutshell. While testing his range of motion and flexibility, I noticed that he was very stiff and his legs were as hard as rocks, even when I asked him to relax them. They had been that way ever since he was wounded when he stepped on a booby trap in Vietnam. When his doctor told him that he needed to relax, he had responded, "Doc, telling me to relax is about as useful as telling me to be a surgeon."

The point is, it didn't do this man any good to be told to relax. He knew he needed to relax more. But he had to learn *how* to relax. He had to experience the process of letting go within his own body and mind. Once he started meditating, he was able to *learn* to relax, and his leg muscles eventually regained a healthy tone.

When something goes wrong with our body or our mind, we have the natural expectation that medicine can make it right, and often it can. But as we will see farther on, our active collaboration is essential in almost all forms of medical therapy. It is particularly vital in the case of chronic diseases or conditions for which medicine has no cures. In such cases the quality of your life may greatly depend on your own ability to know your body and mind well enough to work at optimizing your own health within the bounds, always unknown, of what may be possible. Taking responsibility for learning more about your own body by listening to it carefully and by cultivating your inner resources for healing and for maintaining health is the best way to hold up your end of this collaboration with your doctors and with medicine. This is where the meditation practice comes in. It gives power and substance to such efforts. It catalyzes the work of healing.

◆

The first introduction to the meditation practice in the stress clinic always comes as a surprise to our patients. More often than not, people come with the idea that meditation means doing something unusual, something mystical and out of the ordinary, or at the very least, relaxing. To relieve them of these expectations right off the bat, we give everybody three raisins and we eat them one at a time, paying attention to what we are actually doing and experiencing from moment to moment. You might wish to try it yourself after you see how we do it.

First we bring our attention to seeing the raisin, observing it carefully as if we had never seen one before. We feel its texture between our fingers and notice its colors and surfaces. We are also aware of any thoughts we might be having about raisins or food in general. We note any thoughts and feelings of liking or disliking raisins if they come up while we are looking at it. We then smell it for a while and finally, with awareness, we bring it to our lips, being aware of the arm moving the hand to position it correctly and of salivating as the mind and body anticipate eating. The process continues as we take it into our mouth and chew it slowly, experiencing the actual taste of one raisin. And when we feel ready to swallow, we watch the impulse to swallow as it comes up, so that even that is experienced consciously. We even imagine, or "sense," that now our bodies are one raisin heavier.

The response to this exercise is invariably positive, even among the people who don't like raisins. People report that it is satisfying to eat this way for a change, that they actually experienced what a raisin tasted like for the first time that they could remember, and that even one raisin could be satisfying. Often someone makes the connection that if we ate like that all the time, we would eat less and have more pleasant and satisfying experiences of food. Some people usually comment that they caught themselves automatically moving to eat the other raisins before finishing the one that was in their mouth, and recognized in that moment that that is the way they normally eat.

Since many of us use food for emotional comfort, especially when we feel anxious or depressed, this little exercise in slowing things down and paying careful attention to what we are doing illustrates how powerful and uncontrolled many of our impulses are when it comes to food, and how simple and satisfying it can be and how much more in control we can feel when we bring awareness to what we are actually doing while we are doing it.

The fact is, when you start to pay attention in this way, your relationship to things changes. You see more, and you see more deeply. You may start seeing an intrinsic order and connectedness between things that were not apparent before, such as the connection between impulses that come up in your mind and finding yourself overeating and disregarding the messages your body is giving you. By paying attention, you literally become more awake. It is an emerging from the usual ways in which we all tend to see things and do things mechanically, without full awareness. When you eat mindfully, you are in touch with your food because your mind is not distracted. It is not thinking about other things. It is attending to eating. When you look at the raisin, you really see it. When you chew it, you really taste it.

Knowing what you are doing while you are doing it is the essence of mindfulness practice. We call the raisin-eating exercise "eating meditation." It helps make the point that there is nothing particularly unusual or mystical about meditating or being mindful. All it involves is paying attention to your experience from moment to moment. This leads directly to new ways of seeing and being in your life because the present moment, whenever it is recognized and honored, reveals a very special, indeed magical power: *it is the only time that any of us ever has*. The present is the only time that we have to know anything. It is the only time we have to perceive, to learn, to act, to change, to heal. That is why we value moment-to-moment awareness so highly. While we may have to teach ourselves how to do it through practicing, the effort itself is its own end. It makes our experiences more vivid and our lives more real.

◆

As you will see in the next chapter, to embark on the practice of mindfulness meditation it is helpful to deliberately introduce a note of simplicity into your life. This can be done by setting aside a time during the day for moments of relative peace and quiet; moments which you can use to focus on the basic experiences of living such as your breathing, the sensations you feel in your body, and the flowing movement of thoughts in your mind. It doesn't take long for this "formal" meditation practice to spill over into your daily life in the form of intentionally paying greater attention from one moment to the next, no matter what you are doing. You might find yourself spontaneously paying attention more of the time in your life, not just when you are "meditating."

We practice mindfulness by remembering to be present in all our waking moments. We can practice taking out the garbage mindfully, eating mindfully, driving mindfully. We can practice navigating through all the ups and downs we encounter, the storms of the mind and the storms of our bodies, the storms of the outer life and of the inner life. We learn to be aware of our fears and our pain, yet at the same time stabilized and empowered by a connection to something deeper within ourselves, a discerning wisdom that helps to penetrate and transcend the fear and the pain, and to discover some peace and hope within our situation *as it is*.

We are using the word *practice* here in a special way. It does not mean a "rehearsal" or a perfecting of some skill so that we can put it to use at some other time. In the meditative context practice means "being in the present on purpose." The means and the end of meditation are really the same. We are not trying to get somewhere else, only working at being where we already are and being here fully. Our meditation practice may very well deepen over the years, but actually we are not practicing for this to happen. Our journey toward greater health is really a natural progression. Awareness, insight, and indeed health as well, ripen on their own if we are willing to pay attention in the moment and remember that we have only moments to live.

2

The Foundations of Mindfulness Practice: Attitudes and Commitment

To cultivate the healing power of mindfulness requires much more than mechanically following a recipe or a set of instructions. No real process of learning is like that. It is only when the mind is open and receptive that learning and seeing and change can occur. In practicing mindfulness you will have to bring your whole being to the process. You can't just assume a meditative posture and think something will happen or play a tape and think that the tape is going to "do something" for you.

The attitude with which you undertake the practice of paying attention and being in the present is crucial. It is the soil in which you will be cultivating your ability to calm your mind and to relax your body, to concentrate and to see more clearly. If the attitudinal soil is depleted, that is, if your energy and commitment to practice are low, it will be hard to develop calmness and relaxation with any consistency. If the soil is really polluted, that is, if you are trying to force yourself to feel relaxed and demand of yourself that "something happen," nothing will grow at all and you will quickly conclude that "meditation doesn't work."

To cultivate meditative awareness requires an entirely new way of looking at the process of learning. Since thinking that we know what we need and where we want to get are so ingrained in our minds, we can easily get caught up in trying to control things to make them turn out "our way," the way we want them to. But this

31

attitude is antithetical to the work of awareness and healing. Awareness requires only that we pay attention and see things as they are. It doesn't require that we change anything. And healing requires receptivity and acceptance, a tuning to connectedness and wholeness. None of this can be forced, just as you cannot force yourself to go to sleep. You have to create the right conditions for falling asleep and then you have to let go. The same is true for relaxation. It cannot be achieved through force of will. That kind of effort will only produce tension and frustration.

If you come to the meditation practice thinking to yourself, "This won't work but I'll do it anyway," the chances are it will not be very helpful. The first time you feel any pain or discomfort, you will be able to say to yourself, "See, I knew my pain wouldn't go away," or "I knew I wouldn't be able to concentrate," and that will confirm your suspicion that it wasn't going to work and you will drop it.

If you come as a "true believer," certain that *this* is the right path for you, that meditation is "the answer," the chances are you will soon become disappointed too. As soon as you find that you are the same person you always were and that this work requires effort and consistency and not just a romantic belief in the value of meditation or relaxation, you may find yourself with considerably less enthusiasm than before.

In the stress clinic, we find that those people who come with a skeptical but open attitude do the best. Their attitude is "I don't know whether this will work or not, I have my doubts, but I am going to give it my best shot and see what happens."

So the attitude that we bring to the practice of mindfulness will to a large extent determine its long-term value to us. This is why consciously cultivating certain attitudes can be very helpful in getting the most out of the process of meditation. Your intentions set the stage for what is possible. They remind you from moment to moment of why you are practicing in the first place. Keeping particular attitudes in mind is actually part of the training itself, a way of directing and channeling your energies so that they can be most effectively brought to bear in the work of growing and healing.

Seven attitudinal factors constitute the major pillars of mindfulness practice as we teach it in the stress clinic. They are non-judging, patience, a beginner's mind, trust, non-striving, acceptance, and letting go. These attitudes are to be cultivated consciously when you practice. They are not independent of each other. Each one relies on and influences the degree to which you are able to cultivate the others. Working on any one will rapidly lead you to the others. Since together they constitute the foundation upon which you will be able to build a strong meditation practice of your own, we are introducing them before you encounter the techniques themselves so that you can become familiar with these attitudes from the very beginning. Once you are engaged in the practice itself, this chapter will merit rereading to remind you of ways you might continue to fertilize this attitudinal soil so that your mindfulness practice will flourish.

THE ATTITUDINAL FOUNDATION OF MINDFULNESS PRACTICE

1. Non-judging

Mindfulness is cultivated by assuming the stance of an impartial witness to your own experience. To do this requires that you become aware of the constant stream of judging and reacting to inner and outer experiences that we are all normally caught up in, and learn to step back from it. When we begin practicing paying attention to the activity of our own mind, it is common to discover and to be surprised by the fact that we are constantly generating judgments about our experience. Almost everything we see is labeled and categorized by the mind. We react to everything we experience in terms of what we think its value is to us. Some things, people, and events are judged as "good" because they make us feel good for some reason. Others are equally quickly condemned as "bad" because they make us feel bad. The rest is categorized as "neutral" because we don't think it has much relevance. Neutral things, people, and events are almost completely tuned out of our consciousness. We usually find them the most boring to give attention to.

This habit of categorizing and judging our experience locks us into mechanical reactions that we are not even aware of and that often have no objective basis at all. These judgments tend to dominate our minds, making it difficult for us ever to find any peace within ourselves. It's as if the mind were a yo-yo, going up and down on the string of our own judging thoughts all day long. If you doubt this description of your mind, just observe how much you are preoccupied with liking and disliking, say during a ten-minute period as you go about your business.

If we are to find a more effective way of handling the stress in our lives, the first thing we will need to do is to be aware of these automatic judgments so that we can see through our own prejudices and fears and liberate ourselves from their tyranny.

When practicing mindfulness, it is important to recognize this judging quality of mind when it appears and to intentionally assume the stance of an impartial witness by reminding yourself to just observe it. When you find the mind judging, you don't have to stop it from doing that. All that is required is to be aware of it happening. No need to judge the judging and make matters even more complicated for yourself.

As an example, let's say you are practicing watching your breathing, as you did in the last chapter and as we will do a lot more in the next. At a certain point you may find your mind saying something like, "This is boring," or "This isn't working," or "I can't do this." These are judgments. When they come up in your mind, it is very important to recognize them as judgmental thinking and remind yourself that the practice involves suspending judgment and just watching *whatever* comes up, including your own judging thoughts, without pursuing them or acting on them in any way. Then proceed with watching your breathing.

2. Patience

Patience is a form of wisdom. It demonstrates that we understand and accept the fact that sometimes things must unfold in their own time. A child may try to help a butterfly to emerge by breaking open its chrysalis. Usually the butterfly doesn't benefit from this. Any adult knows that the butterfly can only emerge in its own time, that the process cannot be hurried.

In the same way we cultivate patience toward our own minds and bodies when practicing mindfulness. We intentionally remind ourselves that there is no need to be impatient with ourselves because we find the mind judging all the time, or because we are tense or agitated or frightened, or because we have been practicing for some time and nothing positive seems to have happened. We give ourselves room to have these experiences. Why? Because we are having them anyway! When they come up, they are our reality, they are part of our life unfolding in this moment. So we treat ourselves as well as we would treat the butterfly. Why rush through some moments to get to other, "better" ones? After all, each one is your life in that moment.

When you practice being with yourself in this way, you are bound to find that your mind has "a mind of its own." We have already seen in Chapter 1 that one of its favorite activities is to wander into the past and into the future and lose itself in thinking. Some of its thoughts are pleasant. Others are painful and anxiety producing. In either case thinking itself exerts a strong pull on our awareness. Much of the time our thoughts overwhelm our perception of the present moment. They cause us to lose our connection to the present.

Patience can be a particularly helpful quality to invoke when the mind is agitated. It can help us to accept this wandering tendency of the mind while reminding us that we don't have to get caught up in its travels. Practicing patience reminds us that we don't have to fill up our moments with activity and with more thinking in order for them to be rich. In fact it helps us to remember that quite the opposite is true. To be patient is simply to be completely open to each moment, accepting it in its fullness, knowing that, like the butterfly, things can only unfold in their own time.

3. Beginner's Mind

The richness of present-moment experience is the richness of life itself. Too often we let our thinking and our beliefs about what we "know" prevent us from seeing things as they really are. We tend to take the ordinary for granted and fail to grasp the extraordinariness of the ordinary. To see the richness of the present moment, we need to cultivate what has been called "beginner's mind," a mind that is willing to see everything as if for the first time.

This attitude will be particularly important when we practice the formal meditation techniques described in the following chapters. Whatever the particular technique we might be using, whether it is the body scan or the sitting meditation or the yoga, we should bring our beginner's mind with us each time we practice so that we can be free of our expectations based on our past experiences. An open, "beginner's" mind allows us to be receptive to new possibilities and prevents us from getting stuck in the rut of our own expertise, which often thinks it knows more than it does. No moment is the same as any other. Each is unique and contains unique possibilities. Beginner's mind reminds us of this simple truth.

You might try to cultivate your own beginner's mind in your daily life as an experiment. The next time you see somebody who is familiar to you, ask yourself if you are seeing this person with fresh eyes, as he or she really is, or if you are only seeing the reflection of your own thoughts about this person. Try it with your children, your spouse, your friends and co-workers, with your dog or cat if you have one. Try it with problems when they arise. Try it when you are outdoors in nature. Are you able to see the sky, the stars, the trees and the water and the stones, and really see them as they are right now with a clear and uncluttered mind? Or are you actually only seeing them through the veil of your own thoughts and opinions?

4. Trust

Developing a basic trust in yourself and your feelings is an integral part of meditation training. It is far better to trust in your intuition and your own authority, even if you make some "mistakes" along the way, than always to look outside of yourself for guidance. If at any time something doesn't feel right to you, why not honor your feelings? Why should you discount them or write them off as invalid because some authority or some group of people think or say differently? This attitude of trusting yourself and your own basic wisdom and goodness is very important in all aspects of the meditation practice. It will be particularly useful in the yoga. When practicing yoga, you will have to honor your own feelings when your body tells you to stop or to back off in a particular stretch. If you don't listen, you might injure yourself.

Some people who get involved in meditation get so caught up in the reputation and authority of their teachers that they don't honor their own feelings and intuition. They believe that their teacher must be a much wiser and more advanced person, so they think they should imitate him and do what he says without question and venerate him as a model of perfect wisdom. This attitude is completely contrary to the spirit of meditation, which emphasizes being your own person and understanding what it means to be yourself. Anybody who is imitating somebody else, no matter who it is, is heading in the wrong direction.

It is impossible to become like somebody else. Your only hope is to become more fully yourself. That is the reason for practicing meditation in the first place. Teachers and books and tapes can only be guides, signposts. It is important to be open and receptive to what you can learn from other sources, but ultimately you still have to live your own life, every moment of it. In practicing mindfulness, you are practicing taking responsibility for being yourself and learning to listen to and trust your own being. The more you cultivate this trust in your own being, the easier you will find it will be to trust other people more and to see their basic goodness as well.

5. Non-striving

Almost everything we do we do for a purpose, to get something or somewhere. But in meditation this attitude can be a real obstacle. That is because meditation is different from all other human activities. Although it takes a lot of work and energy of a certain kind, ultimately meditation is a non-doing. It has no goal other than for you to be yourself. The irony is that you already are. This sounds paradoxical and a little crazy. Yet this paradox and craziness may be pointing you toward a new way of seeing yourself, one in which you are trying less and being more. This comes from intentionally cultivating the attitude of non-striving.

For example, if you sit down to meditate and you think, "I am going to get relaxed, or get enlightened, or control my pain, or become a better person," then you have introduced an idea into your mind of where you should be, and along with it comes the notion that you are not okay right now. "If I were only more calm, or more intelligent, or a harder worker, or more this or more that, if only my heart were healthier or my knee were better, then I would be okay. But right now, I am not okay."

This attitude undermines the cultivation of mindfulness, which involves simply paying attention to whatever is happening. If you are tense, then just pay attention to the tension. If you are in pain, then be with the pain as best you can. If you are criticizing yourself, then observe the activity of the judging mind. Just watch. Remember, we are simply allowing anything and everything that we experience from moment to moment to be here, because it already is.

People are sent to the stress clinic by their doctors because something is the matter. The first time they come, we ask them to identify three goals that they want to work toward in the program. But then, often to their surprise, we encourage them not to try to make any progress toward their goals over the eight weeks. In particular, if one of their goals is to lower their blood pressure or to reduce their pain or their anxiety, they are instructed not to *try* to lower their blood pressure nor to *try* to make their pain or their anxiety go away, but simply to stay in the present and carefully follow the meditation instructions.

As you will see shortly, in the meditative domain, the best way to achieve your own goals is to back off from striving for results and instead to start focusing carefully on seeing and accepting things as they are, moment by moment. With patience and regular practice, movement toward your goals will take place by itself. This movement becomes an unfolding that you are inviting to happen within you.

6. Acceptance

Acceptance means seeing things as they actually are in the present. If you have a headache, accept that you have a headache. If you are overweight, why not accept it as a description of your body at this time? Sooner or later we have to come to terms with things as they are and accept them, whether it is a diagnosis of cancer or learning of someone's death. Often acceptance is only reached after we have gone through very emotion-filled periods of denial and then anger. These stages are a natural progression in the process of coming to terms with what is. They are all part of the healing process.

However, putting aside for the moment the major calamities that usually take a great deal of time to heal from, in the course of our daily lives we often waste a lot of energy denying and resisting what is already fact. When we do that, we are basically trying to force situations to be the way we would like them to be, which only makes for more tension. This actually prevents positive change from occurring. We may be so busy denying and forcing and struggling that we have little energy left for healing and growing, and what little we have may be dissipated by our lack of awareness and intentionality.

If you are overweight and feel bad about your body, it's no good to wait until you are the weight you think you should be before you start liking your body and yourself. At a certain point, if you don't want to remain stuck in a frustrating vicious cycle, you might realize that it is all right to love yourself at the weight that you are now because this is the only time you can love yourself. Remember, now is the only time you have for anything. You have to accept yourself as you are before you can really change.

When you start thinking this way, losing weight becomes less important. It also becomes a lot easier. By intentionally cultivating acceptance, you are creating the preconditions for healing.

Acceptance does not mean that you have to like everything or that you have to take a passive attitude toward everything and abandon your principles and values. It does not mean that you are satisfied with things as they are or that you are resigned to tolerating things as they "have to be." It does not mean that you should stop trying to break free of your own self-destructive habits or to give up on your desire to change and grow, or that you should tolerate injustice, for instance, or avoid getting involved in changing the world around you because it is the way it is and therefore hopeless. Acceptance as we are speaking of it simply means that you have come around to a willingness to see things as they are. This attitude sets the stage for acting appropriately in your life, no matter what is happening. You are much more likely to know what to do and have the inner conviction to act when you have a clear picture of what is actually happening than when your vision is clouded by your mind's self-serving judgments and desires or its fears and prejudices.

In the meditation practice, we cultivate acceptance by taking each moment as it comes and being with it fully, as it is. We try not to impose our ideas about what we should be feeling or thinking or seeing on our experience but just remind ourselves to be receptive and open to whatever we are feeling, thinking, or seeing, and to accept it because it is here right now. If we keep our attention focused on the present, we can be sure of one thing, namely that whatever we are attending to in this moment will change, giving us the opportunity to practice accepting whatever it is that will emerge in the next moment. Clearly there is wisdom in cultivating acceptance.

7. Letting Go

They say that in India there is a particularly clever way of catching monkeys. As the story goes, hunters will cut a hole in a coconut that is just big enough for a monkey to put its hand through. Then they will drill two smaller holes in the other end, pass a wire through, and secure the coconut to the base of a tree. Then they put a banana inside the coconut and hide. The monkey comes down, puts his hand in and takes hold of the banana. The hole is crafted so that the open hand can go in but the fist cannot get out. All the monkey has to do to be free is to let go of the banana. But it seems most monkeys don't let go.

Often our minds get us caught in very much the same way in spite of all our intelligence. For this reason, cultivating the attitude of letting go, or non-attachment, is fundamental to the practice of mindfulness. When we start paying attention to our inner experience, we rapidly discover that there are certain thoughts and feelings and situations that the mind seems to want to hold on to. If they are pleasant, we try to prolong these thoughts or feelings or situations, stretch them out, and conjure them up again and again.

Similarly there are many thoughts and feelings and experiences that we try to get rid of or to prevent and protect ourselves from having because they are unpleasant and painful and frightening in one way or another.

In the meditation practice we intentionally put aside the tendency to elevate some aspects of our experience and to reject others. Instead we just let our experience be what it is and practice observing it from moment to moment. Letting go is a way of letting things be, of accepting things as they are. When we observe our own mind grasping and pushing away, we remind ourselves to let go of those impulses on purpose, just to see what will happen if we do. When we find ourselves judging our experience, we let go of those judging thoughts. We recognize them and we just don't pursue them any further. We let them be, and in doing so we let them go. Similarly when thoughts of the past or of the future come up, we let go of them. We just watch.

If we find it particularly difficult to let go of something because it has such a strong hold over our mind, we can direct our attention to what "holding on" feels like. Holding on is the opposite of letting go. We can become an expert on our own attachments, whatever they may be and their consequences in our lives, as well as how it feels in those moments when we finally do let go and what the consequences of that are. Being willing to look at the ways we hold on ultimately shows us a lot about the experience of its opposite. So whether we are "successful" at letting go or not, mindfulness continues to teach us if we are willing to look.

Letting go is not such a foreign experience. We do it every night when we go to sleep. We lie down on a padded surface, with the lights out, in a quiet place, and we let go of our mind and body. If you can't let go, you can't go to sleep.

Most of us have experienced times when the mind would just not shut down when we got into bed. This is one of the first signs of elevated stress. At these times we may be unable to free ourselves from certain thoughts because our involvement in them is just too powerful. If we try to force ourselves to sleep, it just makes things worse. So if you can go to sleep, you are already an expert in letting go. Now you just need to practice applying this skill in waking situations as well.

COMMITMENT, SELF-DISCIPLINE, AND
INTENTIONALITY

Purposefully cultivating the attitudes of non-judging, patience, trust, beginner's mind, non-striving, acceptance, and letting go will greatly support and deepen your practice of the meditation techniques you will be encountering in the following chapters.

In addition to these attitudes, you will also need to bring a particular kind of energy or motivation to your practice. Mindfulness doesn't just come about by itself because you have decided that it is a good idea to be more aware of things. A strong commitment to working on yourself and enough self-discipline to persevere in the process are essential to developing a strong meditation practice and a high degree of mindfulness. We have already seen in Chapter 1 how important self-discipline and regular practice are to the work undertaken by the patients in the stress clinic. Self-discipline and regular practice are vital to developing the power of mindfulness.

In the stress clinic the basic ground rule is that everybody practices. Nobody goes along for the ride. We don't let in any observers or spouses unless they are willing to practice the meditation just as the patients are doing, that is, forty-five minutes per day, six days per week. Doctors, medical students, therapists, nurses, and other health professionals who go through the stress clinic as part of an internship training program all have to agree to practice the meditation on the same schedule as the patients. Without this personal experience, it would not be possible for them really to understand what the patients are going through and how much of an effort it takes to work with the energies of one's own mind and body.

The spirit of engaged commitment we ask of our patients during their eight weeks in the stress clinic is similar to that required in athletic training. The athlete who is training for a particular event doesn't only practice when he or she feels like it, for instance, only when the weather is nice or there are other people to keep him or her company or there is enough time to fit it in. The athlete trains regularly, every day, rain or shine, whether she feels good or not, whether the goal seems worth it or not on any particular day.

We encourage our patients to develop the same attitude. We tell them from the very start, "You don't have to like it; you just have to do it. When the eight weeks are over, then you can tell us whether it was of any use or not. For now just keep practicing."

Their own suffering and the possibility of being able to do something themselves to improve their health are usually motivation enough for the patients in the stress clinic to invest this degree of personal commitment, at least for the eight weeks we require it of them. For most it is a new experience to be in intensive training, to say nothing of working systematically in the domain of being. The discipline requires that they rearrange their lives to a certain extent around the training program. Taking the stress reduction program involves a major life-style change just to make the time every day to practice the formal meditation techniques for forty-five minutes at a stretch. This time does not appear magically in anyone's life. You have to rearrange your schedule and your priorities and plan how you will free it up for practice. This is one of the ways in which taking the stress reduction program can increase the stress in a person's life in the short run.

Those of us who teach in the clinic see meditation practice as an integral part of our own lives and of our own growth as people. So we are not asking our patients to do something that we don't do on a regular basis ourselves. We know what we are asking of them because we do it too. We know the effort that it takes to make space in one's life for meditation practice, and we know the value of living in this way. No one is ever considered for a staff position in the clinic unless he or she has had years of meditation training and has a strong daily meditation practice. The people referred to the stress clinic sense that what they are being asked to do is not something "remedial" but rather "advanced training" in mobilizing their deep inner resources for coping and for healing. Our own commitment to the practice conveys our belief that the journey we are inviting our patients to undertake is a true life adventure, one that we can pursue together. This feeling of being engaged in a common pursuit makes it a lot easier for everyone to keep up the discipline of the daily practice. Ultimately, however, we are asking even more than daily practice of our patients and of ourselves, for it is only by making the meditation a "way of being" that its power can be put to practical use.

To tap this power in your own life, we recommend that you set aside a particular block of time every day, or at least six days per week, for at least eight consecutive weeks to practice. Just making this amount of time every day for yourself will be a very positive life-style change. Our lives are so complex and our minds so busy and agitated most of the time that it is necessary, especially at the beginning, to protect and support your meditation practice by making a special time for it and, if possible, by making a special place in your home where you will feel particularly comfortable and "at home" while practicing.

This needs to be protected from interruptions and from other commitments so that you can just be yourself without having to do or respond to anything. This is not always possible, but it is helpful if you can manage to set things up in this way. One measure of your commitment is whether you can bring yourself to shut off your telephone for the time you will be practicing or to let someone else answer it and take messages. It is a great letting go in and of itself only to be home for yourself at those times, and great peace can follow from this alone.

Once you make the commitment to yourself to practice in this way, the self-discipline comes in carrying it out. Committing yourself to goals that are in your own self-interest is easy. But keeping to the path you have chosen when you run into obstacles and may not see "results" right away is the real measure of your commitment. This is where conscious intentionality comes in, the intention to practice whether you feel like it or not on a particular day, whether it is convenient or not, with the determination of an athlete.

Regular practice is not as hard as you might think once you make up your mind to do it and pick an appropriate time. Most people are inwardly disciplined already to a certain extent. Getting dinner on the table every night requires discipline. Getting up in the morning and going to work requires discipline. And taking time for yourself certainly does too. You are not going to be paid for it, and chances are you will not be enrolled in a stress clinic in which you would know that everybody else is doing it and so feel some social pressure to keep up your end of things. You will have to do it for better reasons than those. Perhaps the ability to function more effectively under pressure or to be healthier and to feel better, or to be more relaxed and self-confident and happy will suffice. Ultimately you have to decide for yourself why you are making such a commitment.

Some people have resistance to the whole idea of taking time for themselves. The Puritan ethic has left a legacy of guilt when we do something for ourselves. Some people discover that they have a little voice inside that tells them that it is selfish or that they are undeserving of this kind of time and energy. Usually they recognize it as a message they were given very early on in their lives: "Live for others, not for yourself." "Help others; don't dwell on yourself."

If you do feel undeserving of taking time for yourself, why not look at *that* as part of your mindfulness practice? Where do such feelings come from? What are the thoughts behind them? Can you observe them with acceptance? Are they accurate?

Even the degree to which you can really be of help to others, if that is what you believe is most important, depends directly on how balanced you are yourself. Taking time to "tune" your own instrument and restore your energy reserves can hardly be considered selfish. *Intelligent* would be a more apt description.

Happily once people start practicing mindfulness, most quickly get over the idea that it is "selfish" and "narcissistic" to take time for themselves as they see the difference that making some time to just be has on the quality of their lives and their self-esteem, as well as on their relationships.

We suggest that everyone find their own best time to practice. Mine is early in the morning. I like to get up an hour or so before I would otherwise and meditate and do yoga. I like the quiet of this time. It feels very good to be up and have nothing to do except to dwell in the present, being with things as they are, my mind open and aware. I know the phone won't ring. I know the rest of my family is asleep, so the meditation is not taking time away from them. Most of the time my children stay asleep now, although for years the littlest one in the family always seemed to sense when there was awake energy in the house, no matter what time it was. There were periods when I had to push my meditation time back as far as 4:00 A.M. to be sure to get some uninterrupted time. Sometimes now, the children meditate or do yoga with me. I don't push it. It's just something Daddy does, so it's natural for them to know about it and to do it with me from time to time.

Practicing meditation and yoga in the early morning has a positive influence on the rest of the day for me. When I start off the day dwelling in stillness, being mindful, nourishing the domain of being, and cultivating calmness and concentration, I seem to be more mindful and relaxed the rest of the day and better able to recognize stress and handle it effectively. When I tune in to my body and work it gently to stretch my joints and feel my muscles, my body feels more alive and vibrant than on the days I don't do it. I also know what state my body is in that day and what I might want to watch out for, such as my low back or my neck if they are particularly stiff or painful that morning.

Some of our patients like to practice early in the morning, but a lot don't or can't. We leave it to each individual to experiment with times to practice and to choose the best one for his or her schedule. Practicing late at night is not recommended in the beginning, however, because it is very hard to keep up the alert attention required when you are tired.

In the first weeks of the stress reduction program, many people have trouble staying awake when they do the body scan (see Chapter 5), even when they do it in the daytime, because they get so relaxed. If I feel groggy when I wake up in the morning, I might splash cold water on my face until I know I am really awake. I don't want to meditate in a daze. I want to be alert. This may seem somewhat extreme, but really it is just knowing the value of being awake before trying to practice. It helps to remember that mindfulness is about being fully awake. It is not cultivated by relaxing to the point where unawareness and sleep take over. So we advocate doing anything necessary to wake up, even taking a cold shower if that is what it takes.

Your meditation practice will only be as powerful as your motivation to dispel the fog of your own lack of awareness. When you are in this fog, it is hard to remember the importance of practicing mindfulness, and it is hard to locate your attitudinal bearings. Confusion, fatigue, depression, and anxiety are powerful mental states that can undermine your best intentions to practice regularly. You can easily get caught up and then stuck in them and not even know it.

That is when your commitment to practice is of greatest value. It keeps you engaged in the process. The momentum of regular practice helps to maintain a certain mental stability and resilience even as you go through states of turmoil, confusion, lack of clarity, and procrastination. These are some of the most fruitful times to practice, not to get rid of your confusion or your feelings but just to be conscious and accepting of them.

◆

Most people who come to the stress clinic, no matter what their medical problem is, tell us that they are really coming to attain peace of mind. This is an understandable goal, given their mental and physical pain. But to achieve peace of mind, people have to kindle a vision of what they really want for themselves and keep that vision alive in the face of inner and outer hardships, obstacles, and setbacks.

I used to think that meditation practice was so powerful in itself and so healing that as long as you did it at all, you would see growth and change. But time has taught me that some kind of personal vision is also necessary. Perhaps it could be a vision of what or who you might be if you were to let go of the fetters of your own mind and the limitations of your own body. This image or ideal will help carry you through the inevitable periods of low motivation and give continuity to your practice.

For some that vision might be one of vibrancy and health, for others it might be one of relaxation or kindness or peacefulness or harmony or wisdom. Your vision should be what is most important to you, what you believe is most fundamental to your ability to be your best self, to be at peace with yourself, to be whole.

The price of wholeness is nothing less than a total commitment to being whole and an unswerving belief in your capacity to embody it in any moment. C. G. Jung put it this way: "The attainment of wholeness requires one to stake one's whole being. Nothing less will do; there can be no easier conditions, no substitutes, no compromises."

With this background to help you to understand the spirit and the attitudes that are most helpful to cultivate in your meditation practice, we are now ready to explore the practice itself.

3

The Power of Breathing: Your Unsuspected Ally in the Healing Process

——

Poets and scientists alike are aware that our organism pulsates with the rhythms of its ancestry. Rhythm and pulsation are intrinsic to all life, from the beating of bacterial cilia to the alternating cycles of photosynthesis and respiration in plants, to the circadian rhythms of our own body and its biochemistry. These rhythms of the living world are embedded within the larger rhythms of the planet itself, the ebb and flow of the tides, the carbon, nitrogen, and oxygen cycles of the biosphere, the cycles of night and day, the seasons. Our very bodies are joined with the planet in a continual rhythmic exchange as matter and energy flow back and forth between our bodies and what we call "the environment." Someone once calculated that, on the average, every seven years all the atoms in our body have come and gone, replaced by others from outside of us. This in itself is interesting to think about. What am I if little of the substance of my body is the same in any decade of my life?

One way this exchange of matter and energy happens is through breathing. With each breath, we exchange carbon dioxide molecules from inside our bodies for oxygen molecules from the surrounding air. Waste disposal with each outbreath, renewal with each inbreath. If this process is interrupted for more than a few minutes, the brain becomes starved for oxygen and undergoes irreversible damage.

The breath has a very important partner in its work, namely the heart. Think of it: This amazing muscle never stops pumping during our entire lifetime. It begins beating in us long before we are born and it just keeps on beating, day in and day out, year in and year out without a pause, without a rest for our entire life. And it can even be kept alive by artificial means for some time after we are dead.

As with the breath, the heartbeat is a fundamental life rhythm. The heart pumps the oxygen-rich blood from the lungs via the arteries and their smaller capillaries to all the cells of the body, supplying them with the oxygen they need to function. As the red blood cells give up their oxygen, they load up with the carbon dioxide that is the major waste product of all living tissue. The carbon dioxide is then transported back to the heart through the veins and from there pumped to the lungs, where it is discharged into the atmosphere on the outbreath. This is followed by another inbreath, which again oxygenates the hemoglobin carrier molecules that will be pumped throughout the body with the next contraction of the heart. This is literally the pulse of life in us, the rhythm of the primordial sea internalized, the ebb and flow of matter and energy in our bodies.

From the moment we are born to the moment we die, we breathe. The rhythm of our breathing varies considerably as a function of our activities and our feelings. It quickens with physical exertion or emotional upset and it slows down during sleep or periods of relaxation. As an experiment you might try to be aware of your breathing when you are excited, angry, surprised, and relaxed and notice how it changes. Sometimes our breathing is very regular. At other times it is irregular, even labored.

We have some measure of conscious control over our breathing. If we choose to, we can hold our breath for a short while or voluntarily control the rate and depth at which we breathe.

But slow or rapid, controlled or left to itself, the breath keeps going, day and night, year in, year out, through all the experiences and stages of life we traverse. Usually we take it completely for granted. We don't pay any attention to our breathing unless something happens to prevent us from breathing normally. That is, unless we start to meditate.

The breath plays an extremely important role in meditation and in healing. Breathing is an incredibly powerful ally and teacher in the work of meditation, although people who have no training in meditation think nothing of it and find it uninteresting.

The fundamental pulsations of the body are particularly fruitful to focus on during meditation because they are so intimately connected with the experience of being alive. While we could theoretically focus on our heart beating instead of on our breathing, the breath is much easier to be aware of. The fact that it is a rhythmic process and that it is constantly changing will make it even more valuable to us. In focusing on the breath when we meditate, we are learning right from the start to get comfortable with change. We see that we will have to be flexible. We will have to train ourselves to attend to a process that not only cycles and flows but that also responds to our emotional state by changing its rhythm, sometimes quite dramatically.

Our breathing also has the virtue of being a very convenient process to support ongoing awareness in our daily lives. As long as we are alive, it is always with us. We can't leave home without it. It is always here to be attended to, no matter what we are doing or feeling or experiencing, no matter where we are. Tuning in to it brings us right into the here and now. It immediately anchors our awareness in the body, in a fundamental, rhythmic, flowing life process.

Some people have trouble breathing when they get anxious. They start to breathe faster and faster and more and more shallowly and wind up *hyperventilating,* that is, not getting enough oxygen and blowing off too much carbon dioxide. This brings on feelings of light-headedness, often accompanied by a feeling of pressure in the chest. When, all of a sudden, you feel like you are not getting in enough air, an overwhelming wave of fear or panic can arise. When you panic, of course, it just makes it that much harder to get control of your breathing.

People who experience episodes of hyperventilation can think they are having a heart attack and are going to die. Actually the worst that can happen is that they will black out, which is dangerous enough. But passing out is the body's way of breaking the vicious cycle, which begins when you feel unable to breathe, which leads to panic, which leads to a stronger feeling of being unable to breathe. When you pass out, your breathing returns to normal on its own. If you are unable to get your breathing under control, your body will do it for you, if necessary by short-circuiting your consciousness for a while.

When patients who suffer from hyperventilation are sent to the stress clinic, they are asked, along with everyone else, to focus on their breathing as the first step in getting into the formal meditation practice. For many of them just the thought of focusing on their breathing produces feelings of anxiety, and they have a lot of trouble *watching* their breath without trying to manipulate it. But with perseverance most people learn to have confidence in their breathing as they get more familiar with it in the meditation practice.

A thirty-seven-year-old firefighter named Gregg came to the stress clinic, referred by a psychiatrist after a year-long history of hyperventilation episodes and unsuccessful drug treatments for anxiety. His problem started when he was overcome by smoke in a burning building. From that day on, every time he tried to put on his gas mask to go into a burning building, his breathing would become rapid and shallow and he would be unable to put on the mask. Several times he was rushed from fires to the emergency room of the local hospital thinking that he was having a heart attack. But it was always diagnosed as hyperventilation. At the time he was referred to the stress clinic, he had been unable to go into buildings to fight fires for over a year.

In the first class Gregg, along with everybody else, was introduced to the basic technique of watching his breathing. As soon as he started focusing on it going in and out, he felt anxiety building. He was reluctant to run out of the room, so he held on and made it through somehow. He also managed to force himself to practice every day that week, mostly out of desperation, in spite of his discomfort and his fear. That first week practicing the body scan, which as you will soon see, involves a lot of focusing on breathing, was torture for him. Every time he would tune in to his breathing, he would feel terrible, as if his breath were an enemy. He saw it as an undependable and potentially uncontrollable force that had already made it impossible for him to work and had thus changed his relationship to his fellow firefighters and his own view of himself as a man.

Yet after two weeks of doggedly working with his breathing while doing the body scan, he discovered that he could put on his mask and go into burning buildings again.

Gregg later described to the class how this dramatic change came about. As he spent time watching it, he became more confident in his breathing. Even though he was unaware of it at first, he was relaxing a little during the body scan, and as he got more relaxed, his feelings about his breathing started to change. By spending time just watching his breath flow in and out as he moved his focus of attention through his body, he began to know what his breathing actually felt like. At the same time he found that he was getting less caught up in his thoughts and fears *about* his breathing. From his own direct experience, he came to see that his breathing was not his enemy and that he could even use it to relax.

It was not a big jump for him to practice being aware of his breathing at other times of the day and to use it in the same way to become calmer wherever he was. One day it occurred to him to try it at a fire. He had been going out with the trucks on occasion but had only been able to do support activities. As he put on the mask, he purposefully focused on his breathing, watching it, letting it be as it was, accepting the feeling of the mask as he put it on his face, just as he worked with accepting his breathing and whatever feelings he was experiencing when he would practice the body scan at home. What he discovered was that it was okay.

From that day on, Gregg was able to put on his mask and go into burning buildings without panicking or hyperventilating. He has had several moments in the three years since he took the program when he experienced fear of being trapped when he was in closed, smoky places. But when this happened, he was able to become aware of his fear, slow down his breathing, and maintain his balance of mind. He has never had another hyperventilation episode.

◆

The easiest and most effective way to begin practicing mindfulness as a formal meditative practice is to simply focus your attention on your breathing and see what happens as you attempt to keep it there, just as we did in Chapter 1 but for longer than three minutes. There are a number of different places in the body where the breath can be observed. Obviously one is the nostrils. If you are watching your breathing from here, you will be focusing on the feeling of the breath as it flows past the nostrils. Another place to focus on is the chest as it expands and contracts, and another is the belly, which moves in and out with each breath if it is relaxed.

No matter which location you choose, the idea is to be aware of the sensations that accompany your breathing at that particular place and to hold them in the forefront of your awareness from moment to moment. Doing this, we *feel* the air as it flows in and out past the nostrils; we *feel* the movement of the muscles associated with breathing; we *feel* the belly as it moves in and out.

Paying attention to your breathing means just paying attention. Nothing more. It doesn't mean that you should "push" or force your breathing, or try to make it deeper, or change its pattern or rhythm. The chances are your breath has been moving in and out of your body very well for years without your having thought about it at all. There is no need to try to *control* it now just because you have decided to pay attention to it. In fact, trying to control it is counterproductive. The effort we make in being mindful of the breathing is simply to be aware of the *feeling* of each inbreath and each outbreath. If you like, you can also be aware of the feeling of the breath as the direction of flow reverses.

Another common mistake that people make when they first hear the meditation instructions about breathing is to assume that we are telling them to *think about* their breathing. But this is absolutely incorrect. Focusing on the breath does not mean you should think about your breathing. It means you should *be aware* of it and *feel* the sensations associated with it and attend to their changing qualities.

In the stress clinic we generally focus on the feelings of the breath at the belly rather than at the nostrils or in the chest. This is partly because doing so tends to be particularly relaxing and calming in the early stages of practice. All professionals who make special use of their breathing as part of their work, such as opera singers, wind-instrument players, dancers, actors, and martial artists, know the value of breathing from the belly and "centering" their awareness in this region. They know from firsthand experience that they will have more breath and better control if the breath comes from the belly.

Focusing on the breath at your belly can be calming. Just as the surface of the ocean tends to be choppy when the wind is blowing, the mind, too, tends to be reactive and agitated when the outside environment is not calm and peaceful. In the case of the ocean, if you go down ten or twenty feet, there is only a gentle swelling; there is calm even when the surface is agitated. Similarly when we focus on our breathing down in the belly, we are tuning to a region of the body that is below the agitations of our thinking mind and is intrinsically calmer. This is a valuable way of reestablishing inner calmness and balance in the face of emotional upset or when you "have a lot on your mind."

In meditation the breath functions as an anchor for our attention. Tuning to it anywhere we feel it in the body allows us to drop below the surface agitations of the mind into relaxation, calmness, and stability. The agitation is still at the surface just as the waves are on the surface of the water. But we are out of the wind and protected from their buffeting action and their tension-producing effects when we shift our attention to the breath for a moment or two. This is an extremely effective way of locating a peaceful center within yourself. It enhances the overall stability of your mind.

When you touch base in any moment with that part of your mind that is calm and stable, your perspective immediately changes. You can see things more clearly and act from inner balance rather than being tossed about by the agitations of your mind. This is one reason why focusing on the breath at your belly is so useful. Your belly is literally the "center of gravity" of your body, far below the head and the turmoil of your thinking mind. For this reason we "befriend" the belly right from the beginning as an ally in establishing calmness and awareness.

Any moment during the day that you bring your attention to your breathing in this way becomes a moment of meditative awareness. It is an effective way of tuning in to the present and orienting yourself to your body and to what you are feeling, not only while you are "meditating" but also while you are going about living your life.

When you practice mindfulness of breathing, you may find it helpful in deepening your concentration to close your eyes. However, it is not always necessary to meditate with your eyes closed. If you decide to keep them open, let your gaze be unfocused on the surface in front of you or on the floor and keep it steady. Bring the same kind of sensitivity to feeling your breathing that we brought to eating the raisins, as described in Chapter 1. In other words, be mindful of what you are actually feeling from moment to moment. Keep your attention on the breath for the full duration of the inbreath and the full duration of the outbreath as best you can, and when you notice that your mind has wandered and is no longer on your breathing, just bring it back.

DIAPHRAGMATIC BREATHING

Many of our patients have found it beneficial to breathe in a particular way that involves relaxing the belly. This is known as diaphragmatic breathing. It may or may not be the way you are already breathing. If it isn't, as you become more aware of your breathing pattern by focusing on your belly, you may find yourself breathing more this way naturally because it is slower and deeper than chest breathing, which tends to be rapid and shallow. If you watch infants breathe, you will see that diaphragmatic breathing is the way we all start out when we are babies.

Diaphragmatic breathing is better described as abdominal or belly breathing, because all respiratory patterns involve the diaphragm. To visualize this particular way of breathing, it helps to know a little about how your body gets air in and out of your lungs in the first place.

The diaphragm is a large, umbrella-shaped sheet of muscle that is attached all around the lower edges of the rib cage. It separates the contents of the chest (the heart and lungs and great blood vessels) from the contents of the abdomen (the stomach and liver, intestines, etc.). When it contracts, it tightens and draws downward (see Figure 1) because it is anchored all along the rim of the rib cage. This downward movement increases the volume of the chest cavity, in which the lungs are located on either side of the heart. The increased volume in the chest produces a decrease in the air pressure in the lungs. Because of the decreased pressure inside the lungs, air from outside the body, which is at a higher pressure, flows into the lungs to equalize the pressure. This is the inbreath.

After the diaphragm contracts, it goes through a relaxation. As the diaphragm muscle relaxes, it gets looser and returns to its original position higher up in the chest, thereby decreasing the volume of the chest cavity. This increases the pressure in the chest, which forces the air in the lungs out through the nose (and mouth if it is open). This is the outbreath. So in all breathing, the air is drawn into the lungs as the diaphragm contracts and lowers and it is expelled as the diaphragm relaxes and comes back up.

Now, suppose the muscles that form the wall of your belly (the abdomen) are tight rather than relaxed when the diaphragm is contracting. As the diaphragm pushes down on the stomach and the liver and the other organs that are in your abdomen, it will meet resistance and will not be able to descend very far. Your breathing will tend to be shallow and rather high up in the chest.

In abdominal or diaphragmatic breathing, the idea is to *relax* your belly as much as you can. Then, as the breath comes in, the belly expands slightly (on its own) in an outward direction as the diaphragm pushes down on the contents of the abdomen from above. The diaphragm can go down farther when this happens so the inbreath is a little longer and the lungs fill with a little more air. Then a little more air is expelled on the outbreath, so that, overall, the full cycle of your breathing will be slower and deeper.

If you are not accustomed to relaxing your belly, you may find your first attempts to breathe in this way to be frustrating and confusing. But if you persevere without forcing it, it soon comes

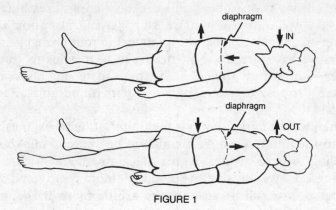

diaphragm

IN

diaphragm

OUT

FIGURE 1

naturally. Babies aren't trying to relax their bellies when they breathe! They are already relaxed. But once our bodies have developed a certain amount of chronic tension, as can happen as we get older, it can take a while to get the hang of relaxing the belly. But it is definitely worth paying attention to.

At the beginning you may find it helpful to lie down on your back or stretch out in a recliner, close your eyes, and put one of your hands over your belly. Bring your attention to your hand and feel it move as the breath flows in and out. If your hand is rising during the inhalation and falling during the exhalation, then you have it. It should not be a violent or forced movement and it should not be very big. It will feel like a balloon, expanding gently on the inbreath, deflating gently on the outbreath. If you feel it now, good. If you don't, that's fine too. It will come with time all by itself as you continue to practice watching your breath. And for the record, keep in mind that there is no balloon in your belly. That's just a way of visualizing the movement. If anything resembles balloons, it's your lungs, and they are in your chest!

◆

When we surveyed several hundred patients who had been out of the stress reduction program for a number of years and asked them what the single most important thing they got out of the program was, the majority said, "The breathing." I find this response amusing since every one of them was breathing long before they came for stress reduction training. Why would breathing, which they were doing before anyway, be so important and so valuable all of a sudden?

The answer is that once you start meditating, breathing is no longer just breathing. When we start paying attention to our breathing on a regular basis, our relationship to it changes dramatically. As we have already seen, tuning in to it helps us to center ourselves. The breath *reminds* us to tune in to our body and to encounter the rest of our experience with mindfulness, in this moment.

When we are mindful of our breathing, it helps us to calm the body and the mind. Then we are able to be aware of our thoughts and feelings with a greater degree of calmness and with a more discerning eye. We are able to see things more clearly and with a larger perspective, all because we are a little more awake, a little more aware. And with this awareness comes a feeling of having more room to move, of having more options, of being free to choose effective and appropriate responses in stressful situations rather than losing our equilibrium and sense of self as a result of feeling overwhelmed, thrown off balance by our own knee-jerk reactions.

This all comes from the simple practice of paying attention to your breathing when you dedicate yourself to practicing it regularly. In addition you will discover that it is possible to direct your breath with great precision to various parts of your body in such a way that it will penetrate and soothe regions that are injured or in pain, at the same time that it calms and stabilizes the mind.

We also can use the breath to deepen our ability to dwell in deep states of calmness and concentrated awareness. Giving the mind *one thing* to keep track of, namely the breath, to replace the whole range of things that it usually finds to preoccupy itself enhances our powers of concentration. Staying with the breath during meditation, no matter what, ultimately leads to deep experiences of calmness and awareness. It is as if the breath contains, folded into itself, a power that we can come to simply by following it as if it were a path.

This power is uncovered when we systematically bring awareness to the breath and sustain it for extended periods. With it comes a growing sense of the breath as a dependable ally. I suspect this is why our patients so often say that "the breathing" is the most important thing they get out of the course. Right in the simple old breath (I won't say "right beneath our noses"), lies a completely overlooked source of power to transform our lives. All we need to do to make use of it is to deepen our attentional skills and our patience.

It is the very simplicity of the practice of mindfulness of breathing that gives it its power to disentangle us from the compulsive and habitual hold of the mind's many preoccupations. Yogis have known this for centuries. Breathing is the universal foundation for meditation practice.

◆

There are two major ways of practicing mindfulness of breathing. One involves the formal discipline of making a specific time in which you stop all activity, assume a special posture, and dwell for some time in moment-to-moment awareness of the inbreath and the outbreath as decribed above. By practicing this way regularly, you naturally deepen your ability to keep your attention on the breath for a sustained period of time. This will improve your ability to concentrate in general as the mind becomes more focused and calmer, less reactive both to its own thoughts and to outside pressures. As you continue practicing, the calmness that comes with just being with your breathing over a period of time develops a stability of its own and becomes much more robust and dependable. Then making time to meditate, whatever technique you use, becomes nothing other than making time to come home to your deeper self, a time of inner peace and renewal.

The second way of practicing using the breath is to be mindful of it from time to time during the day, or even all day long, wherever you are and whatever you are doing. In this way the thread of meditative awareness, including the physical relaxation, the emotional calm, and the insight that come with it, is woven into every aspect of your daily life. We call this "informal" meditation practice. It is at least as valuable as the formal practice, but is easily neglected and loses much of its ability to stabilize the mind if it is not combined with a regular formal meditation practice. The formal and informal practices using the breath complement and enrich one another. It is best to let them work together. Of course, the second way takes no time at all, just remembering.

Mindfulness of breathing is central to all aspects of meditation practice. We will be using it when we practice the sitting meditation, the body scan, the yoga, and the walking meditation, which are all formal meditation practices. We will also be using it throughout the day as we practice developing a continuity of awareness in our lives. If you keep at it, the day will soon come when you will look upon your breathing as an old, familiar friend and a powerful ally in the healing process.

EXERCISE 1

1. Assume a comfortable posture lying on your back or sitting. If you are sitting, keep the spine straight and let your shoulders drop.
2. Close your eyes if it feels comfortable.
3. Bring your attention to your belly, feeling it rise or expand gently on the inbreath and fall or recede on the outbreath.
4. Keep the focus on your breathing, "being with" each inbreath for its full duration and with each outbreath for its full duration, as if you were riding the waves of your own breathing.
5. Every time you notice that your mind has wandered off the breath, notice what it was that took you away and then gently bring your attention back to your belly and the feeling of the breath coming in and out.
6. If your mind wanders away from the breath a thousand times, then your "job" is simply to bring it back to the breath every time, no matter what it becomes preoccupied with.
7. Practice this exercise for fifteen minutes at a convenient time every day, whether you feel like it or not, for one week and see how it feels to incorporate a disciplined meditation practice into your life. Be aware of how it feels to spend some time each day just being with your breath without having to *do* anything.

EXERCISE 2

1. Tune in to your breathing at different times during the day, feeling the belly go through one or two risings and fallings.
2. Become aware of your thoughts and feelings at these moments, just observing them without judging them or yourself.
3. At the same time be aware of any changes in the way you are seeing things and feeling about yourself.

4

Sitting Meditation: Nourishing the Domain of Being

In the first class each person gets a chance to say why he or she has come to the stress clinic and what he or she hopes to accomplish. Last week Linda described feeling as if a large truck were always right on her heels, driving just faster than she can walk. It was an image people could relate to; the vividness of it sent a wave of acknowledging nods and smiles through the room.

"What did she think the truck actually was?" I asked. Her impulses, her cravings (she was very overweight), her desires, she responded. In a word, her mind. Her mind was the truck. It was always right behind her, pushing, driving her, allowing her no rest, no peace.

We have already mentioned how our behavior and our feeling states can be driven by the play of the mind's likes and dislikes, by our addictions and aversions. When you look, is it not accurate to say that your mind is constantly seeking satisfaction, making plans to ensure that things will go your way, trying to get what you want or think you need and at the same time trying to ward off the things you fear, the things you don't want to happen? As a consequence of this common play of our minds, don't we all tend to fill up our days with things that just *have* to be done and then run around desperately trying to do them all, while in the process not really enjoying much of the doing because we are too pressed for time, too rushed, too busy, too anxious? We can feel overwhelmed by our schedules, our responsibilities, and our roles at times even when everything we are doing is important, even when we have chosen to do them all. We live immersed in a world of constant doing. Rarely are we in

59

touch with who is doing the doing or, put otherwise, with the world of being.

To get back in touch with being is not that difficult. We only need to remind ourselves to be mindful. Moments of mindfulness are moments of peace and stillness, even in the midst of activity. When your whole life is driven by doing, formal meditation practice can provide a refuge of sanity and stability that can be used to restore some balance and perspective. It can be a way of stopping the headlong momentum of all the doing and giving yourself some time to dwell in a state of deep relaxation and well-being and to remember who you are. The formal practice can give you the strength and the self-knowledge to go back to the doing and do it from out of your being. Then at least a certain amount of patience and inner stillness, clarity and balance of mind, will infuse what you are doing, and the busyness and pressure will be less onerous. In fact they might just disappear entirely.

Meditation is really a non-doing. It is the only human endeavor I know of that does not involve trying to get somewhere else but, rather, emphasizes being where you already are. Much of the time we are so carried away by all the doing, the striving, the planning, the reacting, the busyness, that when we stop just to feel where we are, it can seem a little peculiar at first. For one thing we tend to have little awareness of the incessant and relentless activity of our own mind and how much we are driven by it. That is not too surprising, given that we hardly ever stop and observe the mind directly to see what it is up to. We seldom look dispassionately at the reactions and habits of our own mind, at its fears and its desires.

It takes a while to get comfortable with the richness of allowing yourself to just *be* with your own mind. It's a little like meeting an old friend for the first time in years. There may be some awkwardness at first, not knowing who this person is anymore, not knowing quite how to be with him or her. It may take some time to reestablish the bond, to refamiliarize yourselves with each other.

Ironically although we all "have" minds, we seem to need to "re-mind" ourselves of who we are from time to time. If we don't, the momentum of all the doing just takes over and can have us living its agenda rather than our own, almost as if we were robots. The momentum of unbridled doing can carry us for decades, even to the grave, without our quite knowing that we are living out our lives and that we have only moments to live.

Given all the momentum behind our doing, getting ourselves to remember the preciousness of the present moment seems to require somewhat unusual and even drastic steps. This is why we make a special time each day for formal meditation practice. It is a way of stopping, a way of "re-minding" ourselves, of nourishing the domain of being for a change.

To make time in your life for being, for non-doing, may at first feel stilted and artificial. Until you actually get into it, it can sound like just one more "thing" to *do*. "Now I have to find time to meditate on top of all the obligations and stresses I already have in my life." And on one level there is no getting around the fact that this is true.

But once you see the critical need to nourish your being, once you see the need to calm your heart and your mind and to find an inner balance with which to face the storms of life, your commitment to make that time a priority and the requisite discipline to make it a reality develop naturally. Making time to meditate becomes easier. After all, if you discover for yourself that it really does nourish what is deepest in you, you will certainly find a way.

♦

We call the heart of the formal meditation practice "sitting meditation" or simply "sitting." As with breathing, sitting is not foreign to anyone. We all sit, nothing special about that. But mindful sitting is different from ordinary sitting in the same way that mindful breathing is different from ordinary breathing. The difference, of course, is your awareness.

To practice sitting, we make a special time and place for non-doing, as suggested in Chapter 2. We consciously adopt an alert and relaxed body posture so that we can feel relatively comfortable without moving, and then we reside with calm acceptance in the present without trying to fill it with anything. You have already tried this in the various exercises in which you have watched your breathing.

It helps a lot to adopt an erect and dignified posture, with your head, neck, and back aligned vertically. This allows the breath to flow most easily. It is also the physical counterpart of the inner attitudes of self-reliance, self-acceptance, and alert attention that we are cultivating.

We usually practice the sitting meditation either on a chair or on the floor. If you choose a chair, the ideal is to use one that has a straight back and that allows your feet to be flat on the floor. We often recommend that if possible you sit away from the back of the chair so that your spine is self-supporting (see Figure 2A). But if you have to, leaning against the back of the chair is also fine. If you choose to sit on the floor, do so on a firm, thick cushion which raises your buttocks off the floor three to six inches (a pillow folded over once or twice does nicely; or you can purchase a meditation cushion, or *zafu*, specifically for sitting).

There are a number of cross-legged sitting postures and kneeling postures that some people use when they sit on the floor. The one I use most is the so-called "Burmese" posture (see Figure 2B), which involves drawing one heel in close to the body and draping the other leg in front of it. Depending on how flexible your hips and knees and ankles are, your knees may or may not be touching the floor. It is somewhat more comfortable when they are. Others use a kneeling posture, placing the cushion between the feet (see Figure 2C).

Sitting on the floor can give you a reassuring feeling of being "grounded" and self-supporting in the meditation posture, but it is not necessary to meditate sitting on the floor or in a cross-legged posture. Some of our patients prefer the floor, but most sit on straight-backed chairs. Ultimately it is not what you are sitting on that matters in meditation but the sincerity of your effort.

Whether you choose the floor or a chair, posture is very important in meditation practice. It can be an outward support in cultivating an inner attitude of dignity, patience, and self-acceptance. The main points to keep in mind about your posture are to try to keep the back, neck, and head aligned in the vertical, to relax the shoulders, and to do something comfortable with your hands. Usually we place them on the knees, as in Figure 2, or we rest them in the lap with the fingers of the left hand above the fingers of the right and the tips of the thumbs just touching each other.

When we have assumed the posture we have selected, we bring our attention to our breathing. We *feel* it come in, we *feel* it go out. We dwell in the present, moment by moment, breath by breath. It sounds simple, and it is. Full awareness on the inbreath, full awareness on the outbreath. Letting the breath just happen, observing it, feeling all the sensations, gross and subtle, associated with it.

It is simple but it is not easy. You can probably sit in front of a TV set or in a car on a trip for hours without giving it a thought. But when you try sitting in your house with nothing to watch but your breath, your body, and your mind, with nothing to entertain you and no place to go, the first thing you will probably notice is that at least part of you doesn't want to stay at this for very long.

FIGURE 2

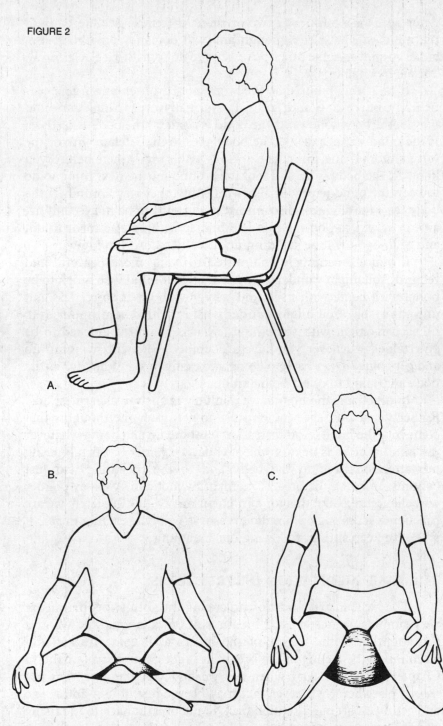

A.

B.

C.

After perhaps a minute or two or three or four, either the body or the mind will have had enough and will demand something else, either to shift to some other posture or to do something else entirely. This is inevitable.

It is at this point that the work of self-observation gets particularly interesting and fruitful. Normally every time the mind moves, the body follows. If the mind is restless, the body is restless. If the mind wants a drink, the body goes to the kitchen sink or the refrigerator. If the mind says, "This is boring," then before you know it, the body is up and looking around for the next thing to do to keep the mind happy. It also works the other way around. If the body feels the slightest discomfort, it will shift to be more comfortable or it will call on the mind to find something else for it to do, and again, you will be standing up literally before you know it.

If you are genuinely committed to being more peaceful and relaxed, you might wonder why it is that your mind is so quick to be bored with being with itself and why your body is so restless and uncomfortable. You might wonder what is behind your impulses to fill each moment with something; what is behind your need to be entertained whenever you have an "empty" moment, to jump up and get going, to get back to doing and being busy? What drives the body and mind to reject being still?

In practicing meditation we don't try to answer such questions. Rather we just observe the impulse to get up or the thoughts that come into the mind. And instead of jumping up and doing whatever the mind decides is next on the agenda, we gently but firmly bring our attention back to the belly and to the breathing and just continue to watch the breath, moment by moment. We may ponder why the mind is like this for a moment or two, but basically we are practicing accepting each moment as it is without reacting to *how* it is. So we keep sitting, following our breathing.

THE BASIC MEDITATION INSTRUCTIONS

The basic instructions for practicing the sitting meditation are very simple. We observe the breath as it flows in and out. We give full attention to the feeling of the breath as it comes in and full attention to the feeling of the breath as it goes out, just as we did in Chapters 1 and 3. And whenever we find that our attention has moved elsewhere, wherever that may be, we just note it and let go and gently escort our attention back to the breath, back to the rising and falling of our own belly.

If you have been trying it, perhaps you will have already noticed that your mind tends to move around a lot. You may have contracted with yourself to keep your attention focused on the breath no matter what. But before long, you will undoubtedly find that the mind is off someplace else . . . it has forgotten the breath, it has been drawn away.

Each time you become aware of this while you are sitting, you gently bring your attention back to your belly and back to your breathing, no matter what carried it away. If it moves off the breath a hundred times, then you just calmly bring it back a hundred times, as soon as you are aware of not being on the breath.

By doing so you are training your mind to be less reactive and more stable. You are making each moment count. You are taking each moment as it comes, not valuing any one above any other. In this way you are cultivating your natural ability to concentrate your mind. By repeatedly bringing your attention back to the breath each time it wanders off, concentration builds and deepens, much as muscles develop by repetitively lifting weights. Working regularly with (not struggling against) the resistance of your own mind builds inner strength. At the same time you are also developing patience and practicing being non-judgmental. You are not giving yourself a hard time because your mind left the breath. You simply and matter-of-factly return it to the breath, gently but firmly.

WHAT TO DO ABOUT YOUR BODY'S DISCOMFORT

As you will quickly see when you sit down to meditate, almost anything can carry your attention away from your breathing. One big source of distracting impulses is your body. As a rule, if you sit still for a while in any position, your body will become uncomfortable. Normally we are continually shifting our position without much awareness of it in response to this discomfort. But when practicing meditation, it is actually useful to resist the first impulse to shift position in response to bodily discomfort. Instead we direct our attention to these sensations of discomfort and mentally welcome them.

Why? Because at the moment they come into awareness, these sensations of discomfort become part of our present-moment experience and thus worthy objects of observation and inquiry in and of themselves. They give us the opportunity to look directly at our automatic reactions and at the whole process of what happens as the mind loses its balance and becomes agitated as it is drawn away from the breath.

In this way the pain in your knee, or the aching in your back, or the tension in your shoulders, rather than being treated as distractions preventing you from staying with your breath, can be included in the field of your awareness and simply accepted without reacting to them as undesirable and trying to make them go away. This approach gives you an alternate way of seeing discomfort. Uncomfortable as they may be, these bodily sensations are now potential teachers and allies in learning about yourself. They can help you to develop your powers of concentration, calmness, and awareness rather than just being frustrating impediments to the goal of trying to stay on your breath.

The cultivation of this kind of flexibility, which allows you to welcome *whatever* comes up and be with it rather than insisting on paying attention to only one thing, say the breath, is one of the most characteristic and valuable features of mindfulness meditation.

What this means in practice is that we make some effort to sit *with* sensations of discomfort when they come up during our attempts to meditate, not necessarily to the point of pain but at least past where we might ordinarily react to them. We breathe *with* them. We welcome them and actually try to maintain a continuity of awareness from moment to moment in their presence. Then, if we have to, we shift our body to reduce the discomfort, but *we do even that mindfully*, with moment-to-moment awareness as we are moving.

It's not that the meditative process considers messages about discomfort and pain that the body produces to be unimportant. On the contrary, as you will see in Chapters 22 and 23, we consider pain and discomfort to be important enough to merit a deeper looking into. The best way of looking into them is to welcome them when they come rather than trying to make them go away because we don't like them. By sitting with some discomfort and accepting it as part of our experience in the moment, even if we don't like it, which we don't, we discover that it is actually possible to relax into physical discomfort. This is one example of how discomfort or even pain can be your teacher and help you to heal.

Relaxing into discomfort sometimes reduces pain intensity. The more you practice, the more skill you can develop in reducing pain or at least becoming more transparent to it. But whether you experience pain reduction or not during the sitting meditation, intentionally working with your reactions to discomfort will help you to develop some degree of calmness and equanimity, qualities which will prove useful in facing many different challenges and stressful situations as well as pain (see Parts II and III).

HOW TO WORK WITH THOUGHTS IN MEDITATION

Aside from physical discomfort and pain, there are numerous other occurrences during meditation that can carry your attention away from the breath. The primary one is thinking. Just because you decide to still your body and observe your breath from moment to moment doesn't mean that your thinking mind is going to cooperate. It doesn't quiet down just because you have decided to meditate!

What does happen as we pay attention to our breathing is that we see that we live immersed in a seemingly never-ending stream of thoughts, coming willy-nilly, one after another in rapid succession. Many people are greatly relieved when they come back after practicing meditation on their own during their first week in the stress clinic and discover that they were not the only ones who found that their thoughts cascaded through their mind like a waterfall, completely beyond their control. They are reassured to learn that everybody in the class has a mind that behaves in this way. It is just the way the mind is.

This discovery amounts to a revelation for many of the people in the stress clinic. It becomes the occasion of or sets the stage for a profound learning experience that many claim is the most valuable thing they get out of their meditation training, namely the realization that they are not their thoughts. This discovery means that they can consciously choose to relate or not to relate to their thoughts in a variety of ways that were not available to them when they were unaware of this simple fact.

In the early stages of meditation practice the activity of thought is constantly pulling our attention away from the primary task we have set ourselves in the developing of calmness and concentration, namely to be with the breath. In order to build continuity and momentum in the meditation practice, you will need to keep reminding yourself to come back to the breath, no matter what the mind is up to from one moment to the next.

The things you find yourself thinking about during meditation may or may not be important to you, but important or not, they do seem to lead a life of their own, as we have seen. If you are in a period of high stress, the mind will tend to obsess about your predicament, what you should do, or should have done, or shouldn't do, or shouldn't have done. At such times your thoughts may be highly charged with anxiety and worry.

At less stressful times the thoughts that go through your mind may be less anxious in nature, but they can be just as powerful in taking your attention away from the breath. You may find yourself thinking about a movie you saw, or fall captive to a song in your head that stubbornly refuses to leave. Or you may be thinking about dinner, or work, or your parents, or your children, or other people, or your vacation, or your health, or death, or your bills, or just about anything else. Thoughts of one kind or another will cascade through the mind as you sit, most of them below the level of your awareness, until finally you realize that you are not watching your breathing anymore and you don't even know how long it's been since you were aware of it, nor how you got to what you are thinking now that you have woken up to the fact that the breath was forgotten.

It's at this point that you say, "Okay, let's just go back to the breath right now and let go of the thoughts I'm having, no matter what they are." It also helps at such moments to check your posture and sit up straight again if your body has slumped over, which it commonly does when your awareness becomes dull.

During meditation we treat all our thoughts as if they are of equal value. We try to be aware of them when they come up and then we intentionally return our attention to the breath as the major focus of observation, *regardless of the content of the thought!* In other words, we intentionally practice letting go of each thought that attracts our attention, whether it seems important and insightful or unimportant and trivial. We just observe them as thoughts, as discrete events that appear in the field of our awareness. We are aware of them because they are there but we intentionally decline getting caught up in the content of the thoughts during meditation, no matter how charged the content may be for us at that moment. Instead we remind ourselves to perceive them simply as thoughts, as seemingly independently occurring events in the field of our awareness. We note their content and the amount of "charge" they have, in other words whether they are weak or strong in their power to dominate the mind at that moment. Then, no matter how charged they are for us at that moment, we intentionally let go and refocus on our breathing once again and on the experience of being "in our body" as we sit.

Letting go of our thoughts, however, does not mean suppressing them. Many people hear it this way and make the mistake of thinking that meditation requires them to shut off their thinking or their feelings. They somehow hear the instructions as meaning that if they are thinking, that is "bad," and that a "good meditation" is one in which there is little or no thinking. So it is important to emphasize that *thinking is not bad nor is it even undesirable during meditation. What matters is whether you are aware of your thoughts and feelings during meditation and how you handle them.* Trying to suppress them will only result in greater tension and frustration and more problems, not in calmness and peace.

Mindfulness does not involve pushing thoughts away or walling yourself off from them to quiet your mind. We are not trying to stop our thoughts as they cascade through the mind. We are simply making room for them, observing them as thoughts, and letting them be, using the breath as our anchor or "home base" for observing, for reminding us to stay focused and calm.

In proceeding in this way, you will find that every meditation is different. Sometimes you may feel relatively calm and relaxed and undisturbed by thoughts or strong feelings. At other times the thoughts and feelings may be so strong and recurrent that all you can do is watch them as best you can and be with your breath as much as you can in between. *Meditation is not so concerned with how much thinking is going on as it is with how much room you are making for it to take place within the field of your awareness from one moment to the next.*

◆

It is remarkable how liberating it feels to be able to see that your thoughts are just thoughts and that they are not "you" or "reality." For instance, if you have the thought that you have to get a certain number of things done today and you don't recognize it as a thought but act as if it's "the truth," then you have created a reality *in that moment* in which you really believe that those things must all be done today.

Peter, who, we saw in Chapter 1, had come because he had had a heart attack and wanted to prevent another one, came to a dramatic realization of this one night when he found himself washing his car at ten o'clock at night with the floodlights on in the driveway. It struck him that he didn't *have* to be doing this. It was just the inevitable result of a whole day spent trying to fit everything in that he *thought* needed doing. As he saw what he was doing to himself, he also saw that he had been unable to question the truth of his original conviction that everything had to get done *today*, because he was already so completely caught up in believing it.

If you find yourself behaving in similar ways, it is likely that you will also feel driven, tense, and anxious without even knowing why, just as Peter did. So if the thought of how much you have to get done today comes up while you are meditating, you will have to be very attentive to it *as a thought* or you may be up and doing things before you know it, without any awareness that you decided to stop sitting simply because a thought came through your mind.

On the other hand, when such a thought comes up, if you are able to step back from it and see it clearly, then you will be able to prioritize things and make sensible decisions about what really does need doing. You will know when to call it quits during the day. So the simple act of recognizing your thoughts *as thoughts* can free you from the distorted reality they often create and allow for more clear-sightedness and a greater sense of manageability in your life.

This liberation from the tyranny of the thinking mind comes directly out of the meditation practice itself. When we spend some time each day in a state of non-doing, observing the flow of the breath and the activity of our mind and body without getting caught up in that activity, we are cultivating calmness and mindfulness hand in hand. As the mind develops stability and is less caught up in the content of thinking, we strengthen the mind's ability to concentrate and to be calm. And each time we recognize a thought as a thought when it arises, and we register its content and discern the strength of its hold on us and the accuracy of its content, each time we then let go of it and come back to our breathing and to a sense of our body, we are strengthening mindfulness. We are coming to know ourselves better and becoming more accepting of ourselves, not as we would like to be but as we actually are.

OTHER OBJECTS OF ATTENTION IN THE SITTING MEDITATION

We introduce the sitting practice in the second class of the stress clinic. People practice it for homework for ten minutes once a day in the second week in addition to the forty-five-minute body scan you will learn in the next chapter. Over the weeks we increase the sitting time until we can sit for up to forty-five minutes at a stretch. As we do, we also expand the range of experiences we attend to in the sitting.

For the first few weeks, we just watch the breath come in and go out. You could practice in this way forever and never come to the end of it. It just gets deeper and deeper. The mind eventually becomes calmer and more relaxed, and mindfulness becomes stronger and stronger.

In the work of meditation the simplest techniques, such as awareness of breathing, are as profoundly healing and liberating as more elaborate methods, which sometimes people mistakenly think are more "advanced." In no sense is being with your breath any less "advanced" than paying attention to other aspects of inner and outer experience. All have a place and value in cultivating mindfulness and wisdom. Fundamentally it is the quality and sincerity of your effort in practicing and the depth of your seeing that are important rather than what "technique" you are using or what you are paying attention to. If you are really paying attention, any object can become a door into direct moment-to-moment awareness. But mindfulness of breathing is a very powerful and effective anchor for all other aspects of meditative awareness. For this reason we will be returning to it over and over again.

Over the weeks, we expand the field of attention in the sitting meditation in a step-wise fashion to include, in addition to breathing, body sensations in particular regions, a sense of the body as a whole, sounds, and finally the thought process itself. Sometimes we just focus on one of these. At other times we may cover all of them sequentially in one sitting and finish by just sitting with awareness of whatever comes up, not looking for anything in particular to focus on, such as sounds or thoughts or even the breath. This is sometimes called *choiceless awareness*. You can think of it as simply being receptive to whatever unfolds in each moment. Simple as it may sound, practicing in this way requires very strong calmness and attentiveness, qualities that are best cultivated, as we have seen, by choosing one object, most commonly the breath, and working with it over a period of months and even years. For this reason some people might benefit most by staying with the breath and a sense of the body as a whole in the early stages of their meditation practice, especially if they are not using the sitting-meditation tape for guidance. For now, we suggest that you practice as described in the exercises at the end of this chapter. Then, in Chapter 10, you will find a comprehensive program for how to develop the meditation practice over an eight-week period, following the schedule we use in the stress clinic.

When we introduce the sitting meditation, there is usually a lot of shifting around and fidgeting and opening and closing of the eyes as people get accustomed to the idea of not doing anything and learn to settle into just being. For those people who come with pain problems or with anxiety, or who are exclusively action-oriented, sitting still may at first seem like an impossibility. They often think that they will be in too much pain or too nervous, or too bored to be able to do it. But after a few weeks the collective stillness in the room is deafening, even though by that time we may be sitting for twenty or thirty minutes at a stretch. There is very little shifting and fidgeting, even among the people with pain and anxiety problems and the "go-getters" who usually never rest for a minute, a clear sign that they are practicing at home and developing some degree of stillness of both body and mind.

Before long, most people in the clinic discover that it can be quite exhilarating to meditate. Sometimes it doesn't even seem like work. It's just an effortless relaxing into the stillness of being, accepting each moment as it unfolds.

These are true moments of wholeness, accessible to all of us. Where do they come from? Nowhere. They are here all the time. Each time you sit in an alert and dignified posture and turn your attention to your breathing, for however long, you are returning to your own wholeness, affirming your intrinsic balance of mind and body, independent of the passing state of either your mind or your body in any moment. Sitting becomes a relaxation into stillness and peace beneath the surface agitations of your mind. It's as easy as seeing and letting go, seeing and letting go, seeing and letting go.

EXERCISE 1
Sitting with the Breath

1. Continue to practice awareness of your breathing in a comfort-able but erect sitting posture for at least ten minutes at least once a day.
2. Each time you notice that your mind is no longer on your breath, just see where it is. Then let go and come back to your belly and to your breathing.
3. Over time try extending the time you sit until you can do it for thirty minutes or more. But remember, when you are really in the present, there is no time, so clock time is not as important as your willingness to pay attention and let go from moment to moment.

EXERCISE 2
Sitting with the Breath and the Body as a Whole

1. When your practice feels strong in the sense that you can maintain some continuity of attention on the breath, try expanding
   the field of your awareness "around" your breathing and
   "around" your belly to include a sense of your body as a whole as
   you are sitting.
2. Maintain this awareness of the body sitting and breathing, and
   when the mind wanders, bring it back to sitting and breathing.

EXERCISE 3
Sitting with Sound

1. If you feel like it, try just listening to sound when you meditate.
   This does not mean listening *for* sounds, rather just hearing what
   is here to be heard, moment by moment, without judging or
   thinking about them. Just hearing them as pure sound. And
   hearing the silences within and between sounds as well.
2. You can practice this with music, too, hearing each note as it
   comes and the spaces between notes. Try breathing the sounds
   into your body and letting them flow out again on the outbreath.
   Imagine that your body is transparent to sounds; that they can
   move in and out of your body through the pores of your skin.

EXERCISE 4
Sitting with Thoughts and Feelings

1. When your attention is relatively stable on the breath, try
   shifting your awareness to the process of thinking itself. Let go
   of the breath and just watch thoughts come into and leave the
   field of your attention.
2. Try to perceive them as "events" in your mind.
3. Note their content and their charge while, if possible, not being
   drawn into thinking about them, or thinking the next thought,
   but just maintaining the "frame" through which you are observing the process of thought.

4. Note that an individual thought does not last long. It is impermanent. If it comes, it will go. Be aware of this.
5. Note how some thoughts keep coming back.
6. Note those thoughts that are "I," "me," or "mine" thoughts, observing carefully how "you," the non-judging observer, feel about them.
7. Note it when the mind creates a "self" to be preoccupied with how well or how badly your life is going.
8. Note thoughts about the past and thoughts about the future.
9. Note thoughts that are about greed, wanting, grasping, clinging.
10. Note thoughts that are about anger, disliking, hatred, aversion, rejection.
11. Note feelings and moods as they come and go.
12. Note what feelings are associated with different thought contents.
13. If you get lost in all this, just go back to your breathing.

This exercise requires great concentration and should only be done for short periods of time, like two to three minutes per sitting in the early stages.

EXERCISE 5
Sitting with Choiceless Awareness

1. Just sit. Don't hold on to anything, don't look for anything. Practice being completely open and receptive to whatever comes into the field of awareness, letting it all come and go, watching, witnessing in stillness.

5

Being in Your Body: The Body-Scan Technique

<hr style="width:10%"/>

It is amazing to me that we can be simultaneously completely preoccupied with the appearance of our own body and at the same time completely out of touch with it as well. This goes for our relationship to other people's bodies too. As a society we seem to be overwhelmingly preoccupied with appearances in general and appearance of bodies in particular. Bodies are used in advertisements to sell everything from cigarettes to cars. Why? Because the advertisers are capitalizing on people's strong identification with particular body images. Images of attractive men and seductive women generate in viewers thoughts about looking a certain way themselves to feel special or better or happy.

Much of our preoccupation with how we look comes from a deep-seated insecurity about our bodies. Many of us grew up feeling awkward and unattractive and disliking our body for one reason or another. Usually it was because there was a particular ideal "look" that someone else had and we didn't, perhaps when we were adolescents, when such preoccupations are at a feverish peak. So if we didn't look a certain way, we were obsessed with what we could do to look that way or to compensate for not looking that way, or we were overwhelmed with the impossibility of "being right." For many people, at one point in their lives, the appearance of their body was elevated to supreme social importance and they felt somehow inadequate and troubled by their appearance. At the other extreme were those who did look "the right way." As a result they were frequently infatuated with themselves or overwhelmed by all the attention they got.

Sooner or later people get over such preoccupations, but the root insecurity can remain about one's body. Many adults feel deep down that their body is either too fat or too short or too tall or too old or too "ugly," as if there were some perfect way that it should be. Sadly we may never feel completely comfortable with the way our body is. We may never feel completely at home in it. This may give rise to problems with touching and with being touched and therefore with intimacy. And as we get older, this malaise may be compounded by the awareness that our body is aging, that it is inexorably losing its youthful appearance and qualities.

Any deep feelings of this kind that you might have about your body can't change until the way you actually experience your body changes. These feelings really stem from a restricted way of looking at your body in the first place. Our *thoughts about* our body can limit drastically the range of feelings we allow ourselves to experience.

When we put energy into actually *experiencing* our body and we refuse to get caught up in the overlay of judgmental *thinking about* it, our whole view of it and of ourself can change dramatically. To begin with, what it does is remarkable! It can walk and talk and sit up and reach for things; it can judge distance and digest food and know things through touch. Usually we take these abilities completely for granted and don't appreciate what our bodies can actually do until we are injured or sick. Then we realize how nice it was when we could do the things we can't do anymore.

So before we convince ourselves that our bodies are *too* this or *too* that, shouldn't we get more in touch with how wonderful it is to have a body in the first place, no matter what it looks or feels like?

The way to do this is to tune in to your body and be mindful of it without judging it. You have already begun this process by becoming mindful of your breathing in the sitting meditation. When you place your attention in your belly and you feel the belly moving, or you place it at the nostrils and you feel the air passing in and out, you are tuning in to the sensations your body generates associated with life itself. These sensations are usually tuned out by us because they are so familiar. When you tune in to them, you are reclaiming your own life in that moment and your own body, literally making yourself more real and more alive.

THE BODY-SCAN MEDITATION

One very powerful technique we use to reestablish contact with the body is known as body scanning. Because of the thorough and minute focus on the body in body scanning, it is an effective technique for developing both concentration and flexibility of attention simultaneously. It involves lying on your back and moving your mind through the different regions of your body.

We start with the toes of the left foot and slowly move up the foot and leg, feeling the sensations as we go and directing the breath in to and out from the different regions. From the pelvis, we go to the toes of the right foot and move up the right leg back to the pelvis. From there, we move up through the torso, through the low back and abdomen, the upper back and chest, and the shoulders.

Then we go to the fingers of both hands and move up simultaneously in both arms, returning to the shoulders. Then we move through the neck and throat, and finally all the regions of the face, the back of the head, and the top of the head.

We wind up breathing through an imaginary "hole" in the very top of the head, as if we were a whale with a blowhole. We let our breathing move through the entire body from one end to the other, as if it were flowing in through the top of the head and out through the toes, and then in through the toes and out through the top of the head.

By the time we have completed the body scan, it can feel as if the entire body has dropped away or has become transparent, as if its substance were in some way erased. It can feel as if there is nothing but breath flowing freely across all the boundaries of the body.

As we complete the body scan, we let ourselves dwell in silence and stillness, in an awareness that may have by this point gone beyond the body altogether. After a time, when we feel ready to, we return to our body, to a sense of it as a whole. We feel it as solid again. We move our hands and feet intentionally. We might also massage the face and rock a little from side to side before opening our eyes and returning to the activities of the day.

The idea in scanning your body is to actually *feel* each region you focus on and linger there with your mind right *on* it or *in* it. You breathe in *to* and out *from* each region a few times and then let go of it in your mind's eye as your attention moves on to the next region. As you let go of the sensations you find in each region and of any of the thoughts and inner images you may have found associated with it, the muscles in that region literally let go too, lengthening and releasing much of the tension they have accumulated. It helps if you can feel or imagine that the tension in your body and the feelings of fatigue associated with it are *flowing out* on each outbreath and that, on each inbreath, you are breathing in energy, vitality, and relaxation.

In the stress clinic we practice the body scan intensively for at least the first four weeks of the program. It is the first formal mindfulness practice that our patients engage in for a sustained period of time. Along with awareness of breathing, it provides the foundation for all the other meditation techniques that they will work with later, including the sitting meditation. It is in the body scan that our patients first learn to keep their attention focused over an extended period of time. It is the first technique they use to develop concentration, calmness, and mindfulness. For many people it is the body scan that brings them to their first experience of well-being and timelessness in the meditation practice. It is an excellent place for anyone to begin formal mindfulness meditation practice, following the schedule outlined in Chapter 10.

In the first two weeks our patients practice the body scan at least once a day, six days per week using the first practice tape. That means forty-five minutes per day scanning slowly through the body! In the next two weeks they do it every other day, alternating with the yoga on the other side of the tape if they are able to do it. If not, they just do the body scan every day. They are using the same tape day after day, and it's the same body day after day too. The challenge, of course, is to bring your beginner's mind to it, to let each time be as if you were encountering your body for the first time. That means taking it moment by moment and letting go of all your expectations and preconceptions.

We start out using the body scan in the early weeks of the stress clinic for a number of reasons. First, it is done lying down. That makes it more comfortable and therefore more doable than sitting up straight for forty-five minutes. Many people find it easier, especially at the beginning, to go into a deep state of relaxation when they are lying down. In addition, the inner work of healing is greatly enhanced if you can develop your ability to place your attention systematically anywhere in your body that you want it to go and to direct energy there. This requires a degree of sensitivity to your body and to the sensations you experience from its various regions. In conjunction with your breathing, the body scan is a perfect vehicle for developing and refining this kind of sensitivity. For many people the body scan provides the first positive experience of their body that they have had for many years.

At the same time, practicing the body scan cultivates moment-to-moment awareness. Each time the mind wanders, we bring it back to the part of the body that we were working with when it drifted off, just as we bring the mind back to the breath when it wanders in the sitting meditation. If you are practicing with the body-scan tape, you bring your mind back to wherever the voice on the tape is when you realize it has wandered off.

When you practice the body scan regularly for a while, you come to notice that your body isn't quite the same every time you do it. You become aware that your body is changing constantly, that even the sensations in, say, your toes, may be different each time you practice using the tape or even from one moment to the next. You may also hear the instructions differently each time. Many people don't hear certain words on the tape until weeks have passed. Such observations can tell people a lot about how they feel about their bodies.

◆

Mary religiously practiced the body scan every day for the first four weeks of the program in a class ten years ago. After four weeks she commented in class that she could do it fine until she got to her neck and head. She reported that she felt "blocked" in this region each time she did it and was unable to get past her neck and up to the top of her head. I suggested that she imagine that her attention and her breathing could flow out of her shoulders and around the blocked region and that she might want to try that. That week she came in to see me to discuss what had happened.

It seems that she had tried the body scan again, intending to flow around the block in the neck. However, when she was scanning through the pelvic region, she had heard the word *genitals* for the first time. Hearing the word triggered a flashback of an experience that Mary immediately realized she had repressed since the age of nine. It reawakened in her a memory of having been frequently molested sexually by her father between the ages of five and nine. When she was nine years old, her father had a heart attack in her presence in the living room and died. As she recounted it to me, she (the little girl) didn't know what to do. It is easy to imagine the conflicted feelings of a child torn between relief at the helplessness of her tormentor and concern for her father. She did nothing.

The flashback concluded with her mother coming downstairs to find her husband dead and Mary sitting in a corner. Her mother blamed her for her father's death because she had not called for help and proceeded to beat her about the head and neck in a fury with a broom.

The entire experience, including the four-year history of sexual abuse, had been repressed for over fifty years and had not emerged during more than five years of psychotherapy. But the connection between the feeling of blockage in the neck during the body scan and the beating she received decades earlier is obvious. One cannot but marvel at her strength as a young girl to repress what she was unable to cope with in any other way. She grew up and raised five children in a reasonably happy marriage. But her body suffered over the years from a number of worsening chronic problems including hypertension, coronary disease, ulcers, arthritis, lupus, and recurrent urinary tract infections. When she came to the stress clinic at age fifty-four, her medical record stood over four feet tall and in it her physicians made reference to her medical problems by using a two-digit numbering system. She was referred to the stress clinic to learn to control her blood pressure, which was not well regulated with drugs, in part because she proved highly allergic to most medications. She had had bypass surgery on one blocked coronary artery the previous year. Several of her other coronary arteries were also blocked but were considered inoperable. She attended the stress clinic with her husband, who also had hypertension. One of her biggest complaints at the time was that she was unable to sleep well and was awake for long stretches in the middle of the night.

By the time she finished the program, she was sleeping through the night routinely (see Figure 3), her blood pressure had come down from 165/105 to 110/70 (see Figure 4), and she was reporting significantly less pain in her back and shoulders (see Figures 5A and B). At the same time the number of *physical* symptoms she complained of in the previous two months had decreased dramatically while the number of *emotional* symptoms that were causing her distress had increased. This was due to the flux of emotions unleashed by her flashback experience. To cope with it, she increased her psychotherapy sessions from one to two per week. At the same time she continued to practice the body scan. She returned for a two-month follow-up after the program ended. At that time the number of emotional symptoms she reported over that period had decreased dramatically as well, a result of articulating and working through some of her feelings. Her neck, shoulder, and back pain had all decreased even further as well (Figure 5C).

Mary had always been extremely shy in groups. She had been

FIGURE 3

MARY'S SLEEP GRAPHS, BEFORE AND AFTER THE PROGRAM

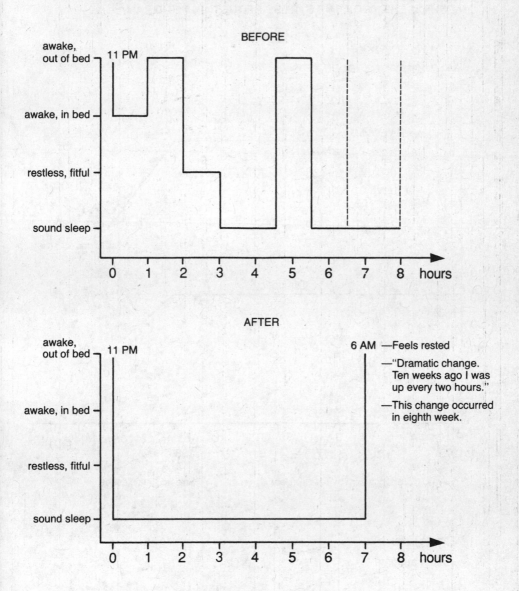

FIGURE 4

**MARY'S BLOOD PRESSURE MEASUREMENTS OVER THE YEAR
IN WHICH SHE TOOK THE STRESS REDUCTION PROGRAM**

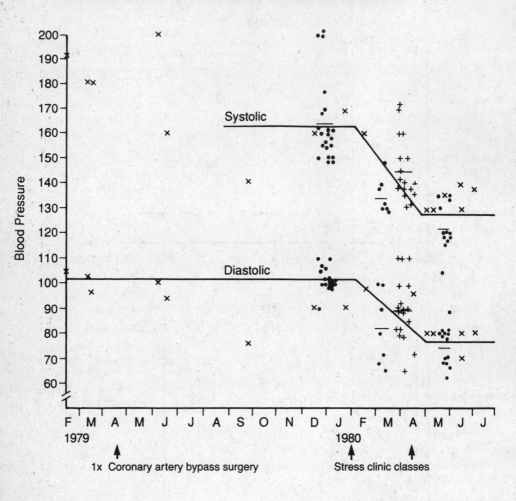

practically incapable of even saying her name when it was her turn to talk in her first class. In the years that followed, she kept up a regular meditation practice, using primarily the body scan. She returned many times to speak to other patients who were just starting out in the clinic, telling them about how it had helped her and recommending that they practice regularly. She fielded questions gracefully and marveled at her newfound ability to speak in front of groups. She was nervous but she wanted to share some of her experience with others. Her discovery also led to her joining an incest survivors' group, in which she was able to share her feelings with people who had had similar experiences.

In the years that followed, Mary was often hospitalized, either for her heart disease or for the lupus. It seemed that she was always going into the hospital for tests, only to wind up having to stay for weeks without anybody being able to tell her when she could go home. On at least one occasion her body swelled up to the point where her face seemed to be twice its normal size. She was almost unrecognizable.

Through it all, Mary managed to maintain a remarkable acceptance and equanimity. She felt she almost *had* to make continual use of her meditation training in order to cope with her spiraling health problems. She amazed the physicians taking care of her with her ability to control her blood pressure and with her ability to handle the very stressful procedures she had to undergo. Sometimes they would say to her before a procedure, "Now, Mary, this may hurt, so you had better do your meditation."

I learned that she had died early one Saturday morning, on a day that we were having our all-day session in the stress clinic (described in Chapter 8). I went to her room to say my good-byes. She had known the end was near for some time and had approached it with a peacefulness that surprised her. She was aware that her suffering would soon be over, but she expressed regret at not having had more than a few years to revel in, as she put it, her "newfound liberated, aware self" outside of the hospital. We dedicated the all-day session to her memory. In the stress clinic we miss her to this day. Many of her doctors came to her funeral and cried openly. She wound up teaching us about what is really important in life.

◆

Over the years, we have seen quite a few people in the clinic with severe medical problems who had similar stories of sexual or

FIGURE 5

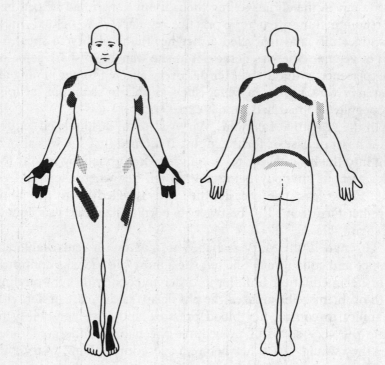

A. Mary's pain drawing before the program started.

solid = intense pain
crosshatch = intermediate pain
dots = dull or aching pain

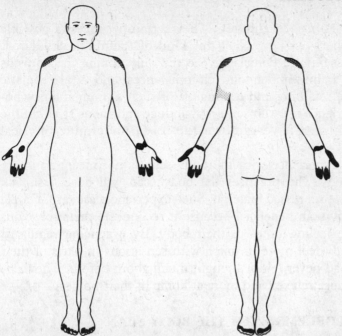

B. Mary's pain drawing ten weeks later.

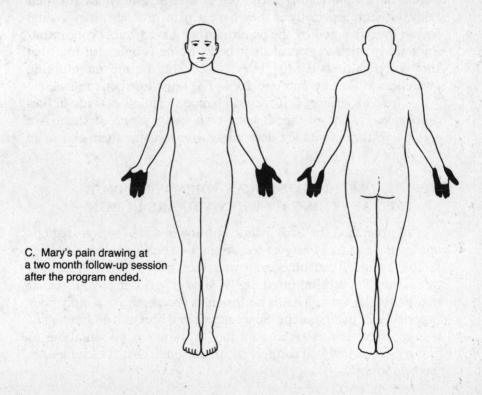

C. Mary's pain drawing at
a two month follow-up session
after the program ended.

psychological abuse as children. They certainly suggest a possible connection between repressing this kind of trauma in childhood, when repression and denial may be the only coping mechanisms available to a child under some circumstances, and future somatic disease. The retaining and walling off of such a traumatic psychological experience must in some way induce enormous stress in the body, which might, years down the road, undermine physical health.

Mary's experience with the body scan is not meant to imply that everybody who practices the body scan will have flashback experiences of repressed material. Such experiences are rare. People find the body scan beneficial because it reconnects their conscious mind to the feeling states of their body. By practicing regularly, people usually feel more in touch with sensations in parts of their body they had never felt or thought much about before. They also feel much more relaxed and more at home in their bodies.

INITIAL PROBLEMS WITH THE BODY SCAN

When some people practice the body scan, they sometimes have a hard time feeling their toes at first or other parts of their body. Others, especially if they have a pain problem, may at first feel so overwhelmed by the pain that they have trouble concentrating on any other region of their body. Some people also find that they keep falling asleep. They have a hard time maintaining awareness as they get more relaxed. They just lose consciousness.

These experiences, if they do happen, can all provide important messages to you about your own body. None of them is a serious obstacle if you are determined to overcome them and to go deeper in the practice.

HOW TO USE THE BODY SCAN WHEN YOU DON'T FEEL ANYTHING OR WHEN YOU ARE IN PAIN

In practicing the body scan, you tune in to the various regions one by one and feel whatever sensations are apparent in each region. If, for instance, you tune in to your toes and you don't feel anything, then "not feeling anything" is your experience of your toes at that particular time. That is neither bad nor good, it's simply your experience in that moment. So we note it and accept it and move on. It is not necessary to wiggle your toes to try to stir up sensations in that region so that you can feel them, although that is okay, too, at the beginning.

The body scan is especially powerful in cases where there is a particular region of your body that is problematic or painful. Take chronic low-back pain as one example. Let's say that when you lie down on your back to do the body scan, you feel considerable pain in your lower back that is not relieved by minor shifts in your position. You start off with awareness of your breathing nevertheless, and then try to move your attention to the left foot, breathing in and out to the toes. But the pain in your back keeps drawing your attention to that region and prevents you from concentrating on the toes or on any other regions. You just keep coming back to your lower back and to the pain.

One way to proceed when this happens is to keep bringing your attention back to your toes and redirecting the breath to that region each time the back captures your attention. You continue to move up systematically through your left leg, then your right leg, then the pelvis, all the while paying meticulous attention to the sensations in the various regions and to whatever thoughts and feelings you become aware of regardless of their content. Of course much of their content may concern your lower back and how it is feeling. As you then move through the pelvis and approach the problem region, you remain open and receptive, noting with precision the sensations you are experiencing as you move into this region, just as you did for all preceding regions.

Now you breathe in to the back and out from the back, at the same time being aware of any thoughts and feelings as they occur. You dwell here, breathing, until when you are ready, you let go of the lower back on purpose and move the focus of your attention to the upper back and the chest. In this way you are practicing *moving through* the region of maximum intensity, experiencing it fully *in its turn* when you come to focus on it. You allow yourself to be open to all the sensations that may be there, in all their intensity, watching them, breathing with them, and then letting them go as you move on.

THE BODY SCAN AS A PURIFICATION PROCESS

The man from whom I learned the body-scan technique had been a chemist before he became a meditation teacher. He liked to describe the body scan as a metaphorical "zone purification" of the body. Zone purification is an industrial technique for purifying certain metals by moving a circular furnace the length of a metal ingot. The heat liquefies the metal in the zone that is in the ring of the furnace, and the impurities become concentrated in the liquid phase. As the zone of melted metal moves along the length of the bar, the impurities stay in the liquid metal. The resolidified metal coming out the back end of the furnace is of much greater purity than it was before the process began. When the whole bar has been treated in this way, the end region of the bar that was the last to melt and resolidify (and that now contains all the impurities) is cut off and thrown away, leaving a purified bar.

Similarly, the body scan can be thought of as an active purification of the body. The moving zone of your attention harvests tension and pain as it passes through various regions and carries them to the top of your head, where, with the aid of your breathing, you allow them to discharge out of your body, leaving it purified. Each time you scan your body in this way, you can think of it or visualize it as a purification or detoxification process, a process that is promoting healing by restoring a feeling of wholeness and integrity to your body.

Although it sounds as if the body scan is being used to achieve a specific end, namely to purify your body, the spirit in which we practice it is still one of non-striving. As you will see in Chapter 13, we let any purification that might occur take care of itself. We just persevere in the practice.

Through repeated practice of the body scan over time, we come to grasp the reality of our body as whole in the present moment. This feeling of wholeness can be experienced no matter what is wrong with your body. One part of your body, or many parts of your body, may be diseased or in pain or even missing, yet you can still cradle them in this experience of wholeness.

Each time you scan your body, you are letting what will flow out flow out. You are not trying to force either "letting go" or purification to happen, which of course is impossible anyway. Letting go is really an act of acceptance of your situation. It is not a surrender to your fears about it. It is a seeing of yourself as larger than your problems and your pain, larger than your cancer, larger than your heart disease, larger than your body, and identifying with the totality of your being rather than with your body or your heart or your back or your fears. The experience of wholeness transcending your problems comes naturally out of regular practice of the body scan. It is nurtured every time you breathe out from a particular region and let it go.

Another way of dealing with pain when it comes up during the body scan is to let your attention go to the region of greatest intensity. This strategy is best when you find it difficult to concentrate on different parts of your body because the pain in one region is so great. Instead of scanning, you just breathe in to and out from the pain itself. Try to imagine or feel the inbreath penetrating into the tissue until it is completely absorbed, and imagine the outbreath as a channel allowing the region to discharge to the outside whatever pain, toxic elements, and "dis-ease" it is willing to or capable of surrendering. As you do this, you continue to pay attention from moment to moment, breath by breath, noticing that even in the most problematic regions of your body the sensations you are attending to from moment to moment change in quality. You may notice that the intensity of the sensations can change as well. If it subsides a little, you can try going back to your toes and scanning the whole body, as described above. In Chapters 22 and 23 you will find further suggestions for how to use mindfulness to work with pain.

ACCEPTANCE AND NON-STRIVING IN THE BODY-SCAN PRACTICE

When practicing the body scan, the key point is to maintain awareness in every moment, a detached witnessing of your breath and your body, region by region, as you scan from your feet to the top of your head. The quality of your attention and your willingness just to feel what is there and be with it no matter what is much more important than imagining the tension leaving your body or the inbreath revitalizing your body. If you just work at getting rid of tension, you may or may not succeed, but you are not practicing mindfulness. But if you are practicing being present in each moment and at the same time you are *allowing* your breathing and your attention to purify the body within this context of awareness and with a willingness to accept whatever happens, then you are truly practicing mindfulness and tapping its power to heal.

The distinction is important. In the introduction to the body-scan practice tape, it says that the best way to get results from the meditation is not to try to get anything from it but just to do it for its own sake. When our patients use the tape, they hear this message every day. Every person has a serious problem for which he or she is seeking some kind of help. Yet these patients are being told that the best way to get something out of the meditation practice is just to practice every day and to let go of their expectations, their goals, even their reasons for coming.

In framing the work of meditation in this way, we are putting them in a paradoxical situation. They have come to the clinic hopeful of having something positive happen, yet they are instructed to practice without trying to get anywhere. Instead, we encourage them to try to be fully where they already are, with acceptance. In addition, we suggest they suspend judgment for the eight weeks that they are in the course and decide only at the end whether it was worthwhile.

Why do we take this approach? Creating this paradoxical situation invites people to explore non-striving and self-acceptance as ways of being. It gives them permission to start from scratch, to tap a new way of seeing and feeling without holding up standards of success and failure based on a habitual and limited way of seeing their problems and their expectations about what they *should* be feeling. We practice the meditation in this way because the effort to try to "get somewhere" is so often the wrong kind of effort for catalyzing change or growth or healing, coming as it usually does from a rejection of present-moment reality without having a full awareness and understanding of that reality.

A desire for things to be other than the way they actually are is simply wishful thinking. It is not a very effective way of bringing about real change. At the first signs of what you think is "failure," when you see that you are not "getting anywhere" or have not gotten where you thought you should be, you are likely to get discouraged or feel overwhelmed, lose hope, blame external forces, and give up. Therefore no real change ever happens.

The meditative view is that it is only through the acceptance of the actuality of the present, no matter how painful or frightening or undesirable it may be that change and growth and healing can come about. As we shall see in the section entitled "The Paradigm," new possibilities can be thought of as already *contained* within present-moment reality. They need only be nurtured in order to unfold and be *dis-covered*.

If this is true, then you don't need to try to get anywhere when you practice the body scan or any of the other techniques. You only need to really be where you already are and *realize* it (make it real). In fact in this way of looking at things *there is no place else to go*, so efforts to get anywhere else are ill conceived. They are bound to lead to frustration and failure. On the other hand, you cannot fail to be where you already are. So you cannot "fail" in your meditation practice if you are willing to be with things as they are.

In its truest expression meditation goes beyond notions of

success and failure, and this is why it is such a powerful vehicle for growth and change and healing. This does not mean that you cannot progress in your meditation practice, nor does it mean that it is impossible to make mistakes that will reduce its value to you. A particular kind of effort *is* necessary in the practice of meditation, but it is not an effort of striving to achieve some special state, whether it be relaxation, freedom from pain, healing, or insight. These come naturally with practice because they are already inherent in the present moment and in every moment. Therefore any moment is as good as any other for experiencing their presence within yourself.

If you see things in this light, it makes perfect sense to take each moment as it comes and accept it as it is, seeing it clearly in its fullness, and letting it go.

If you are unsure of whether you are practicing "correctly" or not, here is a good litmus test: When you notice thoughts in the mind about getting somewhere, about wanting something, or about having gotten somewhere, about "success" or "failure," are you able to honor each one as you observe it as an aspect of present-moment reality? Can you see it clearly as an impulse, a thought, a desire, a judgment, and let it be here and let it go without being drawn into it, without investing it with a power it doesn't have, without losing yourself in the process? This is the way to cultivate mindfulness.

◆

So we scan the body over and over, day by day, ultimately not to purify it, not to get rid of anything, not even to relax. These may be the motives that bring us to practice in the first place and that keep us at it day after day, and we may in fact *feel* more relaxed and better from doing it. But in order to practice correctly *in each moment*, we have to let go of even these motives. Then practicing the body scan is just a way of being with your body and with yourself, a way of being whole right now.

EXERCISE ═══

1. Lie down on your back in a comfortable place, such as on a foam pad on the floor or on your bed (but remember that for this use, you are aiming to "fall awake," not fall asleep). Make sure that you will be warm enough. You might want to cover yourself with a blanket or do it in a sleeping bag if the room is cold.
2. Allow your eyes to gently close.
3. Feel the rising and falling of your belly with each inbreath and outbreath.
4. Take a few moments to feel your body as a "whole," from head to toe, the "envelope" of your skin, the sensations associated with touch in the places you are in contact with the floor or the bed.
5. Bring your attention to the toes of the left foot. As you direct your attention to them, see if you can "direct," or channel, your breathing to them as well, so that it feels as if you are breathing in *to* your toes and out *from* your toes. It may take a while for you to get the hang of this. It may help to just imagine your breath traveling down the body from your nose into the lungs and then continuing through the abdomen and down the left leg all the way to the toes and then back again and out through your nose.
6. Allow yourself to *feel* any and all sensations from your toes, perhaps distinguishing between them and watching the flux of sensations in this region. If you don't feel anything at the moment, that is fine too. Just allow yourself to feel "not feeling anything."
7. When you are ready to leave the toes and move on, take a deeper, more intentional breath in all the way down to the toes and, on the outbreath, allow them to "dissolve" in your "mind's eye." Stay with your breathing for a few breaths at least, and then move on in turn to the sole of the foot, the heel, the top of the foot, and then the ankle, continuing to breathe in *to* and out *from* each region as you observe the sensations that you are experiencing, and then letting go of it and moving on.
8. As with the awareness of breathing exercises (Chapter 3) and the sitting meditation practices (Chapter 4), bring your mind back to the breath and to the region you are focusing on each time you notice that your attention has wandered off.
9. In this way, as described in the body of this chapter, continue to

move slowly up your left leg and through the rest of your body as you maintain the focus on the breath and on the feeling of the particular regions as you come to them, breathe with them, and let go of them. If you are experiencing pain, consult the sections in this chapter that suggest how to work with it, as well as Chapters 22 and 23.

10. Practice the body scan at least once a day. It helps to use the practice tape in the beginning so that the pace is slow enough and to help you remember the instructions accurately.

11. Remember that the body scan is the first formal mindfulness practice that our patients engage in intensively and that they do it forty-five minutes per day, six days per week for *at least* two weeks straight in the beginning of their training.

12. If you have trouble staying awake, try doing the body scan with your eyes open.

6

Cultivating Strength, Balance, and Flexibility: Yoga *Is* Meditation

—

As you have probably gathered by now, bringing mindfulness to any activity transforms it into a kind of meditation. Mindfulness dramatically amplifies the probability that any activity in which you are engaged will result in an expansion of your perspective and of your understanding of who you are. Much of the practice is simply a remembering, a reminding yourself to be fully awake, not lost in waking sleep or enshrouded in the veils of your thinking mind. Intentional practice is crucial to this process because the automatic-pilot mode takes over so quickly when we forget to remember.

I like the words *remember* and *remind* because they imply connections that already exist but need to be acknowledged anew. To remember, then, can be thought of as *reconnecting* with membership, with the set to which what one *already knows* belongs. That which we have forgotten is still here, somewhere within us. It is *access* to it that is temporarily veiled. What has been forgotten needs to renew its membership in consciousness. For instance, when we "re-member" to pay attention, to be in the present, to be in our body, we are already awake right in that moment of remembering. The membership completes itself as we remember our wholeness.

The same can be said for reminding ourselves. It reconnects us with what some people call "big mind," with a mind of wholeness, a mind that sees the whole forest as well as individual trees. Since we are always whole anyway, it's not that we have to *do* anything. We just have to "re-mind" ourself of it.

I believe that a major reason why the people in the stress clinic take so quickly to the meditation and find it healing is that the practice of mindfulness reminds them of what they already knew but somehow didn't know they knew or weren't able to make use of, namely that they are already whole.

We remember wholeness so readily because we don't have far to look for it. It is always within us, usually as a vague feeling or memory left over from when we were children. But it is a deeply familiar memory, one you recognize immediately as soon as you feel it again, like coming home after being away a long time. When you are immersed in doing without being centered, it feels like being away from home. And when you reconnect with being, even for a few moments, you know it immediately. You feel like you are at home no matter where you are and what problems you face.

Part of the feeling in such moments is that you are at home in your body too. So it is a little peculiar that the English language doesn't allow us to "rebody" ourselves. It seems on the face of it to be just as necessary and useful a concept as to remind ourselves. In one way or another all the work we do in the stress clinic involves rebodying.

Bodies are subject to inevitable breakdown. But they do seem to break down sooner and to heal less rapidly and less completely if they are not cared for and listened to in some basic ways. For this reason, taking proper care of your body is of great importance in both the prevention of disease and in the work of healing from illness, disease, or injury.

Step number one in caring for your body, whether you are sick or injured or healthy, is to practice being "in" it. Tuning in to your breathing and to the sensations that you can feel in your body is one very practical way to work at being in your body. It helps you to stay in close touch with it and then to act on what you learn as you listen to its messages. The body scan is a very powerful form of "rebodying," since you are regularly checking in with and listening to and relaxing every region of your body systematically. You can't help developing greater familiarity with and confidence in your body when you do this.

There are many different ways to practice being in your body. All enhance growth and change and healing, especially if they are done with meditative awareness. One of the most powerful in terms of its ability to transform the body, and most wonderful in terms of how good it feels to do it, is *hatha yoga*.

Mindful hatha yoga is the third major formal meditation technique that we practice in the stress clinic, along with the body scan and sitting meditation. It consists of gentle stretching and strengthening exercises, done very slowly, with moment-to-moment awareness of breathing and of the sensations that arise as you put your body into various configurations known as "postures." Many people in the stress clinic swear by the yoga practice and prefer it to the sitting and the body scan. They are drawn to the relaxation and increased musculoskeletal strength and flexibility that come from regular yoga practice. What is more, after enduring the stillness of the sitting and the body scan for several weeks, it allows them at last to move!

But mindful yoga does far more than get you relaxed and help your body to become stronger and more flexible. It is another way in which you can learn about yourself and come to experience yourself as whole, regardless of your physical condition or level of "fitness." Although it looks like exercise and conveys the benefits of exercise, it is far more than exercise. Done mindfully, it is meditation just as much as the sitting or the body scan is.

We practice the yoga with the same attitude that we bring to the sitting meditation or the body scan. We do it without striving and without forcing. We practice accepting our body as we find it, in the present, from one moment to the next. While stretching or lifting or balancing, we learn to work at our limits, maintaining moment-to-moment awareness. We are patient with ourselves. As we carefully move up to our limits in a stretch, for instance, we practice breathing *at that limit*, dwelling in the creative space between not challenging the body at all and pushing it too far.

This is a far cry from most exercise and aerobic classes and even many yoga classes, which only focus on what the body is *doing*. These approaches tend to emphasize *progress*. They like to push, push, push. Not much attention is paid to the art of non-doing and non-striving in exercise classes, nor to the present moment for that matter, nor to the mind. In exercise that is totally body-oriented, there tends to be little explicit care given to the domain of being, which is just as important when working with the body as when doing anything else. Of course anybody can come upon the domain of being on their own, because it is always here. But it is a lot harder to find if the atmosphere and attitude are diametrically opposed to such experiences.

Most of us need to be given permission to switch from the doing to the being mode, mostly because we have been conditioned since we were little to value doing over being. We were never taught how to work with the being mode or even how to find it. So most of us need at least a few pointers on how to let go into it.

It's not all that easy to find the being mode on your own when you are exercising, espccially in a class that is very doing and achievement oriented. On top of that, it is also difficult because we carry our mind's usual agitations, reactivity, and lack of awareness around with us when we are exercising.

To find the domain of being, we need to learn and practice mobilizing our powers of attention and awareness during exercise. Professional and even amateur athletes are now realizing that unless they pay attention to the mind as well as the body, they are disregarding an entire realm of personal power that can make a critical difference in performance.

Even physical therapy, which is specifically oriented toward teaching and prescribing stretching and strengthening exercises for people who are recovering from surgery or who have chronic pain, is usually taught without paying attention to breathing and without enlisting the person's innate ability to relax into the stretching and the strengthening exercises. Often physical therapists undertake to teach people to do healing things for their bodies while neglecting two of the most powerful allies people have for healing; the breath and the mind. Time and again our patients with pain problems report that their physical-therapy sessions go much better when they use awareness of breathing as they perform their exercises. It's as if a whole new dimension of what they are being asked to do is revealed to them. And their physical therapists often comment on the dramatic changes they seem to have undergone.

When the domain of being is actively cultivated during slow and gentle stretching and strengthening exercises, such as yoga or physical therapy, what people think of traditionally as "exercise" is transformed into *meditation*. This allows it to be done and even enjoyed by people who could not tolerate the same level of physical activity in a more accelerated and progress-oriented context.

In the stress clinic, the ground rule is that every individual has to consciously take responsibility for reading his or her own body's signals while doing the yoga. This means listening carefully to what your body is telling you and honoring its messages, *erring on the side of being conservative*. No one can listen to your body for you. If you want to grow and heal, you have to take some responsibility for listening to it yourself. Each person's body is different so each person has to come to know his or her own limits. And the only way to find out about your limits is to explore them carefully and mindfully over an extended period of time.

What you learn from doing this is that, no matter what the

state of your body, when you bring awareness to it and work at your limits, those limits tend to recede over time. You discover that the boundaries of how far your body can stretch or how long you can hold a position are not fixed or static. So your thoughts about what you can and can't do shouldn't be too fixed or static either, because your own body can teach you differently, if you listen carefully to it.

This observation is nothing new. Athletes use this principle all the time to improve their performances. They are always exploring their limits. But they are doing it to get somewhere, whereas we are using it to be where we already are and discover where that is. We will find that we get somewhere, too, but without the relentless striving.

The reason it is so important for people with health problems to work at their limits similar to the way athletes do is that when there is something "wrong" with one part of your body, you tend to back off and not use *any* of it. This is a sensible short-term protection mechanism when you are sick or injured. The body needs periods of rest for recuperation and recovery.

But often the short-term solution evolves into the long-term life-style. Over time, especially if we have an injury or a problem with our body, a restricted body image can creep into our view of ourself and, if we are unaware of this inner process, we can come to identify ourselves that way and believe it. Rather than finding out what our limits and limitations are by directly experiencing them, we declare them to be a certain way, on the basis of what we think or what we were told by the doctor or by family members concerned for our well-being. Unwittingly we may be driving a wedge between ourselves and our own well-being.

Such thinking can lead to a rigid and fixed view of ourself as "out of shape," "over the hill," or as having something "wrong," perhaps even as being "disabled," reasons enough to dwell in inactivity and neglect our body in its entirety. Maybe we have an exaggerated belief that we have to stay in bed just to get through the day or that we can't go out of the house and do things.

Such views lead readily to what is sometimes referred to as "illness behavior." We begin to build our psychological life around our preoccupations with our illness, injury, or disability, while the rest of our life is on hold and unfortunately atrophying, along with the body. In fact even if there is nothing "wrong" with your body, if you do not challenge it much, you may be carrying around a highly restricted image of what it (and you) are capable of doing.

Physical therapists have two wonderful maxims that are extremely relevant for people seeking to take better care of their bodies. One is "If it's physical, it's therapy." The other is "If you don't use it, you lose it." The first implies that it's not so much what you do that is important, it's that you are doing *something* with your body. The second maxim reminds us that the body is never in a fixed state. It is constantly changing, responding to the demands placed upon it. If it is never asked to bend or squat or twist or stretch or run, then its ability to do these things doesn't just stay the same, it actually decreases over time. Sometimes this is called being "out of shape," but being out of shape implies a fixed state. In fact the longer you are "out of shape," the worse shape your body is in. It declines.

This decline is technically known as *disuse atrophy*. When the body is given complete bed rest, say when you are recuperating from surgery in the hospital, it rapidly loses a good deal of muscle mass, especially in the legs. You can actually see the thighs get smaller day by day. When not maintained by constant use, muscle tissue atrophies. It breaks down and is reabsorbed by the body. When you get out of bed and start moving around and exercising your legs, it slowly builds up again.

It's not just the leg muscles that atrophy with disuse. All skeletal muscles do. They also tend to get shorter and lose their tone and become more prone to injury in people who lead a sedentary life-style. Moreover, protracted periods of disuse or underuse probably also affect joints, bones, the blood vessels feeding the regions in question, and even the nerves supplying them. It is likely that with disuse, all these tissues undergo changes in structure and function that are in the direction of degeneration and atrophy.

Twenty-five years ago extended bed rest was the treatment of choice following a heart attack. Now people are out of bed and walking and exercising within days of a heart attack because medicine has come to recognize that inactivity only compounds the heart patient's problems. Even a heart that has atherosclerosis responds to the challenge of regular, graduated exercise and benefits from it by becoming functionally stronger (even more so if the person goes on a very low fat diet, as we shall see in Chapter 31).

Of course, the level of exercise has to be adjusted to the physical state of your body so that you are not pushing beyond your limits at any time but are working in a target range for heart rate that produces what is called a "training effect" on the heart. Then you gradually increase your exercise as your limit recedes, in other words as your heart becomes stronger. Nowadays, it's not unheard of for people who have had a heart attack to build themselves up to the point where they can complete a marathon, that is, run 26.1 miles!

Yoga is a wonderful form of exercise for a number of reasons. To begin with, it is very gentle. It can be beneficial at any level of physical conditioning and, if practiced regularly, counteracts the process of disuse atrophy. It can be practiced in bed, in a chair, or in a wheelchair. It can be done standing up, lying down, or sitting. In fact, the whole point of hatha yoga is that it can be done in any position. Any posture can become a starting place for practice. All that is required is that you are breathing and that some voluntary movement is possible.

Yoga is also good exercise because it is a type of full-body conditioning. It improves strength and flexibility in the entire body. It's like swimming, in that every part of your body is involved and benefits. It can even have cardiovascular benefits when done vigorously. But the way we do it in the clinic is not as cardiovascular exercise. We do it primarily for stretching and strengthening your muscles and joints, to wake up the body to its full range of motion and potential for movement. People who need cardiovascular exercise walk or swim or bike or run or row in addition to doing the yoga.

Perhaps the most remarkable thing about yoga is how much energy you feel *after* you do it. You can be feeling exhausted, do some yoga, and feel completely rejuvenated in a short period of time. Those people who have been practicing the body scan every day for two weeks in a row and found it difficult to feel relaxed are thrilled to discover in the third week of the stress clinic that they can easily achieve a deep state of relaxation with the yoga; it's almost impossible not to unless you have a chronic pain condition, in which case you have to be particularly careful of what you do, as we will see in a moment. At the same time these people find that they stay awake during the yoga and get to taste feelings of stillness and peace that they did not experience in the body scan because they were unable to concentrate, or fell asleep. And once they have had an experience of this kind, many come to feel more positively toward the body scan as well. They understand it better and have an easier time staying relaxed and awake while doing it.

I do yoga almost every day and have for over twenty years. I get out of bed and splash some cold water on my face to make sure I'm awake. Then I work with my body mindfully by doing some yoga. Some days it feels like my body is literally putting itself together as

I practice. Other days it doesn't feel that way. But it always feels like I know how my body is today because I have spent some time with it in the morning, being with it, nourishing it, strengthening it, stretching it, listening to it. This feeling is very reassuring when you have physical problems and limitations and are never quite sure what your body is going to be like on any given day.

Some days I'll do fifteen minutes, just some basic back and leg and shoulder work. Sometimes I'll do half an hour or an hour. My yoga classes are usually two hours long, because I want people to take their time and to luxuriate in the experience of centering themselves in their bodies as they practice exploring their limits in various postures. But even five or ten minutes a day can be very useful as a regular routine. However, if you have embarked on our eight-week training program in mindfulness training or are thinking about doing so, we recommend that you practice for forty-five minutes per day, starting in Week 3, alternating yoga with the body scan daily, as described in Chapter 10.

◆

Yoga is a Sanskrit word that literally means "yoke." The practice of yoga is the practice of yoking together or unifying body and mind, which really means penetrating into the experience of them not being separate in the first place. You can also think of it as experiencing the unity or connectedness between the individual and the universe as a whole. The word has other specialized meanings, which do not concern us here, but the basic thrust is always the same: realizing connectedness, realizing wholeness through disciplined practice. The image of the yoke goes nicely with our notions of re-minding and re-bodying.

The trouble with yoga is that talking about it doesn't help you to do it, and instructions from a book, even under the best of circumstances, can't really convey the feeling of what it is like to practice. One of the most enjoyable and relaxing aspects of doing yoga mindfully is the sense of your body flowing from one posture to the next and through periods of stillness while lying on your back or on your belly. This cannot be achieved when you are going back and forth between the illustrations and descriptions in a book and your body on the floor. It always exasperated me the few times that I tried to learn yoga from a book, no matter how good the book was. That is why we strongly recommend that if you are drawn to the idea of practicing mindful yoga, you use the practice tapes to get started. Then all you have to do is play one of them and let it guide you through the various sequences of postures. This allows you to put all your energy into moment-to-moment awareness of your body, your breath, and your mind. The illustrations and the instructions in this chapter can then be used to clarify any uncertainties you may have and to supplement your own understanding, which will grow mostly out of your personal experiences doing it. Once you know what is involved, you can do it without the tapes and make up different sequences of postures for yourself.

We have already seen that *posture* is very important in the sitting meditation and that positioning your body in certain ways can have immediate effects on your mental and emotional state. Being aware of your body language and what it reveals about your attitudes and feelings can help you to change your attitudes and feelings just by changing your physical posture. Even something as simple as curling up the mouth into a half smile can produce feelings of happiness and relaxation that weren't present before the facial muscles were mobilized to mimic the smile.

This is important to remember when you are practicing yoga. Every time you intentionally assume a different posture, you are literally changing your physical orientation and therefore your inner perspective as well. So you can think of all the positions in which you find yourself while doing yoga as opportunities to practice mindfulness of your thoughts and feelings and mood states as well as of your breathing and of the sensations associated with stretching and lifting different parts of your body.

For example, sometimes rolling up into a fetal position, upside down on the back of your neck and shoulders (position 21 in Figure 6), can provide a welcome change in perspective and can result in a positive mood change. Even such simple things as what you do with your hands when you are sitting, how you position them, whether the palms are open to the ceiling or are facing down on your knees, whether the palms are touching in your lap or not, whether the thumbs are touching or not, can all have an effect on how you feel in a particular posture. They are a very fruitful area for developing an awareness of energy flow in your body.

When you practice the yoga, you should be on the lookout for the many ways, some quite subtle, in which your perspective on your body, your thoughts, and your whole sense of self can change when you adopt different postures on purpose and stay in them for a time, paying full attention from moment to moment. Practicing in this way enriches the inner work enormously and takes it far beyond the physical benefits that come naturally with the stretching and strengthening.

HOW TO GET STARTED ==

1. Lie on your back on a mat or pad that cushions you from the floor. If you can't lie on your back, do it some other way.
2. Become aware of the flow of your breathing and feel the abdomen rising and falling with each inbreath and outbreath.
3. Take a few moments to feel your body as a whole, from head to toe, the "envelope" of your skin, and the sensations associated with touch in the places your body is in contact with the floor.
4. As with the sitting meditation and the body scan, keep your attention focused in the present moment and bring it back when it wanders, noting what drew it away before letting go of it.
5. Position your body as best you can in the various postures illustrated below and try to stay in each one while you focus on your breathing at the abdomen. Figures 6 and 7 give you the sequences of postures we do on the yoga sides of the two mindfulness practice tapes: "Guided Yoga 1" and "Guided Yoga 2." On the tapes some of the postures are repeated at various points. These repeats are not included in the drawings. When a posture is pictured as being on either the right side or the left side, do both, as indicated.
6. While in each posture, be aware of the sensations that you are experiencing in various parts of your body, and if you like, direct your breath in to and out from the region of greatest intensity in a particular stretch or posture. The idea is to relax into each posture as best you can and breathe with what you are feeling.
7. Feel free to skip any of the postures that you know will exacerbate a problem you may have. *Check with your doctor or physical therapist about particular postures if you have a neck problem or a back problem. This is an area in which you have to use your judgment and take responsibility for your own body.* Many of the people in the stress clinic who have back and neck problems report that they can do at least some of these postures, but they do them *very carefully*, not pushing or forcing or pulling. Although these exercises are very gentle and can be healing, they are also deceptively powerful and can lead to muscle pulls

and more serious setbacks if they are not done slowly, mindfully, and gradually over time.

8. Do not get into competing with yourself, and if you do, notice it and let go of it. The spirit of yoga is the spirit of self-acceptance in the present moment. The idea is to explore your limits gently, lovingly, with respect for your body. It is not to try to break through your body's limits because you want to look better or fit into your bathing suit better next summer. That may happen naturally if you keep up the practice, but if you tend to push beyond your limits of the moment instead of relaxing into them, you may wind up injuring yourself. This would just set you back and discourage you about keeping up the practice, in which case you might find yourself blaming the yoga instead of seeing that it was the striving attitude that led to your overdoing it. Certain people tend to get into a vicious cycle of overdoing it when they are feeling good and enthusiastic and then not being able to do anything for a time and becoming discouraged. So it is worth paying careful attention if you have this tendency and erring on the side of being conservative.

9. Although it is not shown in the sequences of postures illustrated in Figures 6 and 7 simply in the interests of space, *you should rest between postures*. Depending on what you are doing, you can do this either lying on your back or in another comfortable posture. At these times be aware of the flow of your breathing from moment to moment, feeling your belly as it gently moves in and out. If you are lying on the floor, feel your muscles let go as you sink more deeply into your mat or pad on each outbreath. Ride the waves of your breathing as you relax and sink more deeply into the floor. You can relax in a similar way as you rest standing up between standing postures; feel the contact your feet make with the floor and let your shoulders drop as you breathe out. In both cases, as your muscles let go and relax, allow yourself to let go of any thoughts you might be having and continue to ride the waves of the breath.

10. There are two general rules that will help you if you keep them in mind as you do the yoga. The first is that you breathe *out* as you do any movements that contract the belly and the front side of your body and you breathe *in* as you do any movements that expand the front side of your body and contract the back. For example, if you are lifting one leg while lying on your back

(see Figure 6, posture 14), you would breathe *out* as you lift it. But if you are lying on your belly and lifting the leg (Figure 6, posture 19), you would breathe *in*. This applies just for the movement itself. Once the leg is up, you just continue observing the natural flow of your breath.

The other rule is to dwell in each posture long enough to let go into it. The idea is to relax into each one. If you find yourself struggling and fighting with it, remind yourself to let go into your breathing. In the beginning you may find that you are unconsciously bracing yourself in many areas while you are in a particular position. After a while your body will realize this in some way, and you will find yourself relaxing and sinking farther into it. Let each inbreath expand the posture out *slightly* in all directions. On each outbreath sink a little more deeply into it, allowing gravity to be your friend and help you to explore your limits. Try not to use any muscles that don't need to be involved in what you are doing. For instance, you might practice relaxing your face when you notice that it is tense.

11. Work at or within your body's limits at all times, with the intention of observing and exploring the boundary between what your body can do and where it says, "Stop for now." Never stretch beyond this limit to the point of pain. Some discomfort is inevitable when you are working at your limits, but you will need to learn how to enter this healthy "stretching zone" slowly and mindfully so that you are nourishing your body, not damaging it as you explore your limits.

FIGURE 6

SEQUENCE OF YOGA POSTURES
(TAPE 1, SIDE 2)

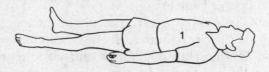

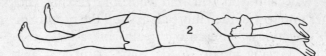

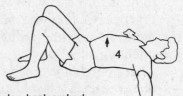

low back pressed against floor

low back arched;
pelvis stays on floor

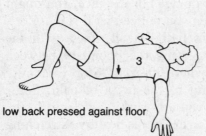

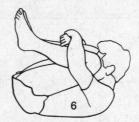

both sides

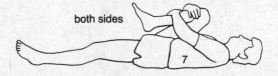

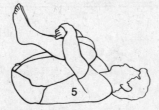

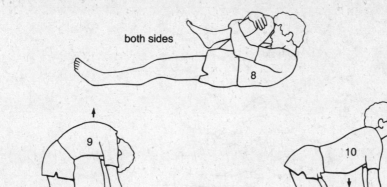

both sides

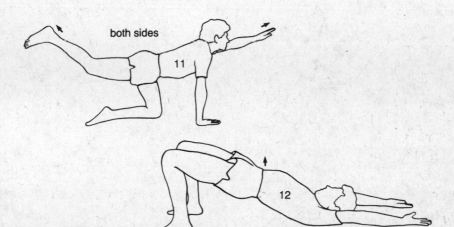

both sides

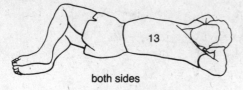

both sides

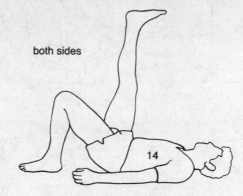

both sides

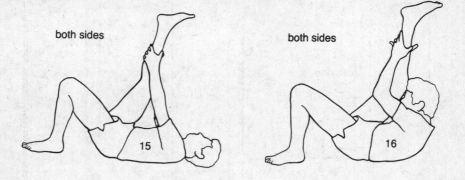

both sides

both sides

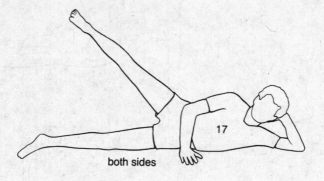

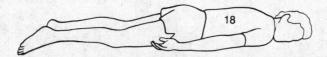

both sides

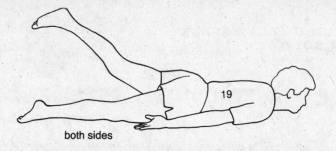

both sides

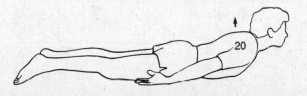

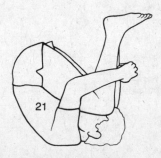

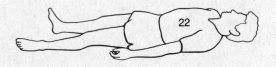

FIGURE 7

**SEQUENCE OF YOGA POSTURES
(TAPE 2, SIDE 2)**

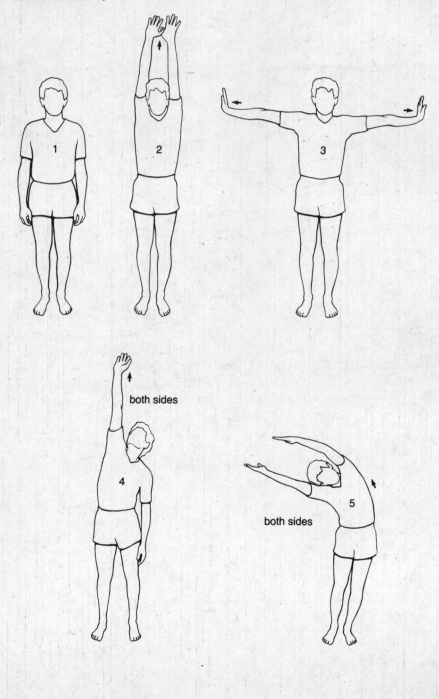

shoulder rolls: do in forward, then backward directions

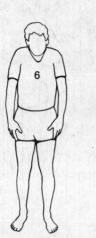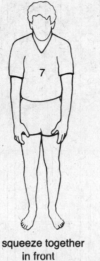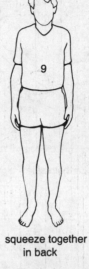

raise up   squeeze together   let drop   squeeze together
in front   in back

neck rolls: do in one direction, then the other

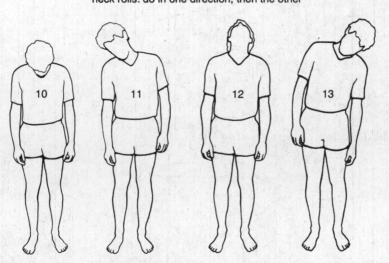

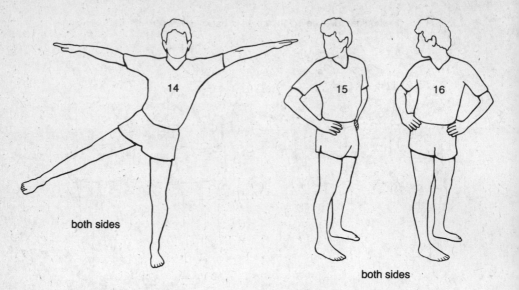

both sides

both sides

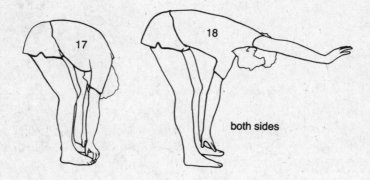

both sides

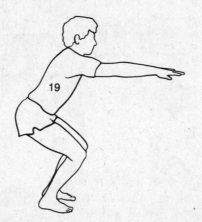

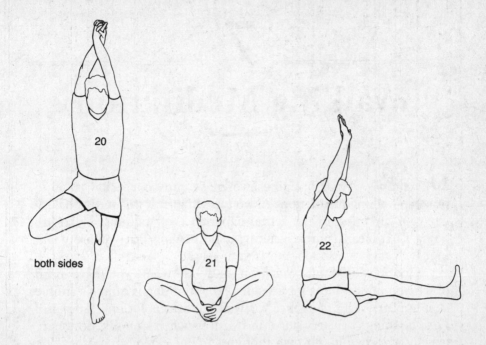

both sides

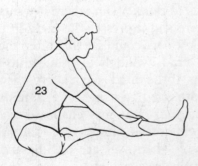

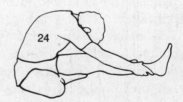

repeat 22 to 24 on other side

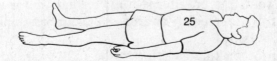

7

Walking Meditation

One simple way of bringing awareness into your daily life is to practice walking meditation. As you might guess, this means bringing your attention to the actual experience of walking as you are doing it. It means simply walking *and* knowing that you are walking. It does *not* mean looking at your feet!

One of the things that you find out when you have been practicing mindfulness for a while is that nothing is quite as simple as it appears. This is as true for walking as it is for anything else. For one thing, we carry our mind with us when we walk, so we are usually absorbed in our own thoughts to one extent or another. We are hardly ever just walking, even when we are "just going for a walk."

Usually we walk for a reason. The most common one is that we want to go from one place to another and walking is how we can best do it. Of course the mind tends to think about where it wants to go and what it is going to do there and it presses the body into service to deliver it there, so to speak. So we could say that often the body is really the chauffeur of the mind, willingly (or reluctantly) transporting it and doing its bidding. If the mind is in a hurry, then the body rushes. If the mind is attracted to something it finds interesting, then the head turns and your body may change direction or stop. And of course, thoughts of all kinds are cascading through the mind just as they are when you are sitting and breathing. All this happens without the least awareness.

Walking meditation involves intentionally attending to the experience of walking itself. It involves focusing on the sensations in your feet or your legs or, alternatively, feeling your whole body moving. You can also integrate awareness of your breathing with the experience of walking.

We begin by making an effort to be fully aware as one foot contacts the ground, as the weight shifts to it, as the other foot lifts and moves ahead and then comes down to make contact with the ground in its turn. As with all the other methods we have been exploring, when the mind wanders away from the feet or the legs or the feeling of the body walking, we simply bring it back when we become aware of it. To deepen our concentration, we do not look around at the sights, but keep our gaze focused in front of us. We also don't look at our feet. They know how to walk quite well on their own. It is an internal observation that is being cultivated, just the felt sensations of walking, nothing more.

Because we tend to live so unconsciously, we take things like the ability to walk very much for granted. When you start paying more attention to it, you will appreciate that it is an amazing balancing act, given the small surface area of our two feet. It took us about a year as a baby to be ready to learn this dynamic balancing act of locomotion.

Although we all know how to walk, if we are conscious of being observed by other people or even when we observe ourselves sometimes, we can feel self-conscious and awkward, even to the point of losing our balance. It's as if, when we look at it closely, we don't really know what we are doing when we are walking. You could say we don't even know how to walk! Aspiring actors have to learn to walk all over again when it comes time to "just walk" across a stage. Even walking is not so simple.

On any given day in the hospital there are many people who are unable to walk because of injury or illness, and some who will never walk again. For all these people, just being able to take one step unassisted—no less walk down the hall or out to a car—is a miracle. Yet we hardly ever appreciate the great wonder of walking.

When we practice walking meditation, we are not trying to get anywhere. It is sufficient to just be with each step, realizing that you are just where you are. The trick is to be there completely.

To reinforce this message, we walk in circles around the room or back and forth in lanes. This helps put the mind to rest because it literally has no place to go and nothing interesting happening to keep it entertained. Either you are going in circles or you are going back and forth; under these circumstances the mind just may grasp that there is no point in hurrying to get somewhere else and it may be willing to just be wherever you actually are in each moment and feel the sensations in your feet.

This doesn't mean that your mind will go along with your intention to just be with each step for very long without a concerted effort to keep it focused. You might soon find it condemning the whole exercise, calling it stupid, useless, idiotic. Or it might start to play games with the pace or with balancing, or have you looking around or thinking of other things. But if your mindfulness is strong, you will quickly become aware of this activity and just return your attention to the feet, legs, and body. It's a good idea to start with awareness of the feet and legs and practice that for a while. Then, when your concentration is stronger, you can expand the field of awareness to include a sense of your whole body walking.

You can practice mindful walking at any pace. We sometimes do it very slowly, so that one step might take a minute. This allows you to really be with each movement from moment to moment. But we also practice it at a more natural pace. During the day-long session in the stress clinic, which is described in the next chapter, there are times when we do the walking meditation at a very fast pace. The point here is to practice being aware even when moving quickly. If you try it, you will find that you won't be able to be with each step so easily, but you can shift your awareness instead to a sense of your body as a whole moving through space. So even rushing, you can be mindful, if you can remember.

◆

To begin walking as a formal meditation practice, you should make the specific intention to do it for a period of time, say ten minutes, in a place where you can walk slowly back and forth in a lane. To keep mindfulness strong, it's a good idea to focus your attention on *one* aspect of your walking rather than changing it all the time. So if you have decided to pay attention to your feet, then you should stay with your feet for that entire walking period, rather than changing to the breath or the legs or the full gait. Since it looks weird to other people to walk back and forth without any apparent purpose, especially if you are doing it slowly, you should do it someplace where you will not be observed, such as your bedroom or living room. Choose a pace that maximizes your ability to pay attention. This might differ from one time to another, but in general it should be slower than your normal pace of walking.

One young woman was so nervous when she started the stress reduction program that she couldn't tolerate any stillness at all. She was unable to keep still and would twitch and pace and pound the walls, or fiddle incessantly with the telephone cord on the desk as we talked. Practicing the body scan and the sitting, even for short periods of time, was out of the question for her. Even the yoga was too static. But in spite of her extreme anxiety, this woman intuitively knew that connecting up with meditation was a route toward sanity for her, if only she could find a way to do it. It turned out that the walking meditation became her lifeline; she used it to anchor her mind as she engaged in working mindfully with her demons at a time when things were totally out of control. Gradually her condition improved over a period of months and years, and she was able to get into the other techniques as well. But it was the walking meditation that came through for her when nothing else was possible. Mindful walking can be just as profound a meditation practice as sitting or doing the body scan or the yoga.

◆

When my children were babies, I did a lot of "enforced" walking meditation. It took place in the house late at night, holding one of them on my shoulder. Back and forth, back and forth. Since I had to be "walking the floors" with them anyway, using it as an occasion to meditate helped me to be present one hundred percent with what was happening.

Of course a lot of the time my mind resisted being up in the middle of the night. It didn't like being sleep-deprived and wanted badly to go back to bed. Every parent knows what this is like, especially when a child is sick.

The reality of the situation was that I had to be up. So it made sense in my mind to decide to be up completely, in other words to practice being fully present holding the baby and walking slowly back and forth, and to work at letting go of whether I wanted to be doing this or not. Sometimes this walking went on for what seemed like hours. The mindfulness practice made it a lot easier to do what had to be done anyway, and it also brought me into much closer contact with my children at those times, since I would include in the field of my awareness the sense of the little body snuggled over my shoulder or in my arms and of our bodies breathing together. When a parent is in a meditative state, it is very reassuring and comforting for the child, who feels the calmness and love coming in through his or her own body.

There are probably circumstances of one kind or another in your life in which you have to be walking, whether you like it or not. These can be wonderful occasions to bring awareness to your walking and thereby transform it from a dull, mostly unconscious chore into something rich and nurturing.

◆

Once you have practiced walking mindfully as a formal exercise and you have some experience of what is involved, you will find that you can easily practice a more informal mindfulness of walking in many different circumstances. For instance when you park your car and go into stores to do errands or shopping, that is a good occasion to try walking to where you are going with a continuity of awareness. So often, when we have routine errands to do, we feel impelled to rush from one to the next until we get them all done. This can be exhausting, even depressing, because of the monotony of what we are doing if the places we go are the same old places we find ourselves all the time. The mind craves something new. But if we bring awareness to our walking during these routine tasks, it will short-circuit the automatic-pilot mode and make our routine experiences more vivid and actually more interesting and leave us calmer and less exhausted at the end.

I usually do it with a sense of the whole body walking and breathing. You can walk at a normal pace or you can decide to just "take the edge off" your pace to be more attentive. No one will notice anything unusual if you do this, but it might make a great deal of difference in your state of mind.

Many of our patients walk for exercise on a regular basis. They find that they enjoy it much more when they intentionally practice being aware of their breathing and of their feet and legs with every step. Some do this early every morning as a regular discipline. John, a forty-four-year-old stockbroker and father of two who had been referred to the stress clinic with idiopathic cardiomyopathy (a poorly understood and very dangerous disease involving the heart muscle itself that causes the heart to dilate and perform poorly) was, by his own description, a wreck when he came to the stress clinic. His diagnosis two years earlier, after experiencing severe problems with his heart, sent him into a deep depression and self-destructive behaviors. His attitude then had been "I'm going to die anyway, why bother trying to take care of myself." He loved all the things that were bad for him; alcohol and high-sodium and high-fat foods. His wild mood swings would trigger a vicious cycle of anxiety followed by shortness of breath, and he would eat things he knew he shouldn't. These behaviors would often bring on severe pulmonary edema (a dangerous condition in which the lungs fill up with fluid) requiring hospitalization.

At a three-month follow-up session we held for his class, he reported that when he had started in the stress clinic, he had been incapable of walking for more than five minutes. By the time it ended, he was getting up at 5:15 A.M. and walking mindfully for forty-five minutes every day before going to work. And now, three months later, he was still doing it. His pulse rate was down below 70, and his cardiologist had told him his heart had decreased in size, a very good sign.

John called me six months later to let me know that his practice was going well and was still "working for him." He said he knew it was because he had had a lot of stress in his life recently and had handled it, he thought, very well. His mother had died several weeks before, and he felt he had been able to accept it and be conscious during that entire time and help his family with it. He had also just come out of a very intense period of studying for a professional exam, during which he was getting only three hours of sleep a night. He said the meditation practice helped him to get through this time without resorting to any drugs for anxiety. He is continuing to practice the body scan with the tape about three nights per week. On those days, as soon as he gets home from work, he goes upstairs and does it immediately. Before the stress reduction program he said he spent two years just feeling sorry for himself. He would just sit home and say, "Oh God, I'm dying." Now he is out walking every morning—even in the cold New England winter— and he is feeling healthier every day. His cardiologist told me recently that mindfulness is the perfect thing for John. According to him, John *has* to be mindful in his life. When he really pays attention to every aspect of his life, he does very well. When he doesn't, he brings severe medical emergencies on himself.

At that same three-month follow-up session several other people commented about how the meditation had improved their ability to walk and increased their enjoyment of it. Rose said that she has been doing the walking meditation regularly since the classes ended and that she usually does it focusing on sensations of touch, such as the warmth of the sun on her skin or the feeling of the wind. Karen, a woman in her mid-forties, reported that she is walking three to four miles every night as part of her meditation practice. For twenty-two years she went without doing any regular exercise and she is thrilled to be "using her body" again.

In summary, any time you find yourself walking is a good time to practice mindfulness. But sometimes it's good to find an isolated spot and do it formally as well, back and forth, step by step, moment by moment, walking gently on the earth, in step with your life, being exactly where you are.

8

A Day of Mindfulness

It is a beautiful New England morning in early June. The sky is blue and cloudless. At 8:15 A.M. people start arriving at the hospital, carrying sleeping bags and pillows and blankets and lunch, looking much more like a group of campers than medical patients. The Faculty Conference Room is set up with blue straight-backed plastic and metal chairs in a large circle around the room. By 8:45 A.M. there are 120 people in the large, friendly, sunny room, stowing their coats and shoes and purses and lunches under the seats and sitting on the chairs or on the colorful meditation cushions scattered around the room. About 15 people who have already been through the stress reduction program are returning to do the day again, or because they missed it the first time. Sam, seventy-four years old, comes in with his son, Ken, forty. Both had taken the program in previous years and decided to come back for a "booster." They thought it would be fun to do it together.

Sam looks terrific. A retired truck driver, he is grinning from ear to ear as he comes over to hug me and to say how happy he is to be back. He is short, lean, and appears relaxed and jovial. He looks so different from the drawn, tense, angry man who first entered my class two years ago with his face knotted and his jaw characteristically clenched. I marvel at the transformation as I recall momentarily his Type-A diagnosis and his problems with anger, the story of how hard he was on his wife and children, by his own admission "impossible to live with" since his retirement, "a real son of a bitch" around the house, a total "nice guy" to everybody else.

I comment on how good he looks, and he says, "Jon, I'm a different person." His son, Ken, nods his agreement, saying that Sam is no longer hostile and cantankerous and hard to reach. He is getting along well with his family now, happy and relaxed at home, even easygoing. We banter a little before the session gets down to business at nine o'clock sharp.

120

As the staff of the clinic gets ready to start the day rolling, we look around the room. Aside from the "graduates" like Sam and Ken, the rest of the people are currently in their sixth week of the stress reduction program. They have two more weeks to go to finish it after today. We have combined all the separate stress clinic classes this Saturday for our all-day session. It is an integral and required part of the course and always takes place between the sixth and seventh classes.

There are a number of physicians in the room, all of whom are enrolled in the program. One is a senior cardiologist who decided to take the program himself after sending a number of his patients. He is wearing a cutoff football jersey and sweatpants and has his shoes off, as we all do. This is quite a change from his usual hospital attire, with the necktie, the white coat, and the stethoscope hanging out of the pocket. Today the doctors in the room are just regular people, even though they work here. Today they are here for themselves.

Norma Rosiello is here too. She first took the program nine years ago as a pain patient and is now finishing her sixth year working as a secretary and receptionist in the stress clinic office. In many ways Norma is the heart of the clinic. She is the first person the patients usually talk with about the program after they are referred by their doctor, so she has spoken with most of the people in the room at one time or another, often providing them with comfort and reassurance and hope. She does her work with such grace and poise and independence that we hardly notice how much work she actually does and how critical her work is in ensuring that things run smoothly.

When she first came as a patient with facial pain and head-aches, she was winding up in the emergency room like clockwork, at least once a month, with pain that she could not bear and had no way of relieving. She was working as a hairdresser a few times a week but was constantly missing work because of her pain problem, which she had had for fifteen years and for which she had sought help from many specialists. In the stress clinic, over a relatively short period of time, she was able to get her pain under control using meditation instead of hospital visits and medications. Then she started working with us as a volunteer, coming in from time to time to help out. I finally persuaded her to take on the job as our secretary and receptionist even though she was a hairdresser and couldn't type and knew nothing about working in an office. I thought she would be the perfect person for the job because she had been through the clinic herself and would be able to talk with the patients in a way that someone doing the work as "a job" wouldn't be able to do. I figured she could learn to type and to do the other things the job required. And she has. Moreover in the past six years she has been out from work maybe six days because of headaches and facial pain and none in the past two years. As I look over at her now, I marvel at her and am happy to see her here. She has come on her own time to practice with us today.

As I look around the room, I see a mix of ages. Some people have shining white hair while others look about twenty or twenty-five years old. Most are between thirty and fifty. Some come on crutches or with canes. Amy, a graduate of the stress clinic who has cerebral palsy and who has come to each one of our all-day sessions in her wheelchair since she took the program several years ago, is not here, and I feel her absence. She moved to Boston recently, where she is in graduate school. She called yesterday to say she wouldn't be coming because she couldn't find someone who could come with her for the whole day. She has her own van, which has a special wheelchair lift, but she needs another person to drive her. As I look around the circle of faces, I find myself recalling her determination to participate fully in the activities of the day each time she came, even though it meant letting one of us feed her her lunch and wipe her mouth and take her to the bathroom. Her courage and perseverance and lack of self-consciousness about her condition had become part of the meaning of the all-day session for me and I am sorry she isn't able to come this time because she always taught us a lot through her being and through her speech. Although it is sometimes difficult to understand her when she talks, her willingness and courage to speak out, to ask questions and to share her experiences at the end of the day in such a large group had been inspiring to all of us.

At nine o'clock my colleague and friend Saki Santorelli welcomes the group and invites us to sit, that is, to begin meditating. The sounds in the room from everybody talking quiet some when he speaks, but they disappear completely as he suggests that we sit up in our chairs or on the floor and come to our breathing. You can actually hear a wave of silence rise in the room as 120 people bring their attention to their breathing. It is a crescendo of stillness. I am always moved by it.

So begin six hours of silent mindfulness practice on this beautiful Saturday. All of us have other things we might be doing today, yet we have all chosen to be here together, working on the mind and the body, practicing paying attention from moment to moment for an entire day, working at deepening our ability to concentrate and be still, relaxing into just being ourselves.

We have drastically simplified our lives for today just by coming, as Saki explains after our first sitting. By being here we have made the choice not to run around doing the usual things we do on the weekend, such as errands, cleaning the house, going away, or working. To simplify things even further so that we can benefit the most from this very special day, Saki now reviews certain "ground rules" for the day, among which are no talking and no eye contact. He explains that these rules will allow us to go more deeply into the meditation practice and to conserve our energy for the work of mindfulness. In six very concentrated hours of "non-doing," just sitting and walking and lying down and eating and stretching, a lot of different feelings can come up. Many of these feelings can be quite intense, especially when all of our usual outlets such as talking, doing things, moving around, reading, or listening to the radio are intentionally suspended. While many people find the all-day session enjoyable from the very start, for others the moments of relaxation and peace, if any, may be interspersed with other experiences that may be a lot less enjoyable. Physical pain can well up for extended stretches; so can emotional pain or discomfort in the form of anxiety or boredom or guilt feelings about being here rather than someplace else, especially if someone had to give up a lot to come today.

Rather than commenting on such feelings to a neighbor and perhaps disturbing someone else's concentration as well as compounding our own reactions, Saki counsels us for today just to watch whatever comes up and simply to accept our feelings and our experiences in each moment. The silence and ban on eye contact will support this process of looking into and accepting ourselves, he says. They will help us to become more intimate and familiar with the actual comings and goings of our own minds and bodies, even those that are sad or painful. We can't talk with our neighbor about them, we can't complain or comment about how things are going or what we are feeling. What we can do is practice just being with things as they are. We can practice being calm. We can practice in the exact same way that we have been practicing the meditation over the past six weeks in the stress clinic, only now over a more extended period of time and under more intense, perhaps even stressful circumstances.

Saki reminds us we are intentionally making time for this very process to occur. This is to be a day of mindfulness, a day to be with ourselves in a way we usually don't have time for because of all our obligations and entanglements and busyness, and also because, when you come right down to it, a lot of the time we don't feel like paying too much attention to our being, especially if we are hurting, and because in general we would prefer not being still and quiet. So, when we do have some "free" time, ordinarily we tend to want to fill it up right away with something to keep us occupied. We entertain or distract ourselves to "pass" the time.

Today will be different, he concludes. Today we will have no props to pass the time and distract us. The idea is to be with whatever we are feeling in any moment and to accept it as we practice staying with our breathing, with walking, with stretching, with whatever the instructors are guiding us through. He points out that today is not a day for trying to feel a certain way but for just letting things unfold. So he counsels us to let go of all our expectations, including that we should have a relaxing and pleasant day and to practice being fully awake and aware of whatever happens, moment by moment.

Elana Rosenbaum and Kacey Carmichael, the other instructors in the stress clinic, guide the flow of the day along with Saki and myself. After Saki's talk we all get down on the floor on our mats to do an hour of yoga. We do it slowly, gently, mindfully, listening to our bodies. As I begin to guide this part of the day, I emphasize the importance of remembering to listen to our own bodies carefully and honoring them by not doing anything that we know to be inappropriate for a particular condition we might have. Some of the patients, particularly those with low-back or neck problems don't do the yoga at all but just sit on the side of the room and watch or meditate. Others do a little but only what they know they can handle. The heart patients are monitoring their pulse as they learned to do in cardiac rehabilitation and only hold the postures as long as their pulse rate is in the appropriate range. Then they rest and do repetitions as the rest of us hold the postures a little longer, going "behind" the intensity of sensations, which grows and changes as we maintain each pose.

Everybody is doing as much or as little as he or she feels comfortable with. We are working at our limits, moment by moment, as we go through a slow sequence of yoga postures. We are breathing in to our limits and feeling the sensations in various parts of our body as we lift, stretch, tense, roll, move, bend, and rest. At the same time we are noting our thoughts and feelings as they arise and practicing seeing them and letting them be, seeing them and letting them go, bringing the mind back to the breath every time it wanders off.

After the yoga we sit for thirty minutes. Then we walk mindfully in a circle around the room for ten minutes or so. Then we sit again for twenty minutes. Everything we do this day we do with awareness and in silence. Even lunch is in silence so that we can eat our food knowing that we are eating, chewing, tasting, swallowing, pausing. It is not so easy to do this. It requires a lot of energy to stay focused and concentrated in the present.

During lunch I notice one man who is reading a newspaper in spite of the spirit of the day and our explicit ground rule to the contrary. Our hope is that everyone will see the value, at least as an experiment, of going along with the ground rules and taking responsibility for keeping them. But perhaps it's too much intensity for him to handle eating mindfully right now. So I smile to myself, observing my own self-righteous impulse to insist he do it "our way" today, and let it go. After all he is here, isn't he? Perhaps that is enough. Who knows what his morning was like?

Last year we had a group of district court judges, for whom we ran a special stress reduction program. They were in a class by themselves so that they could speak freely about their unique stresses and problems. Since the job description for judges is that they "sit" on the bench, it seemed fitting that they were getting some formal training in how to sit and also in how to cultivate being intentionally non-judgmental. Some were strongly drawn to the concept of mindfulness when we first discussed the possibility of a program for them. To do their job well requires enormous concentration and patience and both compassion and dispassion. They have to listen to a steady stream of sometimes painful and repugnant but mostly boring and predictable testimony while maintaining equanimity and dispassion and above all paying careful attention to what is actually happening in the courtroom. Having a systematic way of handling one's own intrusive thoughts and feelings and reactions might be particularly useful professionally for a judge, in addition to being an aid in reducing his or her own stress levels.

When they came for the all-day session, the judges were anonymous in the large group of patients. I noticed that they sat next to each other and that they ate lunch together out on the lawn. They commented later that they had felt a special closeness to each other during lunch as they sat together without talking or looking at each other, a very unusual experience for them.

◆

The energy in the room today feels very crisp. Most people are clearly awake and focused during the sitting and the walking. You can feel the efforts being made to concentrate. The stillness up to now has been exquisite.

After a period of silent walking in which people are on their own to walk where they please for a half hour, we start off the afternoon program with a lovingkindness-and-forgiveness meditation. This simple meditation (see Chapter 13) often has people sobbing with sadness or joy. Following it, we move into quietly sitting and then more slow walking.

We do "crazy walking" in the middle of the afternoon to keep the energy up. Almost everybody enjoys the change of pace, although some people have to sit this one out and just watch. The crazy walking involves walking very quickly, changing direction every seven steps, then every four, then three, with our jaws and fists clenched, not making eye contact, all done with moment-to-moment awareness. Then we do it with eye contact, at the same pace, minding the differences this time. Then we walk backward, very slowly, with our eyes closed, changing direction when we bump into someone, after we allow ourselves to feel the bump, the contact with another body. The crazy-walking period ends with everybody backing up slowing into what they think is the center of the room with their eyes closed, until we are all in one big mass. Then we lean our heads on whatever is available for support. There is a lot of laughing at this point. It eases some of the intensity that builds as the level of concentration deepens during the afternoon.

The longest sitting of the afternoon starts off with what we call the *mountain meditation*. We use the image of a mountain to help people remember what the sitting is all about as the day goes on and a certain fatigue sets in. The image is uplifting, suggesting as it does that we sit like mountains, feeling rooted, massive, and unmoving in our posture. Our arms are the sloping sides of the mountain, our head the lofty peak, the whole body majestic and magnificent, as mountains tend to be. We are sitting in stillness, just being what we are, just as a mountain "sits there," unmoved by the changing of day into night and the changes of the weather and of the seasons. The mountain is always grounded, rooted in the earth, always still, always beautiful. It is beautiful just being what it is, seen or unseen, snow-covered or green, rained on or wrapped in clouds.

This image sometimes helps us to remember our own strength and intentionality as the sunlight begins to wane in the room in the late afternoon. It reminds us that we might look upon some of the changes we are observing in our own minds and bodies as internal "weather." The mountain reminds us that we can remain stable and balanced in our sitting in the face of the storms of our own minds and bodies.

People like the mountain meditation because it gives them an image that they can use to anchor themselves in the sitting practice and deepen their calmness and equanimity. But the image has its limits too, since we are the kind of "mountain" that can walk and talk and think and act as well as just be still.

◆

And so the day unfolds, moment by moment, breath by breath. Many people had come in this morning anxious about whether they would be able to make it through six hours of silence, whether they would be able to endure just sitting and walking and breathing in silence for much of a day. But here it is three o'clock already, and everybody is still here and seemingly very much with it.

Now we suspend the silence and the injunction against making eye contact. We start talking, 120 people in a circle holding an intimate conversation about our experiences, asking questions and sharing how we felt and what we saw and learned. The calmness and peacefulness in the room are such that it really feels intimate, even with so many people. It almost feels as if we are sharing one big mind together around the circle and mirroring different aspects of it back and forth to each other.

One woman said that during the lovingkindness-and-forgiveness meditation she had been able to direct some love and kindness toward herself and that she found she was able to forgive her husband just a little for years of violence and physical abuse that she said had almost killed her. She said it felt good to let go of it in this way, just the little bit that she had, that it felt as if something was being healed inside of her by forgiving him. She said she saw that she didn't have to carry her anger around with her like an enormous weight forever and that she could move on with her life as she let this be behind her.

At this, another woman wondered for herself whether it is always appropriate to forgive. She said she didn't think it was healthy for her to practice forgiveness right now; that she had been a "professional victim" most of her adult life and was always forgiving people and making herself the object of other people's needs at the expense of her own. She said that what she thought she needed was to *feel* her anger. She said she had gotten in touch with it today for the first time and saw that she had been unwilling to face it in the past. She was realizing today that she needs to pay attention to and honor the dominant feeling that she has at this time, which is a lot of anger, and that "forgiveness can wait."

Several graduates said that they had come to "recharge their batteries," as a way of getting back into a daily meditation routine, which some had moved away from. Janet said that it reminded her of how much better she feels when she meditates regularly. Mark said that his regular sitting practice helps him to trust his body and listen to it too rather than exclusively to his doctors. He said his doctors had told him that he would never be able to do all sorts of things anymore because of his worsening spinal condition, known as *ankylosing spondylosis,* in which the vertebrae fuse together to form a rodlike structure; but he finds he is now able to do many of them again.

During the hour-long discussion there are frequent stretches of silence in the group, as if we have collectively gone into a state beyond the need for talk. It feels as if the silence is communicating something deeper than what we are able to express with words. It binds us together. We feel peaceful in it, comfortable.

And so the day comes to an end. We sit for a final fifteen minutes and then say our good-byes. Sam still has a big grin on his face. It is obvious that he has had a good day. We hug once more and promise to keep in touch. Some people help us roll up the mats and put them away.

Later in the week, in our regular classes, we discussed the all-day session some more. Bernice said she was so nervous about coming that she got practically no sleep the night before. Around five in the morning she did the body scan on her own, without the tape for the first time, in a last-ditch attempt to relax enough to feel able to come. To her surprise it worked. But she said she was still in a somewhat deranged state from lack of sleep and almost decided that it would be too hard for her to sit for a whole day with so many people without talking. For some reason that she could not really explain, at some point she decided that she might be able to do it.

She got into her car and played the body-scan tape the whole way to the medical center, using the sound of my voice to reassure her. She said this sheepishly and laughed along with the rest of the class, because everybody knew that they were not supposed to use the meditation tapes while driving.

During the morning, Bernice went on, there had been three separate times that she almost bolted from the room in a state of sheer panic. But she didn't. Each time she told herself that she could always leave if she had to, that there was nothing holding her prisoner in the room. Reframing the situation this way was enough to help her stay with her anxious feelings and breathe with them when they welled up. In the afternoon she experienced no feelings of panic at all. Instead she felt peaceful. She discovered for the first time in her life, she said, that she could actually "stay with" her feelings and watch them without running from them.

Not only did she discover that they eventually subside by themselves, she also discovered a new feeling of confidence in her ability to handle such episodes. She saw that she could have long stretches of relaxation and peace in the afternoon, even though she had had almost no sleep the night before and therefore had every "reason" to expect things to be "bad." She was thrilled to make this discovery and feels that it is going to have relevance to other situations in which, in the past, she has been controlled by her fears.

Bernice was particularly pleased with this discovery because she suffers from Crohn's disease, a chronic ulcerative disorder of the intestines that gives rise to intense abdominal pain whenever she is tense and stressed. She had had none of her usual symptoms during the all-day session, as she managed to ride out and regulate her feelings of panic that morning.

Ralph then told a story about jumping out of his parents' car as a child when it was stuck in traffic in a long tunnel and running toward the end of the tunnel, driven by an uncontrollable fear. This recollection struck a chord in Bernice, who confessed that she won't go to the airport in Boston because she has to go through the Callahan Tunnel. But later, before the class ended, she said that going through a tunnel would probably be similar to making it through the all-day session. Since she did that, she decided she can probably go through the Callahan Tunnel. It seems she is thinking about doing it now, almost as a homework assignment for herself, a rite of passage to test her growth in the stress clinic.

Fran said that her experience of the all-day session was one of having a "funny" feeling that she didn't want to call relaxation or peace, it was more like feeling "solid" and "free." She said that even lying down on the grass outside after lunch felt special. She hadn't lain on grass and just looked at the sky since she was a little girl. Now she is forty-seven. Her first thought after she realized how good she was feeling was "What a waste!" meaning all those years she had felt out of touch with herself. I suggested that those years were what led up to this present experience of freedom and solidity and that she bring her awareness to the impulse to label them as "bad" or "a waste" just as she would if we were meditating. Perhaps then she could see those years with greater acceptance, as what she was able to do then, seeing things as she did at that time.

The cardiologist said he realized that his whole life was spent trying to get somewhere else, using the present to achieve results that would bring him what he wanted sometime later. During the all-day session he had seen that nothing bad would happen to him if he started living in the present and appreciating it *for itself.* He also expressed amazement at how effortless the crazy walking had been. He said if he had thought about it, he would have predicted that people would bang into each other and actually get hurt with so many people moving so quickly and changing directions at random every two steps. But he found that he hardly brushed or was brushed by anyone and he said he thought this was because all the meditating we did in the morning had refined everybody's concentration and awareness to the point where they could be much more sensitive at high speed, all without overt communication or eye contact.

A young psychiatrist spoke of how discouraged she had felt on Saturday doing the meditation. She had had a hard time keeping her attention focused on her breath or on her body. She described it as feeling just like "slogging through mud." She said she kept having to "start over, again and again, from the bottom."

This image became the subject of some discussion, since there is a big difference between "starting over" and "starting from the bottom." Starting over implies just being in the moment, the possibility of a fresh beginning with each breath. Seeing things this way, coming back to the breath in each moment that the mind wanders would be relatively effortless, or at least neutral. Each breath really *is* a new beginning of the rest of our lives. But the words she used carried a strong negative judgment. "Starting from the bottom" implies that she feels she has lost ground, is submerged, has to rise up. Taken with the weight and resistance of the mud image, it is easy to see why she might have felt discouraged about bringing her mind back to her breathing when it wandered.

When she saw this, she laughed good-naturedly. The meditation practice is a perfect mirror. It allows us to look at the problems our thinking creates for us, those little or not-so-little traps that our own minds set for us and in which we get caught and sometimes stuck. What we ourselves have made laborious and difficult becomes easier the moment we see the reflection of our own mind in the mirror of mindfulness. In a moment of insight, her confusion and difficulty dissolved, leaving the mirror empty, at least for a moment. And laughing.

9

Really Doing What You're Doing: Mindfulness in Daily Life

Jackie returned home from the all-day stress reduction intensive late in the afternoon on Saturday. Although she was tired from the effort she had put in, she felt it had been a good day. She had made it through and had enjoyed being silent and alone with all those people. In fact she was pleasantly surprised by how good she felt about herself after seven and a half hours of just sitting and walking, seven and a half hours of doing nothing really.

Arriving home, she discovered a note from her husband saying he had gone off overnight to take care of things at their summer home in a neighboring state. He had mentioned that he might do this, but she had not taken it seriously because he knew very well that she would not want to be alone that night. Had she known in advance that he was going to be away, she could have arranged not to be alone, as she had always done in the past. In fact Jackie had spent very little time alone in her life and she was well aware that the prospect frightened her. When her daughters were younger and still living at home, she had always encouraged them to get out of the house and do things, to get together with friends, anything rather than being along in the house, to which they had always responded, "But Mom, we *like* being alone." Jackie could never understand how they could like being alone. The prospect simply terrified her.

When she got home and found the note from her husband, her first impulse was to reach for the telephone and invite a friend over

132

for dinner and to spend the night. In mid-dialing, she stopped herself and thought, "Why am I in such a rush to fill up this time? Why not really take seriously what those people in the stress clinic are saying about living your moments fully?" She hung up and decided just to let the momentum of her day of mindfulness that had begun that morning at the hospital continue. Then she decided she would allow herself to be in her house all alone for the first time in her adult life and just feel it.

As she described it to me a few days later, it turned out to be a special time. Rather than experiencing loneliness and anxiety, she was filled with a feeling of joy that lasted all evening. With some effort she moved her mattress and box spring to another room where she knew she would feel more secure keeping her windows open on a Saturday night alone. She stayed up late, enjoying herself in her own house. She got up early the next morning, before sunrise, still feeling exuberant, and watched the sun come up.

Jackie had made a very important discovery. In her mid-fifties she had discovered that all her time is really her own. Her experience that night and the next morning helped her to see that she is really living her own life all the time, that all her moments are hers, available to be felt and lived if she chooses to. When we talked, she expressed concern that she wouldn't be able to duplicate the feeling of peace that she had had that night and the next day. I reminded her that that very concern was itself just another worried thought about the future, and she agreed, mindful that it had been her willingness to be in the present that night that had brought about her experience of inner peace in the first place and that having such a positive experience under such conditions was in itself a breakthrough for her.

The discovery that she could be happy by herself came about because she had chosen to use the momentum she had built up in her meditation practice during the day-long session. We reviewed how she had kept the "being mode" alive when she got home and encountered the unexpected. She had caught herself thinking first of filling up that time to escape from being with herself and had chosen instead, quite intentionally, to dwell in the present, to accept it as it was at that moment. This being the case, we discussed the possibility that perhaps she didn't need to worry about either *duplicating* her experience or *losing* it. The happiness she experienced came from inside herself in the first place. It was released by her courage and her intention to bring awareness to her situation and to be mindful in the face of her insecurities. As we talked, she began to see that she can tap this dimension of her being at any time, that it is a part of her; that all it really takes is a willingness to be mindful and to adjust her priorities so that time by herself is valued and protected.

◆

The peacefulness Jackie experienced that night is something that can be felt in any moment, under any circumstances, if the commitment to practice mindfulness is strong. It is a great gift we can give to ourself. It means we can reclaim our entire life rather than just living for our vacations or the other "special" times when everything will be "perfectly arranged" to bring on those hoped-for feelings of inner peace and serenity. Of course it hardly ever works out that way anyway, even on vacation.

The challenge is to make calmness, inner balance, and clear seeing a part of everyday life. In the same way that it is possible to be mindful *whenever* we are walking, not just when we are practicing walking meditation, we can attempt to bring moment-to-moment attention to the tasks, experiences, and encounters of ordinary living, such as setting the table, eating, washing the dishes, doing the laundry, cleaning the house, taking out the garbage, working in the garden, mowing the lawn, brushing our teeth, shaving, taking a shower or a bath, drying off with the towel, playing with the children, cleaning out the garage, taking the car in to be fixed or fixing it ourselves, riding a bike, taking the subway, getting on a bus, talking on the phone, hugging, kissing, touching, making love, taking care of people who depend on us, going to work, working, or just sitting on the front steps or in the backyard.

If you can name something or even feel it, you can be mindful of it. As we have already seen a number of times, in bringing mindfulness to an activity or an experience, whatever it may be, you flesh it out. It becomes more vivid, more bright, more real for you. In part things become more vivid because the stream of your thinking subsides a little and is less likely to interpose itself between you and what is actually happening. This greater clarity and fullness can be experienced in the activities of daily living in the very same way that we have felt it practicing the body scan and the sitting and the yoga. Your formal mindfulness practice heightens your ability to encounter the whole of your life with moment-to-moment awareness. When you are practicing regularly, mindfulness will tend naturally to spill over into all the various contours of your daily life. You might find your mind altogether calmer and less reactive.

As encountering each moment with awareness becomes more familiar to you, you will find that it is not only possible but even enjoyable to be in the moment, even with ordinary tasks such as washing the dishes. You come to see that you don't have to rush to get through with the dishes so that you can get on to something better or more important because, at the moment that you are doing the dishes, that *is* your life. As we have seen, if you miss these moments because your mind is somewhere else, in an important way you are shortchanging your life. So try taking each pot and each cup and each plate as it comes, being aware of the movements of your body in holding and scrubbing and rinsing, the movements of the breath, and the movements of your mind.

You can follow a similar approach with anything and everything you find yourself doing, whether it be alone or with other people. As long as you are doing it, doesn't it make sense to do it with your full being? If you choose to do things mindfully, then your doing will be coming out of non-doing. It will feel more meaningful and requires less effort.

If you are able to be present while doing routine daily activities, if you are willing to remember that those moments can be moments of calm and alert attention as well as times of doing things that have to be done, you may find that not only do you enjoy the process more but you are also more likely to have insights into yourself and your life while you are doing these routine activities.

For instance, in doing the dishes mindfully, you may come to see with great vividness the reality of impermanence. Here you are, doing the dishes again. How many times have you done the dishes? How many more times will you do them in your life? What *is* this activity we call doing the dishes? Who is doing them? Why?

By inquiring in this way, by looking deeply into this ordinary routine of "doing the dishes," you may find that the whole world is represented in it, that you can learn a lot about yourself and the world by doing the dishes with your whole being, with alert interest and an inquiring mind. The dishes can teach you something important in this way. They become a mirror of your own mind.

We are not talking about simply seeing that life is a stream of dirty dishes, after which you go back to doing the dishes mechanically. The point is to really *do* the dishes when you are doing them, to be awake and alive as you do them, mindful of the tendency to slip back into autopilot and do them unconsciously, perhaps also aware of your resistance to get to them, to procrastinate, to resent other people who you want to help you but who don't. Mindfulness can also lead to decisions to make changes in your life based on your insights. Perhaps you might even get others to do their fair share of the dishes!

Take cleaning the house as another example. If you have got to clean your house, why not clean it mindfully? So many people tell me that their houses are spotless, that they cannot live with mess, with disorder, that they are *always* cleaning and picking up and straightening and dusting. But how much of the time are they doing it with awareness? How much of the time are they aware of their bodies as they are cleaning? And are they inquiring at all about how clean is clean? About their attachment to the house looking a certain way? About what they get out of doing it? Or whether they resent doing it? Are they inquiring about when they should stop? Or about what else they might be doing with their energy instead of keeping the house like a showpiece? About why they are driven to clean compulsively? About who will clean their house after they are dead twenty years, or whether it will matter to them?

By making cleaning the house into part of your meditation practice, this routine chore can become an entirely new experience. You may also wind up doing it differently, or less, and not because you have stopped caring about order and cleanliness. These do not need to be sacrificed. But you may change how you clean the house because you have seen more deeply into your relationship to order and cleanliness and into yourself and your own needs and priorities. Inquiry here means simply non-judgmental awareness, a penetration behind the veil of unawareness that usually covers our activities, especially those that we do routinely.

Perhaps these suggestions for how to do the dishes mindfully or to clean your house mindfully will give you some ideas for ways to do whatever you find yourself doing with greater awareness and for ways to nurture a clearer seeing into your own mind and life situation. The important point to keep in mind is that each moment that you are alive is a moment that you can live fully, a moment not to be missed.

◆

George does the grocery shopping for himself and his wife every week. He does it mindfully. He has to. With his condition, almost anything he does can send him into a severe episode of shortness of breath. Moment-to-moment awareness helps him to keep his body and his breathing under control.

George has chronic obstructive pulmonary disease (COPD). He cannot work, so he at least tries to help out with things around the house while his wife is at work. He is sixty-six years old and has had the disease for the past six years. He was a smoker, on top of which he had worked his whole adult life in a poorly ventilated machine shop, continually breathing chemicals and abrasive dust. Recently he has had to go on oxygen twenty-four hours a day. He has a portable oxygen canister on wheels that he pulls along. A tube brings the oxygen to his nostrils. He is able to get around this way.

George learned to practice mindfulness when he took the pulmonary rehabilitation program in our hospital four years ago. Part of the program involves using mindfulness of breathing to control shortness of breath and the panic that occurs when you find you can't get the next breath into your lungs. For the past four years he has been practicing faithfully four or five mornings per week for fifteen minutes. While he is meditating, his breathing is unlabored and he doesn't feel he needs the oxygen, although he still uses it.

For George, practicing the meditation has made a big difference in the quality of his life. For one thing he has learned to reduce the frequency of the episodes of shortness of breath by bringing awareness to his breathing. "My breathing is not so hard, let's put it that way. It sort of lets down a little bit and I don't have to go after it, it just stabilizes itself." Although he knows that his condition will not get better and that there are many things he cannot do, George has come to accept this and has learned that he can move along at the slow pace he is capable of and still be happy. He is acutely aware of his limits and tries to be mindful of his body and his breathing throughout the day.

When he came in to the hospital today, he parked his car, walked slowly into the building, and then stopped in the men's room to rest and breathe for a few minutes. Then he went to the elevator and rested for another few minutes. He consciously paces himself and takes his time everywhere he goes. He has to. Otherwise he would be in the emergency room all the time.

It took him a while to adjust psychologically to needing the oxygen twenty-four hours per day. At first he had stopped going to stores because he felt self-conscious and embarrassed by his oxygen tank, but finally he said to himself, "This is crazy! I am only hurting myself." So now he is back doing the grocery shopping again. He gets everything put in small plastic bags with handles. He can lift these smaller bags and put them into the trunk of his car if he does everything slowly, with awareness.

When he gets home, he has to walk about fifty feet from the car to the side of the house. He can pull his oxygen bottle and carry a few bags if they are not too heavy. The heavy ones he leaves in the car for his wife to bring in later. He says, "The folks in the store know me now and they give me the plastic bags with no problem. So I kind of licked that problem. That is the routine; there's a way to cut corners, ya know. I say to myself 'If I can do it, I'm going to do it. If I can't, I'm going to leave it,' and that's the general idea."

By doing the shopping for the family, George is contributing to the work that needs to be done to keep the household going as well as saving his wife from having to do it on top of working. This helps him to continue to feel engaged in his own life. Within the limits of his disease, he is actively meeting life's challenges rather than sitting at home and bemoaning his fate. He takes each moment as it comes and figures out how he can work with it and stay relaxed and aware. By living this way, by exploring his limits and by pacing himself, staying with his breathing right through the day, George is functioning extremely well in his life at a level of physiological lung impairment that might completely disable somebody else. For in this disease in particular, the degree of disability at a given level of lung damage depends more on psychological factors than on anything else once the person is receiving proper medical treatment.

Just as George found a way to make use of mindfulness in his day-to-day life and adapt it to his situation and physical condition, so might each one of us begin to take some responsibility for cultivating mindfulness in our own daily lives, whatever our circumstances. As we will see in the chapter on time and time stress (Chapter 26), bringing full awareness to each moment is a particularly effective way to make the best use of the time that we have. Living in this way, life naturally becomes more balanced and the mind more steady and calm.

◆

When it comes right down to it, the challenge of mindfulness is to realize that "*this is it.*" Right now *is* my life. The question is, What is my relationship to it going to be? Does my life just automatically "happen" to me? Am I a total prisoner of my circumstances or my obligations, of my body or my illness, or of my history? Do I become hostile or defensive or depressed if certain buttons get pushed, happy if other buttons are pushed, and frightened if something else happens? What are my choices? Do I have any options?

We will be looking into these questions more deeply when we take up the subject of our reactions to stress and how our emotions affect our health. For now the important point is to grasp the value of bringing the practice of mindfulness into the conduct of our daily lives. Is there any waking moment of your life that would not be richer and more alive for you if you were more fully awake while it was happening?

10

Getting Started in the Practice

—

If you are interested in establishing a formal mindfulness-meditation practice yourself and have tried the various techniques as we have discussed them, perhaps you are wondering what the best way to proceed might be at this time. Should you start with the sitting or the body scan? What about the yoga? Where do the recommendations about the breathing fit in, and the instructions in Chapter 4 about sitting? How often should you practice and at what times and for how long? What about the walking meditation and practicing mindfulness in daily life?

We have already given some indications about how we combine the various aspects of the formal practice in the stress clinic as we have gone along. In this chapter we provide you with specific recommendations for getting started in your own daily mindfulness practice based on exactly what we do with the patients in the clinic. In this way, as you continue to move through the rest of the book, you can also be practicing as you would if you were enrolled in the clinic. Or, alternatively, you may wish to read through to the end before you decide whether to engage in the practice itself in a regular way. You will find further details about developing and maintaining a regular meditation practice in Chapters 34 and 35.

It is not a bad idea for you to start practicing at this point if what has come before speaks to you. This is certainly what you would have to do were you to enroll in the stress clinic. All the talk *about* the practice, the instructions for how to practice, the discussion of the applications of mindfulness in the case of specific illnesses and problems and people, and what its relationship is to the larger areas of medicine and health and illness, mind and body, and stress—all these considerations and discusions are secondary to the

actual practice of the meditation. Doing it is what is most fundamental.

In the clinic we begin practicing in the very first class. The
material you will be encountering in the following sections of this
book will be richer and make more sense to you if you are already at
work cultivating mindfulness in your own life. So if you feel inclined at this point to get started on a structured program, this
chapter will give you guidelines for how to proceed over the next
eight weeks. You may only get as far as the first two weeks before
you complete the book. That is fine. There is no need to take eight
weeks to read the book. The important thing is just to get started if
you are ready to make that commitment to yourself. Hopefully once
you start, you will keep it up and proceed through the entire eight
weeks. That is certainly what we would recommend. Remember,
we tell our patients, "You don't have to like it, you just have to do
it." By the time you have been practicing for eight weeks, you will
have enough momentum and direct personal experience with the
practice to keep going with it for years if you choose to.

The place to start, of course, is with your breathing. If you
haven't done the three-minute experiment on paying attention to
your breathing (see Chapter 1) and watching what your mind does,
then you might want to do that now, just to make sure you know
what we mean about keeping the mind on the breath and bringing it
back when it wanders. We recommend that, at the very least, you
do this every day for five or ten minutes, either sitting or lying
down, at a time that is convenient for you. Review the chapter on
breathing (Chapter 3) and start getting comfortable with feeling
your belly expand and deflate (rise and fall) as you breathe, then
follow the instructions in exercises 1 and 2 at the end of that
chapter.

The most important thing to remember is to practice every day.
Even if you can make only five minutes to practice during your day,
five minutes of mindfulness can be very restorative and healing. But
as we have pointed out, we require the people in the stress clinic to
commit to between forty-five minutes and an hour of practice per
day, six days per week for at least eight weeks, and we strongly
recommend that you commit yourself to a similar schedule. The
mindfulness practice tapes can be of considerable help in getting
started, and you will find in the following pages indications for
which side of which tape to use at various times. However, as we
pointed out before, there are ample instructions in this section of
the book for you to develop a formal mindfulness practice without

the tapes. We recommend that you study all the chapters in this section from time to time to review the descriptions and suggestions that they contain, whether you are using the practice tapes or not.

WEEKS 1 AND 2

For the first two weeks of your formal practice, we recommend that you do the body scan as described in Chapter 5 (tape 1, side 1). Do it every day, whether you feel like it or not, for approximately forty-five minutes. As we have seen, you will have to experiment with what the best time of day is for you to practice, but remember, the idea is to "fall awake," not to fall asleep. If you have a lot of trouble with sleepiness, do it with your eyes open. In addition to the body scan, practice mindfulness of breathing while sitting for ten minutes at some other time during the day.

To cultivate mindfulness in your daily life—what we have been calling "informal practice"—you might try bringing moment-to-moment awareness to routine activities such as waking up in the morning, brushing your teeth, showering, drying your body, getting dressed, eating, driving, taking out the garbage, shopping. The list is endless, but the point is simply to zero in on *knowing what you are doing as you are actually doing it* and on what you are thinking and feeling from moment to moment as well. If this seems too overwhelming, just pick out one routine activity each week, such as taking a shower, and see if you can remember to just be fully there when you take your shower, every time. And you might try to eat at least one meal a week mindfully as well.

WEEKS 3 AND 4

After practicing in this way for two weeks, start alternating the body scan one day with the first sequence of hatha yoga postures (tape 1, side 2) the next, and keep this up during weeks 3 and 4. Follow the recommendations for the yoga as described in chapter 6. Remember only to do what you feel your body is capable of and always to err on the side of being conservative, listening carefully to your body's messages as you practice. Remember also to check with your doctor or physical therapist if you have chronic pain or some kind of musculoskeletal problem, or lung or heart disease. Continue to practice mindfulness of breathing in the sitting posture, now for fifteen to twenty minutes per day.

For informal practice in week 3, try to be aware of *one pleasant event* per day in your life *as it is happening*. Keep a calendar for the week, jotting down what the experience was, whether you were actually aware of it at the time it was happening (that's the assignment but it doesn't always work out that way), how your body felt at the time, what thoughts and feelings were present, and what it means to you at the time you write it down. A sample calendar is provided in the appendix. In week 4, do the same thing for *one unpleasant or stressful event* per day, again bringing awareness to it *as it is happening*.

WEEKS 5 AND 6

In weeks 5 and 6 we recommend that you stop doing the body scan for a while and replace it with longer sittings (up to forty-five minutes at a time) (tape 2, side 1). Practice the sitting meditation as described in the exercises at the end of Chapter 4. You can sit the whole time just focusing on your breathing (exercise 1) or you can gradually expand the field of your awareness to include other objects such as bodily sensations (exercise 2), sounds (exercise 3), thoughts and feelings (exercise 4) or no particular object (exercise 5). Remember to let your breathing serve as the anchor for your attention in all of these practices.

In the long run you might benefit most from the sitting meditation, especially if you are not using the sitting tape for guidance, if you stay with the breath as the primary object of attention for weeks, even months. In the early stages of the sitting practice it is possible to be uncertain as to where to focus your attention when, and to worry inordinately about whether you are doing it "right." For the record, if your energy is continually going into patient self-observation from moment to moment, whether your attention is on the breathing or on other objects, and you are bringing it back each time it wanders without giving yourself a hard time, then you are doing it right. If you are looking for a special feeling to occur, whether it be relaxation or calmness or concentration, or insight, then you are trying to get somewhere else other than where you already are and you need to remind yourself to just be with the breath in the present. Paradoxically, as we have seen, this is the most effective way to "get somewhere" and to nurture relaxation, calmness, concentration, and insight. They will come by themselves in time if you keep up the daily discipline and practice according to these guidelines.

In weeks 5 and 6 the people in the stress clinic alternate a forty-five-minute sitting one day with the yoga practice the next. If you aren't doing the yoga, then you might like to alternate the sitting with the body scan during these weeks or to just sit every day. This is also a good time to start practicing some walking meditation as described in Chapter 7.

By this time you will probably want to be making the decisions about when and what to practice and for how long for yourself. After four or five weeks many people feel ready to start crafting and personalizing their own meditation practice more and more, using our guidelines merely as suggestions. By the end of the eight weeks our goal is for you to have made the practice your own by adapting it to suit your schedule, your body's needs and capabilities, and your personality in terms of which combination of formal and informal techniques you find most effective.

WEEK 7

To encourage self-directed practice, week 7 in the stress clinic is dedicated to practicing without the tapes if at all possible. People devote a total of forty-five minutes per day to a combination of sitting, yoga, and body scanning, but they have to decide on the mix themselves. They are encouraged to experiment, perhaps by using two or even three of the techniques together on the same day, say thirty minutes of yoga followed by fifteen minutes of sitting, or twenty minutes of sitting followed by yoga either right after it or at another time of day entirely.

Some people find they do not feel ready for practicing in this way at this point. They prefer to continue using the tapes. They find the guidance comforting and reassuring and don't get the same degree of relaxation on their own when it is up to them to decide what to do next, particularly in the body scan and the yoga. From our point of view this is not a problem. Our hope is that, with time, people will internalize the practice and be comfortable practicing on their own, without tapes or books for guidance. However, the development of this kind of confidence and faith in your own capacity to guide the meditation does take time, and it varies from one individual to another. Many of our patients can meditate quite well on their own but still prefer to use their tapes even years after they complete the program.

WEEK 8

In week 8 in the stress clinic we come back to the tapes. Leaving them and coming back to them in this way can be quite revealing. You are likely to hear things on the tape you never heard before and to perceive the deeper structure of the meditation practice in a new way. In this week you are encouraged to practice with the tapes even if you prefer doing it without them. By this point *you* are deciding what technique or techniques you wish to use. You may just be practicing the sitting meditation or the yoga or the body scan, depending on your situation, or you may be combining two or three in various ways.

Whether you realize it or not, it is important that you now have some familiarity with all three formal techniques. You are likely to find this knowledge beneficial in very practical ways. For instance, you may find yourself drawn from time to time to practice yoga or the body scan even if your daily practice is mainly sitting. The body scan can be particularly useful when you are sick in bed, or in acute pain, or unable to sleep, even if it is not your regular practice. Likewise, a little yoga can be particularly helpful at certain times, such as when you are very tired and need to revitalize yourself, or when there is stiffness in particular regions of your body.

The eighth week, being the end of our formal recommendations for practice, is also the first week of practicing on your own. We tell our patients that the eighth week lasts the rest of their lives. We see it as a beginning much more than an ending. The practice doesn't end just because we have stopped telling you what to do. By this point you will be firmly in the driver's seat yourself and, one would hope, if you have been practicing in a regular, disciplined way, you will have enough skill and experience to keep up the momentum you have developed to guide your own mindfulness practice. At the end of the book you will find more suggestions for how to keep up the momentum of mindfulness practice and deepen it over the years. This includes not only a review of the formal practice but more suggestions for bringing mindfulness into daily life and using it to help you to cope with the situations you might be facing. But in all likelihood, by the time you get there, you will probably have invented better ones for yourself.

In the next section we will be looking at a new way of thinking about health and illness and how it relates directly to your own efforts to develop a personal mindfulness-meditation practice. From there we will go on to explore ways of looking at stress and change from a meditative perspective, as well as specific applications of mindfulness for different medical problems and for handling stress in its many different guises. As we proceed, we recommend that you keep to the practice schedule outlined above, so that as you read more *about* the process and its ramifications, it is actually unfolding simultaneously in your own life and in your own heart.

II

THE PARADIGM:
A NEW WAY OF
THINKING ABOUT
HEALTH AND
ILLNESS

11

Introduction to the Paradigm

In order for the meditation practice to take root in your life and flourish, you will have to know why you are practicing. How else will you be able to sustain non-doing in a world where only doing seems to count? What will get you up early in the morning to sit and follow your breathing when everybody else is snug in bed? What will motivate you to practice when the wheels of the doing world are turning, your obligations and responsibilities are beckoning, and a part of you decides or remembers to take some time for "just being"? What will motivate you to bring moment-to-moment awareness into your daily life? What will prevent your practice from losing energy and becoming stale or from petering out altogether after an initial burst of enthusiasm?

To sustain your commitment and keep your meditation practice fresh over a period of months and years, it is important to develop your own personal vision that can guide you in your efforts and remind you at critical times of the value of charting such an unusual course in your life. There may be times when your vision will be the only support you will have in keeping up your practice.

In part your vision will be molded by your unique life circumstances, by your personal beliefs and values. Another part will develop from your experience of the meditation practice itself, from letting everything become your teacher: your body, your attitudes, your mind, your pain, your joy, other people, your mistakes, your failures, your successes, nature, in short, all your moments. If you are cultivating mindfulness in your life, there is not one thing that you do or experience that cannot teach you about yourself by mirroring back to you the reflections of your own mind and body.

But still another element of your vision will have to come from your knowledge of the world and from your beliefs about where and how you fit into it. If your health is a major part of your motivation for coming to meditation practice, then your knowledge of and respect for your own body and how it works, your perspective on what medicine can and cannot do for you, and your understanding of the role of the mind in health and healing may be important elements of your vision. The strength of your personal vision will depend in great measure on what you know in these areas and on how much you are willing to learn. As with the meditation practice itself, this kind of learning requires a lifelong commitment to continual inquiry and a willingness to modify your perspective as you acquire new knowledge and arrive at new levels of understanding and insight.

In the stress clinic we try to stimulate people to learn more about their own bodies and about the role of the mind in health and illness as a fundamental part of their adventure in growth and healing. We do this by touching on the ways in which new scientific research and thinking are transforming the practice of medicine itself, and by exploring the direct relevance of these new developments to our lives as individuals and to the meditation practice.

The stress clinic does not exist in a vacuum. It is a behavioral-medicine clinic in the department of medicine at a major medical center. Behavioral medicine represents a new current within medicine itself, one that is rapidly expanding our ideas and knowledge about health and illness. New research findings and new ways of thinking about health and illness in behavioral medicine are rapidly producing a more comprehensive perspective within medicine, one that recognizes the fundamental unity of mind and body. This perspective explicitly recognizes that people need to be active participants whenever possible in their own health care by learning more about health and how to maintain and optimize it. It also recognizes the importance of people learning to communicate more effectively with their doctors in order to ensure that they understand as much as they want to about what their doctor is telling them, that they are in turn understood by their doctor, and that their needs will be acknowledged and honored. In this spirit we introduce the participants in the stress clinic to some of the research developments in behavioral medicine and to the new perspective developing in medicine so that they will have a better understanding of what we are asking of them and why it is so important.

Perhaps the most fundamental development in behavioral medicine is the recognition that we can no longer think about health as being solely a characteristic of the body or the mind because body and mind are interconnected. The new perspective acknowledges the central importance of thinking in terms of *wholeness* and *interconnectedness* and the need to pay attention to the interactions of mind, body, and behavior in efforts to understand and treat illness. This view emphasizes that science will never be able fully to describe a complex dynamic process such as health or even a relatively simple chronic disease without looking at the functioning of the whole organism and not *restricting* itself to an analysis of parts and components, no matter how important that may be as well.

Medicine is presently expanding its own working model of what health and illness are and how life-style, patterns of thinking and feeling, relationships, and environmental factors all interact to influence health. The new model explicitly rejects the view that mind and body are fundamentally and inexorably separate. In its place medicine is presently seeking to articulate an alternative, more encompassing vision for understanding what we actually mean by "mind" and "body," "health" and "disease."

This transformation in medicine is sometimes referred to as a *paradigm shift*, a movement from one entire worldview to another. There is little doubt that not only medicine but all of science is going through such a shift as the implications of the revolutionary changes in our understanding of nature and of ourselves that have come about in the twentieth century become clearer. For the most part our day-to-day thinking about physical reality—our tacit assumptions about the world, the body, matter and energy—is based on an outmoded view of reality, one that has changed little in the past three hundred years. Science is now searching for more comprehensive models that are truer to our understanding of the interconnectedness of space and time, mass and energy, mind and body, even consciousness and the universe.

In this section you will encounter some of these new ways of looking at the world based on the principles of wholeness and connectedness and their implications in medicine and health care. We will follow two major threads, both of which are intimately related to the meditation practice and to each other. The first has to do with the whole process of paying attention. In the next chapter we will take a closer look at how we see things (or don't see things) and how we think about them and represent them to ourselves. This has direct bearing on how we conceptualize our problems and on our ability to cope with stress and illness. We will explore what we mean by wholeness and interconnectedness and why they are so important for health and healing. We return to this theme in the last chapter in this section.

The second thread we will follow has to do with the new perspective that is developing based on research in behavioral medicine. It addresses the question of how the mind and body interact to influence health and illness, what the implications of this new understanding are for health care, and what we mean when we speak of "health" and "healing" in the first place.

Taken together, both threads may help you to expand your perspective on the meditation practice. They underscore the importance of paying attention to both personal experience *and* current developments in medical research if you hope to enhance your own health.

However, if the information and the perspective presented in this section are only assimilated by your thinking mind, they will be of little practical value. This section and the following one on stress are meant to stimulate in you a growing interest, respect, and appreciation for the exquisite beauty and complexity of your own body and its remarkable ability to self-regulate and heal. Their aim is not to give you detailed information about specialized disciplines such as physiology or psychology or psychoneuroimmunology, but rather to expand your perspective and your beliefs about yourself and your relationship to the world as a thinking, feeling, and socially interacting being, stimulating you to think more deeply about and develop greater confidence in your own body and mind. It is hoped that the views and information presented here will help you to develop your own view of why you might undertake to practice meditation regularly, a vision within which you can put the healing power of mindfulness to practical use in your own life.

12

Glimpses of Wholeness, Delusions of Separateness

Have you ever looked at a dog and really seen it in its total "dogness"? A dog is quite miraculous when you really see it. What is it? Where did it come from? Where is it going? What is it doing here? Why is it shaped the way it is? What is its "view" of things, of the neighborhood? What are its feelings?

Children tend to think about things this way. Their vision is fresh. They see things as if for the first time every time. Sometimes our seeing gets tired. We just see a dog. "If you've seen one, you've seen them all." So we barely see it at all. We tend to see more through our thoughts and opinions than through our eyes. Our thoughts act as a kind of veil preventing us from seeing things with fresh eyes. What comes into view is identified by the thinking, categorizing mind and quickly framed: a dog. This mind actually prevents us from seeing the dog in its fullness. It processes and categorizes the "dog" signal very quickly in our brain and then moves on to do the same to the next perception or thought.

When my son was two years old, he wanted to know if there was a person inside of our dog. It warmed my heart to see through his eyes in that moment. I knew why he was asking. Sage was a real family member. He had his rightful place. His presence was felt, he participated in the psychic space of the house, he was a complete being, as much a "personality" as any of the people in the family. What could I say to him?

Never mind dogs. What about a bird, or a cat, or a tree, or a flower, or a rhinoceros?! They are all quite miraculous really. When you really look at one, you can hardly believe it exists; there it is, this perfect thing, just being what it is, complete in itself. Any imaginative child could have dreamed up a rhinoceros, or an elephant, or a giraffe. But they didn't get here as the product of a child's imagination. The universe is spinning these dreams. They come out of the universe, as do we.

It doesn't hurt to keep this in mind on a daily basis. It would help us to be more mindful. All life is fascinating and beautiful when the veil of our routinized thinking lifts, even for a moment.

There are many different ways of looking at any thing or event or process. A dog is just a dog. In one way there is nothing special about it; at the same time it is extraordinary, even miraculous. It all depends on how you are looking at it. We might say that it is both ordinary *and* extraordinary. The dog doesn't change when you change the way you look. It is always just what it is. That is why dogs and flowers and mountains and the sea are such great teachers. They reflect your own mind. It is your mind that changes.

When your mind changes, new possibilities tend to arise. In fact everything changes when you can see things on different levels simultaneously, when you can *see* fullness and connectedness as well as individuality and separateness. Your thinking expands in scope. This can be a profoundly liberating experience. It can take you beyond your limited preoccupations with yourself. It can put things in a larger perspective. It will certainly change the way you relate to the dog.

When you observe things through the lens of mindfulness, whether it be during formal meditation practice or in daily living, you invariably begin to appreciate things in a new way because your very perceptions change. Ordinary experiences may suddenly be seen as extraordinary. This does not mean that they stop being ordinary. Each is still just what it is. It's just that now you are appreciating them more in their fullness.

Let's take eating once again as an example. Eating is an ordinary activity. We do it all the time, usually without much awareness and without thinking much about it. We have seen this already in the eating-meditation exercise with the raisins. But the fact that your body can digest your food and derive energy from it is extraordinary. The process by which this is accomplished is exquisitely organized and regulated at every level, from the ability of your tongue and cheeks to keep the food between your teeth so that it can be chewed to the stepwise biochemical processes by which it is broken down and absorbed and used to fuel your body and rebuild

its cells and tissues, to the effective elimination of the waste products of this process so that toxins do not accumulate and the body
remains in metabolic and biochemical balance.

In fact everything your body normally does is quite wonderful
and extraordinary, though you may hardly ever think of it this way.
Walking is another good example. If you have ever been unable to
walk, you will know how precious and miraculous walking is. It is
an extraordinary capability. So are seeing and talking, thinking and
breathing, being able to turn over in bed, and anything else you
choose to focus on that your body does.

A little reflection on your body will easily lead you to conclude
that it does wondrous things, all of which you probably take completely for granted. When was the last time you gave some thought
to the remarkable job your liver is doing, for instance? It is the
largest internal organ in your body, performing over thirty thousand
enzymatic reactions per second to ensure metabolic harmony. Dr.
Lewis Thomas, chancellor of Memorial Sloan-Kettering Cancer
Center, wrote in *The Lives of a Cell* that he would rather be given
the controls of a 747, knowing nothing about how to fly, than to be
responsible for the functioning of his liver.

And what about your heart or your brain and the rest of your
nervous system? Do you ever think about them when they are doing
their job well? If you do, do you see them as ordinary or extraordinary? What about your eyes' ability to see, your ears' ability to hear,
your arms and legs' ability to move just where you want them to, the
ability of your feet to keep your whole body balanced when standing. These functions are quite extraordinary. Our well-being depends on the integrated functioning of our sense organs and our
muscles and nerves, our cells, organs, and organ systems at all
times. Yet we tend not to see and think in this way and so we forget
or are ignorant of the fact that our body is truly wondrous. It is a
"universe" in itself, consisting of more than ten million million
million cells, all derived from one single cell, all organized into
tissues and organs and systems and structures with a built-in ability
to regulate itself as a whole to maintain internal balance and order.
In a word our bodies are undeniably self-organizing and self-heal-
ing.

The body accomplishes this inner balance through finely tuned
feedback loops that interconnect all aspects of the organism. For
instance, when you exert yourself, as in running or climbing stairs,
your heart will automatically pump more blood to provide more

oxygen to your muscles so that they can perform the task. When the exertion is over, the output of the heart returns to a resting level, and the muscles rest and recuperate. The exertion may also have generated a lot of heat if it lasted a while. This might have caused you to sweat. This is your body's way of cooling off. If you did sweat a lot, you will feel thirsty and drink something, your body's way of ensuring that the lost fluid will be replaced. All these are interconnected regulatory processes, which operate through feedback loops.

Such interconnections are built into living systems. When the skin is cut, biochemical signals are sent out and cellular blood-clotting processes set in motion that stop the bleeding and heal the wound. When the body is infected by microorganisms such as bacteria and viruses, the immune system goes into action to isolate and neutralize them. If any of our own cells lose their feedback loops that control cell growth and become cancerous, a healthy immune system will mobilize specific types of lymphocytes, called natural killer cells, that can recognize structural changes on the surface of the cancerous cells and destroy them before they can cause damage.

On every level of organization, from the molecular biology of our cells to the functioning of whole organs and larger systems, our biology is regulated by information flow, which connects each part of the system to those other parts that are important for its functioning. The incredible network of interconnections by which the nervous system monitors and regulates all of our organ functions, the countless hormones and neurotransmitters released by glands and by the nervous system itself that transmit chemical messages to targets throughout the body via the bloodstream and nerve fibers, and the panoply of specialized cells in the immune system all play crucial and varied roles in organizing and regulating this flow of information in the body so that you can function as an integrated, coherent, whole being.

If connectedness is crucial for physical integration and health, it is equally important psychologically and socially. Our senses allow us to connect with external reality as well as with our internal states. They give us essential information about the environment and about other people that allows us to organize a coherent impression of the world, to function in "psychological space," to learn, to remember things, to reason. Without these coherent impressions, we would be unable to function in even the most basic ways in the world. So the organization of the body allows for a psychological order that arises out of the physical order and also contains it. At each level of our being there is a wholeness that is itself embedded in a larger wholeness.

The web of interconnectedness goes beyond our individual psychological self. While we are whole ourselves as individual beings, we are also part of a larger whole, interconnected through our family and our friends and acquaintances to the larger society and ultimately to the whole of humanity and life on the planet. Beyond the ways in which we can perceive through our senses and through our emotions that we are connected with the world, there are also the countless ways in which our being is intimately woven into the larger patterns and cycles of nature that we only know about through science and thinking (although even here traditional peoples always knew and respected these aspects of interconnectedness in their own ways as natural laws). To mention just a few, we depend on the ozone layer in the atmosphere to protect us from lethal ultraviolet radiation; we depend on the rain forests and oceans to recycle the oxygen we breathe; we depend on a relatively stable carbon dioxide content in the atmosphere to buffer global temperature changes. In fact one scientific view, known as the Gaia hypothesis, is that the earth as a whole behaves as one self-regulating living organism, given the name Gaia after the Greek goddess of the earth. This hypothesis affirms a view based on scientific reasoning that was, in essence, also held by all traditional cultures and peoples, a world in which humans were interconnected and interdependent with all beings and with the earth itself.

The ability to perceive interconnectedness and wholeness in addition to separateness and fragmentation can be cultivated through mindfulness practice. Partly it comes from recognizing how quick our mind is to jump to a particular way of seeing things out of habit or out of unawareness, how easily our views of events and of ourselves are shaped by prejudices and beliefs and likes and dislikes that we acquired at earlier times. If we hope to see things more clearly as they actually are and thereby perceive their intrinsic wholeness and interconnectedness, we have to be mindful of the ruts our thinking gets us into, and we have to learn to see and approach things differently.

To illustrate the automatic nature of our patterns of seeing and thinking, as well as the power inherent in keeping wholeness in mind, we give the following exercise to the people in the stress clinic as a homework "problem" in the very first class. It usually generates a good deal of stress during the week because some people invariably think that they are going to be judged by their answers.

By design we don't say anything until the next class about how this puzzle relates to what they are doing in the clinic. We call it the problem of the nine dots. You may know it from your own childhood. It is a vivid and easily grasped example of how the way we perceive a problem tends to limit our ability to see solutions to it. I am indebted to Dr. Ilan Kutz for his suggestion to use it in our classes.

    The problem is as follows: Below is an arrangement of nine dots. You are to connect up all the dots by making four straight lines without lifting your pencil and without retracing along any line. Before you turn the page, try to solve this puzzle yourself for five or ten minutes if you don't already know the answer.

FIGURE 8

•   •   •

•   •   •

A.   •   •   •

    What invariably happens with most people is that they start out in one corner and draw three lines around the square, and then the light dawns! One of the dots will be left out this way.

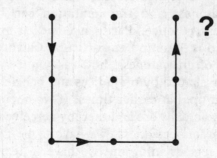

B.

    At this point the mind can experience distress. The more solutions you try that don't work, the more frustrated you can become. When we go over it in class the following week, we ask all those people who do not know the answer to watch carefully what their reaction is when all of a sudden they "see" the solution when a volunteer draws it on the blackboard.

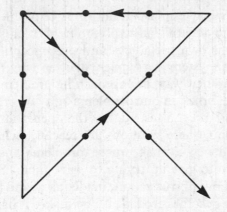

C.

When you see or discover for yourself the solution to this problem, especially after you have been struggling with it for a while, there is usually an "aha!" experience at the moment of discovery. This is associated with the realization that the solution lies in extending the lines you draw *beyond* the imaginary square that the dots make. The problem as stated does not prevent you from going outside the dots, but the "normal" tendency is to see the nine-dot square pattern as the field of the problem rather than seeing the dots in the context of the paper and recognizing that the field of the problem is the whole surface that contains the dots.

If you isolate the nine dots by themselves as the domain of the problem because of the automatic way in which you perceive things and think about them, you will never find a satisfactory solution to this problem. As a consequence, you may wind up blaming yourself for being stupid or getting angry at the problem and proclaiming it impossible or foolish. All the while you are putting your energy in the wrong place. You are not seeing the full domain of the problem. You are missing the larger context.

The problem of the nine dots suggests that we may need to take a broader view of certain problems if we hope to solve them. This approach involves asking ourselves what the extent of the problem actually is and discerning the relationship between the various isolated parts of the problem and the problem as a whole. This is called taking a "systems view." If we do not identify the system correctly in its entirety, we will never be able to come to a satisfactory solution of the problem because a key domain will always be missing, the domain of the whole.

The problem of the nine dots teaches us that we may have to expand beyond our habitual ways of seeing and thinking and acting in order to solve or resolve certain kinds of problems. If we don't, our attempts to identify and solve our problems will usually be thwarted by our own prejudices and preconceptions. Our lack of awareness of the system as a whole will often prevent us from seeing new options and new ways of approaching problems. We will have a tendency to get stuck in our problems and our crises and to make faulty decisions and choices. Rather than penetrating *through* problems to the point where solutions are reached, when we get stuck, there is a tendency to make more problems and to make them worse, and also to give up trying to solve them. Such experiences can lead to feelings of frustration, inadequacy, and insecurity. When self-confidence becomes eroded, it just makes it harder to solve any other problems that come along. Our doubts about our own abilities become self-fulfilling prophecies. They can come to dominate our lives. In this way, we effectively make our own limits by our own thought processes. Then, too often, we forget that we have created these boundaries ourself. Consequently we get stuck and feel we can't get beyond them.

You can get a closer look at this process on a day-to-day level by being mindful of your own inner dialogue and beliefs and how they affect what you wind up doing in certain situations. Unless we are practicing mindfulness, we rarely observe our inner dialogue with any detachment and ponder its validity, especially when it concerns our thoughts and beliefs about ourselves. For instance, if you have the habit of saying to yourself "I could never do that" when you encounter some kind of problem or dilemma, such as learning to use a tool or fixing a mechanical device or speaking up for yourself in front of a group of people or in any other situation, one thing is pretty certain—you won't be able to do it. At that moment your thought fulfills or makes real its own content. Saying "I can't" or "I could never . . ." is a self-fulfilling prophecy.

If you are in the habit of thinking about yourself in this way in such situations, by the time you have a chance to act or to do something to solve the problem, you will have already put yourself in a box of your own creation and limited your possibilities. The fact is you really do not know in many situations what you are capable of doing at any particular moment. You might surprise yourself if you took on a problem, just for fun, and tried something new, even if you didn't know what you were doing and even if you inwardly doubted your ability to do it. I have fixed many a clock and car door that way, sometimes learning about clocks and doors but sometimes managing to fix it just by fiddling with it without having the foggiest idea about how it got fixed.

The point is that we don't always know what our true limits are. However if your beliefs and attitudes, your thoughts and feelings are always producing reasons for not taking on new challenges, for not taking risks, for not exploring what might be possible for you at the limits of your understanding and your beliefs, for not looking at what the entire scope of a problem might be and at your relationship to it, then you may be severely and unnecessarily limiting your own learning, your own growth, and your ability to make changes in your life. Whether it is losing weight, or giving up cigarettes once and for all, or not yelling at your kids all the time, or going back to school, or starting your own business, or finding out what there is to live for when you have experienced a deep personal loss or are in the middle of a momentous change in your life that threatens your well-being and that of everything you hold dear, what you can do will very strongly depend on how you see things, on your beliefs about your own limits and resources, and on your beliefs about life itself. As we will see in Chapter 15, our beliefs and attitudes, our thoughts and emotions, can actually have a major influence on our health. In the stress clinic, most people rise to the challenge and take on the risks of facing the full catastrophe with mindfulness. And they often surprise themselves and their families with their newfound courage and clarity. In the process they discover their limits receding and they find themselves capable of doing things they never thought they could do, buoyed up by a new sense of wholeness and connectedness within themselves.

◆

Wholeness and connectedness are what are most fundamental in our nature as living beings. No matter how many scars we carry about from what we have gone through and suffered in the past, our intrinsic wholeness is still here: what else contains the scars? None of us has to be a helpless victim of what was done to us or what was not done for us in the past, nor do we have to be helpless in the face of what we may be suffering now. We are also what was present before the scarring, our original wholeness, what was born whole. And we can reconnect up with our intrinsic wholeness at any time because its very nature is that it is always present. So when we make contact with the domain of being in the meditation practice, we are already beyond the scarring, beyond the isolation and fragmentation and suffering we may be experiencing. This means that it will always be possible to transcend fragmentation, fear, vulnerability, and insecurity, even despair, if you come to see differently, to see with eyes of wholeness.

Perhaps more than anything else, the work in the stress clinic involves helping people to see and feel and believe in their wholeness, helping them to mend the wounds of disconnectedness and the pain of feeling isolated, fragmented, and separate, to discover an underlying fabric of wholeness and connectedness *within themselves*. Obviously this is the work of a lifetime. For our patients the stress clinic is often the first conscious, intentional step as an adult in this lifelong process.

Clearly the body is an ideal place to begin. In the first place, as we have seen, it is convenient. It is also a door to the larger world, in that what we see in the workings of our body teaches us many lessons that apply in other domains of our lives. What's more, our bodies usually require some healing. We all carry around at least some physical and psychological tension and armor. Our body has a lot to teach us about stress and pain, illness and health.

These are some of the reasons why we focus our attention on our breathing and why we start out in the clinic with two weeks of practicing the body scan every day. This is why we tune in to sensations in different regions of our body, why we cultivate a sense of our body as a whole, why we pay attention to such basics as eating, walking, moving, and stretching in the meditation practice. All these facets of our body's experience are doors through which at first we can catch glimpses of our own wholeness in any moment. In time and through daily practice we can walk through those doors more and more frequently. Through practice we can come to live in a more integrated way from day to day and from moment to moment, in touch with our own wholeness and connectedness and aware of our *interconnectedness* as well. Feeling whole, even for brief moments, nourishes us on a deep level. It is a source of healing and wisdom when faced with stress and pain.

◆

You probably won't be too surprised to learn that the very word *health* itself means "whole." *Whole* implies integration, an interconnectedness of all parts of a system or organism, a completeness. The nature of wholeness is that it is always present.

Someone who has had an arm amputated or has lost some other part of the body or who faces death from an incurable disease is still fundamentally whole. Yet he or she will have to *come to terms* with the physical loss or the meaning of the prognosis to experience that wholeness. This will certainly entail profound changes in one's view of oneself and of the world and of time, even of life itself. It is this process of coming to terms with things as they are that embodies the process of healing.

While every living organism is whole in itself, it is also embedded in a larger wholeness. We are whole in our bodies, but as we have already seen, our bodies are constantly exchanging matter and energy with the environment. So although our bodies are complete, they are also constantly changing. Our bodies are literally immersed in a larger whole, namely the environment, the planet, the universe. Looked at in this way, health is a dynamic process. It is not a fixed state that you "get" and then hold on to.

The notion of wholeness is found not only in the meaning of the words *health* and *healing* (and, of course, also in the word *holy*); we also find it embedded in the deep meaning of the words *meditation* and *medicine*, words that are obviously related to each other in some way. According to David Bohm, a theoretical physicist whose work involves exploring wholeness as a fundamental property of nature, the words *medicine* and *meditation* come from the Latin *mederi*, which means "to cure." *Mederi* itself derives from an earlier Indo-European root meaning "to measure."

Now what might the concept of measure have to do with either meditation or medicine? Nothing, if we are thinking of measure in the usual way, as the process of comparing the dimensions of an object to an external standard. But the concept of "measure" has another, more Platonic meaning. This is the notion that all things have, in Bohm's words, their own "right inward measure" that makes them what they are, that gives them their properties. "Medicine," seen in this light, is basically the means by which right inward measure is restored when it is disturbed by disease or illness or injury. "Meditation," by the same token, is the process of perceiving directly the right inward measure of one's own being through careful, non-judgmental self-observation. Right inward measure in this context is another way of saying wholeness. So it may not be as farfetched as it may first appear to have a clinic based on meditation in a medical center.

The choice of meditation training as the central and unifying practice in the stress clinic was not arbitrary. Meditation training has unique characteristics that distinguish it from the many relaxation and stress reduction techniques in common use. The most important is that it is a door into direct experiences of wholeness, experiences not so easily tapped and deepened by methods that focus on doing and getting somewhere rather than non-doing and being. Meditation is what is called a *consciousness discipline* by Dr. Roger Walsh, professor of psychiatry and behavioral sciences at the School of Medicine of the University of California at Irvine and a student of the interface between Eastern and Western psychologies. Dr. Walsh emphasizes that the consciousness disciplines are based on a profoundly different paradigm from that of mainstream Western psychology. From the perspective of the consciousness disciplines, our ordinary state of waking consciousness is severely *suboptimal*. Rather than contradicting the Western paradigm, it is rather an extension of it beyond Western psychology's dominant concern with pathology and with therapies aimed at restoring people to "normal" functioning in the usual waking state of consciousness. At the heart of this perspective lies the conviction that it is essential for a person to engage in a personal, intensive, and systematic training of the mind through the discipline of meditation practice to free him or herself from the incessant distortions characteristic of our everyday emotional and thought processes, distortions that, as we have seen, can continually undermine the experiencing of our intrinsic wholeness.

Many great minds have been preoccupied with the notion of wholeness and how to realize it in one's own life. Carl Jung, the great Swiss psychiatrist, held the meditative traditions of the Orient in very high regard in this connection. He wrote, "This question [coming to wholeness] has occupied the most adventurous minds of the East for more than two thousand years, and in this respect, methods and philosophical doctrines have been developed that simply put all Western attempts along these lines into the shade." Jung well understood the relationship between meditation practice and the realization of wholeness.

Albert Einstein also clearly articulated the importance of seeing with eyes of wholeness. At the end of the stress reduction program, we give our patients a booklet that closes with the following quotation from a letter of Einstein's that appeared in *The New York Times* on March 29, 1972. This statement is particularly meaningful, in part because it captures so well the spirit of the meditation practice and also because it was said by the scientist who, more than any other, revolutionized our concepts of physical reality and demonstrated the unity of space and time and of matter and energy.

When Einstein was living in Princeton, working at the Institute of Advanced Study, he used to receive letters from people from all over the world asking for his advice about their personal problems. He had a unique reputation for wisdom among laypeople throughout the world because of his scientific achievements, which few understood but most people knew were revolutionary. But he also had a profound reputation for compassion because of his kindly face and his outspoken involvement in humanitarian causes. He was thought of by many people as "the smartest man in the world," although he himself could never understand the big fuss made over him. The following passage comes from a letter he wrote in response to a rabbi who had written explaining that he had sought in vain to comfort his nineteen-year-old daughter over the death of her sister, a "sinless, beautiful, sixteen-year-old child." The letter to Einstein was clearly a cry for help, coming out of one of the most painful of human experiences, the death of a child. Einstein replied,

> A human being is a part of the whole, called by us "Universe," a part limited in time and space. He experiences himself, his thoughts and feelings as something separated from the rest—a kind of optical delusion of his consciousness. This delusion is a kind of prison for us, restricting us to our personal desires and to affection for a few persons nearest to us. Our task must be to free ourselves from this prison by widening our circle of compassion to embrace all living creatures and the whole nature in its beauty. Nobody is able to achieve this completely, but the striving for such achievement is in itself a part of the liberation, and a foundation for inner security.

In his reply Einstein is suggesting that we can easily become imprisoned in and blinded by our own thoughts and feelings because they are concerned solely with the particulars of our lives and our desires as separate beings. He is not belittling the suffering we experience at such a loss. But he is saying that our overwhelming preoccupation with our own separate lives ignores another, more fundamental level of reality. In his view we all come into and go out of this world as passing gatherings of structured energy. Einstein is reminding us to see wholeness as more fundamental than separateness. He is reminding us that our experience of ourselves as separate and enduring is a delusion, and ultimately, imprisoning.

Of course we *are* separate in the sense that our lives are localized in time (a lifetime) and space (a body). We *do* have particular thoughts and feelings and unique, wonderful, love-filled relationships, and we suffer greatly and understandably when those bonds and connections are broken, especially when death comes to the young. But at the same time, is it not equally true that we are all here and gone in an instant, little eddies or whirlpools in a flowing current, waves briefly rising on an ocean of wholeness? As eddies and waves, our lives do have a certain uniqueness, but they are also the stuff of a larger whole expressing itself in ways that ultimately surpass our comprehension.

Einstein is reminding us that when we neglect the perspective of wholeness and connectedness, we only see one side of being alive. This view inflates the sense of *my* life, *my* problems, *my* loss, *my* pain as what is supremely important and prevents us from seeing another, very real dimension of our own being that is not so separate or so unique. When we identify ourselves with a permanent, solid "self," it is a delusion of consciousness, a form of self-imprisonment, according to Einstein. Elsewhere he wrote that "the true value of a human being is determined primarily by the measure and sense in which he has attained liberation from the self."

Einstein's remedy for this dilemma of the delusion and tyranny of what we might call the small self, which he exemplified in large measure in his own life, is for us to break out of this "optical delusion" of consciousness by intentionally cultivating compassion for all life and an appreciation of ourselves and of "all living creatures" as part of the natural world in its beauty. In suggesting this as a way to freedom and inner security, Einstein was not merely speaking romantically or philosophically. He understood that it took a certain kind of *work* to achieve liberation from the prison of our own thought habits. He also knew that this work is intrinsically healing.

Coming back to the nine dots, we have seen that how we perceive a problem, and by extension how we perceive the world and also ourselves, can have a profound influence over what we are capable of doing. Seeing with eyes of wholeness means recognizing that nothing occurs in isolation, that problems need to be seen within the context of whole systems. Seeing in this way, we can perceive the intrinsic web of interconnectedness underlying our experience and merge with it. Seeing in this way is healing. It helps us to acknowledge the ways in which we are extraordinary and miraculous, without losing sight of the ways in which we are simultaneously nothing special, just part of a larger whole unfolding, waves on the sea, rising up and falling back in brief moments we call life spans.

13

On Healing

—

When we use the word *healing* to describe the experiences of people in the stress clinic, what we mean above all is that they are undergoing a profound transformation of view. This transformation is brought about by the encounter with one's own wholeness, catalyzed by the meditation practice. When we glimpse our own completeness in the stillness of any moment, when we directly experience ourself during the body scan or the sitting or while practicing the yoga as whole in that moment and also as part of a larger whole, a new and profound coming to terms with our problems and our suffering begins to take place. We begin to see both ourselves and our problems differently, namely from a perspective of wholeness. This transformation of view creates an entirely different context within which we can see and work with our problems, however serious they may be. It is a perceptual shift away from fragmentation and isolation toward wholeness and connectedness. With this change of perspective comes a shift from feeling out of control and beyond help (helpless and pessimistic) to a sense of the possible, a sense of acceptance and inner peace and control. Healing always involves an attitudinal and emotional transformation. Sometimes, but not always, it is also accompanied by a major reduction in physical symptoms and by improvement in a person's physical condition.

This transformation of view comes about in many different ways as people immerse themselves in mindfulness-meditation practice. In the stress clinic, sometimes people have sudden and dramatic experiences during meditation that lead them to new ways of seeing. More frequently people speak of moments of simply feeling deeply relaxed or confident. Many times they don't even recognize such experiences at the time they are happening as being particularly important, although they often can't remember having had such an experience before. These incremental transformations can be quite subtle. Yet they can be as profound or even more so than the more dramatic ones. Dramatic or subtle, such shifts in perspective are signs of seeing with eyes of wholeness. Out of this shift in perspective comes an ability to act with greater balance and inner security in the world, especially when encountering stress or pain.

◆

In the first week of the program Phil, a forty-seven-year-old French-Canadian truck driver who had injured his back three years previously in a lifting accident and who was referred to the stress clinic by his doctors in the pain clinic, had a breakthrough while practicing the body scan. He started out listening to the tape lying on his back. He was in a lot of pain and he said to himself, "Oh my god, I don't know if I can do this." But because he had made the commitment to "do it right" in spite of his pain, he stayed with the tape. After about twenty minutes he started feeling his breathing "all over his body" and he found himself completely focused on that extraordinary feeling of his body breathing. He said to himself, "Wow, you know, this is great!" Then he realized something else. He wasn't feeling any pain at all. Phil found that he was able to achieve this experience with the body scan each day that week. He came to the second class ecstatic.

The second week turned out to be just the opposite. Nothing he did worked. He practiced the body scan with the tape every day, and his pain was just as bad as ever. Nothing he did could bring back the feelings he had had the first week. I suggested that perhaps he was trying too hard to bring back his experiences of the first week. Perhaps he was fighting with his pain now, trying to get rid of it so that he could regain those good feelings. He went home determined to look into what I had suggested. He made up his mind that he would try just to let whatever was going to happen happen during the body scan and not try to get anywhere. After that things went more smoothly. He was able to concentrate and be calm during the body scan when he ceased fighting with his pain. He found that the pain would diminish as his concentration deepened. On the average, he said it would be about 40 to 50 percent less severe, sometimes even more by the end of the forty-five minutes.

◆

Joyce came to the stress clinic in 1980, referred by her oncologist, shortly after having been diagnosed and treated for a cancerous tumor on her leg. At the time she was fifty years old. Her husband had died from esophageal cancer two years earlier, a "horrendous and painful death," and on the day he died, her mother also died unexpectedly. Her own medical problems had started while she was taking care of her husband. With increasing frequency, she felt pain in her right thigh that would travel down her leg. She consulted several doctors, who said that it was nothing serious, either varicose veins or just part of getting older. One day, two years after the death of her husband and her mother, as she was picking out a Christmas tree with her son, her thighbone broke. When she was operated on, a tumor called a *plasmacytoma* was discovered that had eaten away the bone to the point where it had just crumbled. They removed the tumor and rebuilt the bone with a bone graft. During the surgery Joyce bled so much that the surgeon had told her children that he did not expect her to make it. But she did survive. She then underwent six weeks of radiation therapy and, soon after, came to the stress clinic.

When Joyce took the tape home from her first class, she said to herself that she was going to do everything that she was told to do in the course and that she was really going to get into it. The first time she did the body scan, she had what she described as "a very powerful experience of some otherness." This feeling came up toward the end of the tape, during a long stretch of silence. She remembers saying to herself at the time, "Oh, so this is what God is." In describing it, she said "it felt like a nothingness and an everything at the same time. It wasn't any kind of person or anything that I had ever thought of as God."

Joyce still remembers this feeling ten years later and says it is what kept her going through very difficult times, which have included multiple surgeries to repair her bone graft, a hip replacement, and severe family stresses. She is convinced that her meditation practice is responsible for keeping her plasmacytoma in remission for the past ten years, preventing it from progressing to become multiple myeloma, which it does in almost all cases over a five-year period. Her oncologist says that he has never seen another case in which a plasmacytoma did not cross over to become multiple myeloma in that period of time. He is not sure that it is Joyce's meditating that is responsible for her remission, but he admits that he doesn't have any idea why the disease has not progressed. Whatever the reason, he is happy about it and hopes things continue that way. So he supports Joyce in doing everything positive that she believes in to keep mind and body in harmony.

◆

Both Phil and Joyce had strong experiences with the body scan right off the bat. Others sometimes go for weeks before experiencing even a little relaxation or change in perspective. Yet we find that something positive is usually happening beneath the surface for most people as a result of practicing the body scan regularly in the first two weeks if we probe deeply enough, even if it is not so dramatic. Sometimes these stirrings don't manifest fully until the person switches over and starts doing the yoga. The change to a more active use of the body can trigger a change in perspective that has been slowly building below the person's level of awareness during weeks of working with the body scan.

Ultimately the process of healing will be different in its details for each individual. Healing is always a unique and deeply personal experience. Each of us, whether well or ill, has to face our own particular life circumstances and cope with them. The meditation practice, taken on in the spirit of self-exploration and self-inquiry, can transform our capacity to face, embrace, and work with and within the full catastrophe. But to make this transformation a reality in your life requires that you take responsibility for adapting the basic practice so that it becomes *yours,* so that you "own" it, so that it fits with *your* life and *your* needs! The particular choices you make will depend on your unique life circumstances and on your temperament.

Here is where your own imagination and creativity come in. As we have seen, meditation practice is, more than anything, a way of being. It is not a set of techniques for healing. Healing comes out of the practice itself when it is engaged in *as a way of being.* Meditation is much less likely to be healing if you are using it as a way of getting somewhere, even to wholeness. From this perspective, you already are whole, so what is the point of trying to become what you already are? What is required above all is that we *let go into* the domain of being. This is what is fundamentally healing.

◆

In the stress clinic we are constantly astonished at the ways in which our patients come to adapt the practice in their own lives and the effects that the practice comes to have on them. These effects are completely unpredictable. Most people come to the clinic because they want to learn to relax. But they often leave transformed beyond anything they had hoped to accomplish in the first place. For example, Hector was a wrestler from Puerto Rico who came with frequent angry outbursts and chest pain and left having found control over both and having discovered a deep strain of gentleness he never knew he had. Bill was a butcher who came years ago at the urging of his psychiatrist when he was left to father six children after his wife committed suicide; Bill became a vegetarian and told me recently, "Jon, the practice has deepened in me to the point that I can't even lie anymore"; he is now starting his own meditation-practice group. Edith learned the meditation in the pulmonary rehabilitation program in order to control her shortness of breath; she kept up the practice on her own, and proudly told me at a reunion several years later how she had used it during cataract surgery to successfully control pain when told by her doctors at the last minute that they couldn't use anesthesia because of her lung disease, and then proceeded to stick needles into her eye. Henry came with anxiety, heart disease, and high blood pressure, and in the fourth week of the program had an episode of vomiting blood due to ulcers. Taken to the ICU thinking he might very well die, Henry calmed himself down using his breathing as he lay in bed with tubes coming out of his arms and nose. Nat was a middle-aged businessman who was in an extreme state of distress due to a combination of severe high blood pressure, even on medication (he had been fired from his job two weeks earlier) and from having tested positive for the HIV virus after his wife contracted AIDS (presumably from a blood transfusion she received during an appendectomy) and died; he was in such bad shape that the nurse in the primary-care clinic personally marched him down to the stress clinic office to make sure he enrolled; eight weeks later Nat had his blood pressure back to normal, had gotten his bad temper under control, was relating much better with his only child, and was looking at his life optimistically in spite of his positive HIV test. Edward is a young man who has AIDS; he has not missed a day of meditation practice in six months now and finds he is no longer a "nervous wreck" at work; he thought to use his breathing to let go of his fear of the pain when he had another bone marrow test and found that he didn't feel any pain. None of these "results" was predictable. But they all grew directly out of the meditation practice.

Of course part of making the practice your own, as we will see farther on, will include paying attention to the particulars in your life that may directly or indirectly influence your health, such as diet; exercise; negative health habits including smoking, and alcohol and drug abuse; negative attitudes, especially hostility and cynicism; and the unique constellation of stresses and difficulties you face. Cultivating mindfulness in these areas enhances the process of personal transformation that grows out of dwelling regularly in the domain of being.

◆

Healing, as we are using the word here, does not mean "curing," although the two words are often used interchangeably. As we shall see in the next chapter, there are few if any outright *cures* for chronic diseases or for stress-related disorders. While it may not be possible for us to *cure* ourselves or to find someone who can, it is possible for us to *heal* ourselves. Healing implies the possibility for us to relate differently to illness, disability, even death as we learn to see with eyes of wholeness. As we have seen, this comes from practicing such basic skills as going into and dwelling in states of deep physiological relaxation and seeing and transcending our fears and our boundaries of body and mind. In moments of stillness you come to realize that you are already whole, already complete in your being, even if your body has cancer or heart disease or AIDS or pain, even if you don't know how long you will live or what will happen to you.

Experiences of wholeness are as accessible to people with chronic illness or stress-related problems as they are to anyone else. Moments of experiencing wholeness, moments when you connect with the domain of your own being, often include a palpable sense of being larger than your illness or your problems and in a much better position to come to terms with them. Thus to think that you are a "failure" if you "still" have pain or heart disease or cancer or AIDS after you have been meditating for a while is to completely misunderstand the practice of mindfulness. *We are not meditating to make anything go away.* Whether we are basically healthy at the moment or have a terminal illness, none of us knows how long we have to live. Life only unfolds in moments. The healing power of mindfulness lies in living each one as fully as we can.

One woman who had breast cancer had the insight while she was meditating one day that *she* was not her cancer. She saw vividly in one moment that she was a whole person and that the cancer was a process that was going on within her body. Prior to that her life had been consumed with identification with the disease and with being a "cancer patient." Realizing that she was not her cancer made her feel freer. She was able to think more clearly about her life and decided that she could use having cancer as an opportunity to grow and to live more fully, for however long she had to live. In making the commitment to live each moment of her life as fully as possible and to use her cancer to help her rather than to shower blame on herself for having it, she was setting the stage for healing, for the dissolving of boundaries, for coming to terms with things as they are. She understood that although she had hope that this approach might influence the cancer itself, there was no guarantee that the tumor would shrink or that she would live any longer. Her commitment to live with greater awareness was not chosen for those reasons. It was chosen because she wished to live life as fully as possible no matter what. At the same time she wanted to remain open to the possibility that the course of the disease might be positively influenced by her total state of mind-body integration.

◆

There is mounting evidence that this might be possible. A whole new field has emerged in the past ten years, known as *psychoneuroimmunology,* or PNI, beautifully described for the layperson in the book *The Healer Within* by Dr. Steven Locke of the Harvard Medical School, and Douglas Colligan. Simply put, studies in this new field are showing that our body's many exquisite cellular and molecular defense mechanisms against infection and disease, known collectively as the immune system, do not operate in a vacuum to keep us healthy. As the term *psychoneuroimmunology* suggests, the immune system is now known to be regulated in part at least by the nervous system, which integrates all the organ systems of the body so that we can function harmoniously as a unified organism. And of course, the nervous system makes the life of the mind possible. So there appear to be important interconnections, as yet only poorly understood, between the brain and the immune system. This means that science now has at least a plausible working model to explain how our thoughts and emotions and life experiences might, under some circumstances, influence our susceptibility or resistance to disease.

Numerous recent studies have shown that stressful life experiences can influence immune system activity. Drs. Janice Kielcot-Glaser and Ron Glaser of Ohio State University College of Medicine and their colleagues showed that the natural killer (NK) cell activity of medical students went down and then back up as a function of how much pressure they were under. During exams, NK activity and other immune functions were diminished compared to their levels during periods when they did not have examinations. These researchers and others have also shown that loneliness, separation, and divorce are sometimes associated with reduced immune functions and that the practice of relaxation techniques can have enhancing effects. Some of the immune functions measured in studies of this kind (such as natural killer cell activity) are thought to play an important role in the body's defense mechanisms against cancer and viral infections.

A remarkable series of experiments conducted by Drs. Robert Ader and Nicholas Cohen at Rochester University Medical School, starting in the mid 1970s, contributed profoundly to the explosion of research and interest in PNI. They uncovered a dramatic relationship between the brain and the immune system. They showed that immunosuppression (a lowering of the immune response) in rats could actually be *conditioned* by pairing treatment of the animals with a drug having the property of reducing immune system functions (called an immunosuppressant) with exposure to a sweet-tasting chemical (saccharin) in their drinking water. After receiving this combination of an immunosuppressant injection and saccharin in their water, when saccharin alone was readministered in their drinking water at a later time, these animals once again showed immunosuppression, this time *without the immunosuppressing drug*. It appeared that their bodies had somehow *learned* to suppress immune functioning in response to tasting the saccharin when it had been given with the immunosuppressing drug. Control animals did not show this conditioned response. This suggested that in the conditioned animals, their immune functioning was affected by a kind of psychological learning, which could only have come through the nervous system.

Many experiments have now been conducted which suggest that experiences of uncontrollable stress in animals produce deficits in immune function and decrease natural resistance to cancers and tumor growth. Recent studies with people are also showing intriguing connections between stress, feelings of helplessness, immune system deficits, and diseases such as cancer. Ultimately, a major question for future research is the extent to which the mind might influence the *healing* of specific diseases, not simply indirectly by changing life-style, important as such changes are, but also by directly influencing the functioning of the immune system. However, according to Dr. Ader, at present there is no firm evidence that the changes observed in immune functioning in any of the studies on people that have been conducted to date are related to an increase or decrease in a specific disease process. So caution needs to be exercised in jumping to conclusions about the ultimate meaning of the changes now being measured. It will be interesting to see what future research in this rapidly growing field uncovers.

At the University of Massachusetts Medical School we have been conducting an experiment to look at the question of whether the mind can be shown to have a direct effect on a well-recognized healing end point. In collaboration with Dr. Jeffrey Bernhard and his colleagues in the division of dermatology, and Dr. Jean Kristeller of behavioral medicine, we are studying people who have the skin disease known as psoriasis. People who have psoriasis suffer from an increased rate of growth of their skin cells that produce scaly patches. The extent of the disease fluctuates and is thought to be related to emotional stress as well as to other factors.

The standard therapy for psoriasis is ultraviolet light treatment, known as *phototherapy*. Ultraviolet light is used because it slows down the growth of the cells in the scaly patches of skin. Treatment requires the patient to stand naked in a round light box, much like a telephone booth, the walls of which have head-to-toe ultraviolet light bulbs, for increasing periods of time. Treatments are usually three times a week. It can take quite a few treatments for the skin to clear completely.

In our study of this healing process, twenty-three people prescribed ultraviolet light treatments in the phototherapy clinic were randomly assigned to two groups. One group practiced mindfulness meditation, focusing on their breathing and body sensations while they were in the light booth. People in the other group received the standard light treatment without engaging in any particular mental training. As the treatment sessions got longer, the meditators also visualized that the ultraviolet light was slowing down the growth of their skin cells by "jamming" the machinery those cells depend on to divide.

What we found was that, over a 12-week treatment period the meditators' skin patches cleared up much more rapidly than the skin patches of the people who were not meditating, even though both groups were receiving the same standard phototherapy treatment. Of the thirteen people in the meditation group, ten had clear skin by the end of forty sessions while the skin of only two people out of the ten receiving phototherapy by itself had cleared in the same period of time. While this experiment is just preliminary, it suggests that something that the meditators were doing was affecting their rate of healing above and beyond the effect of the light itself. This experiment needs to be repeated and similar ones conducted before we can say with certainty that it is an example of a direct effect of the mind on healing. At present it is an intriguing and promising finding.

◆

Psychoneuroimmunology has received widespread coverage in the popular press. Having heard about thc various experimental results of research studies, many people with cancer or AIDS now want to learn meditation to control their stress, with the expectation that by doing so they will be able to stimulate their immune system to combat their disease more effectively. But while it is entirely possible that practicing meditation and specific visualizations might significantly influence immune function, as we have noted, that conjecture is far from proven at this time.

From our point of view, an individual who comes to the stress clinic with the strong expectation that his or her immune system can be strengthened by meditating might actually be creating impediments to his or her own healing. Too strong an investment in making your immune system respond the way you want it to might be more of a problem than a help because the quality and the spirit of the meditation practice can be easily undermined by *any* goal orientation. If the essence of meditation is non-doing, then trying to work it around to getting what you want can distort and undermine those very qualities of letting go and acceptance that allow you to experience wholeness, in our view the foundation for healing. This would be true even if it is ultimately shown that meditation can lead to positive changes in immune function that result in an increased ability of the body to heal disease processes.

This is not to say that you cannot use meditation for specific ends. There are countless ways of incorporating specific visualizations and goals into meditation practice, as in the use of the mountain meditation described in Chapter 9, in the psoriasis experiment just mentioned, and in the lovingkindness meditation we will discuss shortly. In all the meditative traditions of the world, visualizations and imagery are used to invoke particular states of mind. There are meditations on love, God, lovingkindness, peace, forgiveness, selflessness, impermanence, and suffering. There are meditations on energy, body states, particular emotions, compassion, generosity, wisdom, death, and of course healing. Imagery and specific channeling of one's energy and attention are integral to these practices.

However, it is important to emphasize that they are all *practices*, engaged in with a systematic discipline and commitment, and always within the larger context of meditation *as a way of being*. When we take them up as isolated techniques that we invoke only when we feel bad or when we want something, we invariably ignore or discard this greater context. In fact we may not even realize that it exists. In any event, the great wisdom and power inherent in the non-doing perspective can be easily lost or overlooked and, with it, the deeper power of the particular visualization. There is little wisdom in this approach, and potentially a great deal of frustration, disappointment, and wasted energy.

In order to be effective for healing, we believe that the use of visualization and imagery needs to be embedded in a larger context, one that understands and honors non-doing and non-striving. Otherwise, visualization exercises can too easily degenerate from meditation into wishful thinking, and the intrinsic healing power and wisdom of the simple mindfulness practice itself can remain untapped or be trivialized in the quest for something more elaborate and goal oriented. Even in the simple case of lowering blood pressure, which meditation has been shown to do in numerous clinical studies, it is not wise to meditate primarily for that purpose. It tends to make the meditation mechanical and too success and failure oriented. We believe that it is far more effective just to practice the meditation regularly and let your blood pressure take care of itself.

When you are practicing meditation as a way of being and not as a means to a particular end, then the use of specific visualizations to work on particular areas of concern within that larger context can sometimes be very helpful. Not enough research has yet been done to be able to determine the relative importance of specific visualizations in the healing process compared with the simple practice of moment-to-moment awareness. The psoriasis experiment may lead to studies of this kind.

From our experiences in the clinic, we believe that symptom reduction and a transformation of perspective are more likely to occur if you actively cultivate non-doing in the meditation practice rather than preoccupy yourself with what your blood pressure, particular symptoms, or your immune system is doing.

We tell our patients in the stress clinic, whether they have high blood pressure or cancer or AIDS, that it is fine to come with the hope of controlling their blood pressure or improving their immune function, just as it is fine to come wanting to learn to relax and be calmer. But once they decide to take the program, they need to let go of their goals for the moment and just practice for its own sake. Then, if their blood pressure comes down or if their natural killer cells or helper T-cells increase in number and activity, or if their pain lessens, so much the better. We want our patients to experiment with what their bodies and minds are capable of without feeling they have to perform a specific physiologic task by a specific time. To bring calmness to the mind and body requires that at a certain point we be willing to let go of wanting anything at all to happen and just accept things as they are and ourselves as we are with an open, receptive heart. This inner peace and acceptance lie at the heart of both health and wisdom.

◆

Ideally hospitals should be environments in which there is an appreciation and nourishing of a person's own inner capacity for healing as a complement to the medical management of his or her problems. Many doctors and nurses honor this domain and try to work within it as best they can, given the less-than-ideal conditions in which they often work and in which the patients find themselves.

To provide a resource for the individual patient to participate more directly in his or her own healing while in the hospital, and to give physicians and nurses a resource that they could offer to their patients, the stress clinic developed a television "outreach" program to teach hospitalized patients how to meditate. Our hope was that inpatients lying in bed would be able to engage in a similar kind of work on themselves as do the people who come to the stress clinic as outpatients.

Ordinarily, television functions to carry us away from ourselves and away from the moment, in ways that are discussed in Chapter 32. We attempted to use the medium in a new way, which you might think of as interactive television.

Many patients have their televisions on most of the time while they are in the hospital. When I visit people on the wards, usually there is a game show on or the news, a soap opera, or a movie. Often the person isn't even watching. Nonetheless, the TV is on. This is hardly conducive to relaxation and healing. Silence would be better, especially if people knew what to do with it, knew *how* to be in silence, *how* to concentrate their energies for being in the moment and for dwelling in calmness and stillness.

If you are hospitalized in a room with another person, you might have to put up with whatever is on your roommate's set, even if your own is off. For people in pain, or who are dying or who are in a crisis, it can be degrading and demoralizing to have to tolerate soap operas and game shows as the backdrop to their real-life problems. It is hardly a dignified atmosphere in which to die, or suffer and hardly the best conditions under which to try to recuperate.

The idea of our TV program, which we call *The World of Relaxation*, is to reach out to the patient from the television up on the wall and say, "Look, as long as you are lying here in the hospital with time on your hands, perhaps you might be interested in using some of this time to learn how to go into and dwell in deep states of relaxation. This might at least give you a feeling of being able to control and reduce some of the stress, pain, and anxiety that you might be experiencing; and what is more, it might also enhance the healing process itself."

The World of Relaxation is an unusual use of television. Visually it is simply my face on the screen for an hour—not exactly high drama or entertainment. Even worse, after a brief introduction I ask the viewer to close his or her eyes, and then I close my eyes too. So for most of the hour the picture is just my face on the screen with my eyes closed. I am meditating and guiding the listener in an extended healing-oriented meditation that includes mindfulness of breathing, a modified body scan, and directing the breath to the regions the patient feels require the most attention. The verbal guidance is entwined with soothing harp music composed and played by Georgia Kelly, a musician and composer committed to using music and sound for healing.

You might ask, "Why a television program at all if the patient has his or her eyes closed for most of it?" The answer is, "Because the image of another person is there, and that itself may contribute to a feeling of trust and acceptance on the part of the patient." If the person gets disoriented or bored, he or she can always open his or her eyes and see someone up on the screen and perhaps be reassured that it is possible to become calm and focused and so be encouraged to return to his or her breath once again, to the present moment, and to the sounds of the music.

We encourage people to tune in and out of what is being said as they feel like it and to just flow with the sounds of the harp, an instrument that has been associated with healing since biblical times. The notes of the harp in this piece of music sound as if they are coming out of nowhere and going back into nowhere. They have a timeless quality, rather than giving a feeling of going somewhere. The music provides an effective background for meditation practice, especially for someone attempting it for the very first time, mirroring as it does the way in which thoughts and feelings and perceptions also appear to rise out of nowhere and dissolve back into nowhere, moment by moment.

The World of Relaxation plays on the in-house cable channel in our hospital seven times each twenty-four hours. Doctors can "prescribe" it for their patients to help them with pain, anxiety, or sleep problems or to enhance relaxation and well-being and reduce the stress of hospitalization. To do this, they give their patients a little flyer with the times when the program is on and a few suggestions for how to use it and suggest they "do" it twice a day during their hospital stay. In our view, regular meditation practice using this program is a far better diet for patients in the hospital than the usual fare they are served up on TV. We hear numerous reports from the patients who discover it that bear this out. The program has now been purchased by over a hundred hospitals in the United States and Canada and, hopefully, these hospitals are also using it on their in-house patient television channels.

I was recently contacted by a woman who used *The World of Relaxation* when she was a patient at New York University Medical Center. We had a long talk, during which I asked if she would be willing to write down the circumstances under which she used it. This is how she described her experience:

October 31, 1988

Dear Dr. Kabat-Zinn:

"There is more right with you than wrong with you"—those words of yours have stayed with me through two frightening

cancer surgeries. So many other comforting thoughts that you offer on your video have helped me keep my sanity.

At night, when alone after my visitors were gone, I couldn't wait to turn on the NYU Medical Center in-house channel because, somehow, I became dependent on the comfort you would offer. I can still see your face before me, almost as though my experience was a personal one. You offer a meaningful philosophy that puts everything into perspective for a frightened human being. Thank you so much for that. I tried so hard to remember how to practice the relaxation technique, but I still need the help that the tape provides.

So many other patients during my hospital stay were taking comfort from your voice. When I took my required walks along the hospital corridor, I could hear the tape coming out of different rooms. Whenever I had the chance to talk to a patient who was suffering, I told them to put the tape on and was thanked. (My first hospital stay was for twenty-three days. I had lots of time to meet others.)

I am still hurting from my most recent surgery, and I am still scared, but I have so many good, in fact wonderful, moments because of your help. I am really very grateful.

LOVINGKINDNESS MEDITATION

Healing energy can be directed toward others and toward your relationships as well as toward your own body. This is a very effective way of healing yourself, because the process of generating strong feelings of empathy, compassion, and love toward others has its own purifying effect on the mind. When such strong positive feelings are invoked in a mind that has become relatively calm and stable through intensive meditation practice, these feelings can then be effectively directed toward others.

We do a lovingkindness meditation in the all-day session to give people a taste of the power a concentrated and calm mind can generate when evoking feelings of kindness, generosity, goodwill, love, and forgiveness. The response is invariably moving; a great many tears are shed, both in joy and in sorrow. This type of meditation strikes a deep chord in many people. It can help us to cultivate strong positive emotions within ourselves, and to let go of ill will and resentment. Some of the feelings of the participants in the all-day session about this form of meditation have already been voiced in Chapter 8.

To practice lovingkindness meditation, we begin by stabilizing the mind and calming it with mindfulness of breathing. Then we consciously invoke feelings of love and kindness *toward ourselves*, perhaps by saying inwardly to ourselves "May I be free from anger, may I be free from hatred; may I be filled with compassion, may I feel kindness toward myself."

Then we can go on to invoke someone else, perhaps a particular person we care about. We can visualize that person in our mind's eye or hold the feeling of the person in our heart as we wish that person well: "May he or she be happy, may he (she) be free from pain and suffering, may he (she) experience love and joy." We may then include others we know and love: parents, children, friends.

Then we identify a person we may have a particularly difficult time with, perhaps someone we do *not* like to feel sympathy for. We intentionally cultivate feelings of kindness, generosity, and compassion toward this person, letting go of our feelings of resentment and dislike for that person and reminding ourself instead to see that person as a whole being, as deserving of love and kindness, as having feelings, as someone who feels pain and anxiety, someone who is suffering. If that person has caused us harm, we purposefully forgive him or her in our heart, letting go of our own anger and resentment and hurt, letting go of our feelings of righteousness, of our justifications for our lack of empathy. We also ask that that person forgive us if we have caused him or her hurt, knowingly or unknowingly. This can be done with people whether they are alive or have already died, and there can be a strong release of long-carried negative emotions as you ask for forgiveness and forgive them. It is a profound process of coming to terms in your own heart and mind with the way things are in this moment, a deep letting go of past feelings and hurt.

We can continue to direct lovingkindness to others, perhaps those who we feel may be in need of positive energy, who are not as fortunate as we are. Then we can expand our scope still further, radiating our feelings of lovingkindness to all people who are suffering, oppressed, in need of kindness and caring. The meditation can be carried even further, expanding the field of lovingkindness out from our own heart in all directions until it includes all life on the planet, not just people, and the living planet itself if we like.

Finally we return to our own body, we come back to the breathing, and end cradling our feelings of warmth and generosity and love for all beings in our own hearts.

I always thought this was a little strange and contrived until I saw the power it had. When practiced regularly, lovingkindness meditation has a softening effect on the heart. It can help you to be kinder to yourself and to others in your own mind, to see all beings as deserving of kindness and compassion, so that, even if disputes do arise, your mind can see clearly and your heart does not close down and become lost in self-serving yet ultimately self-destructive negative feeling states.

◆

In summary, healing is a transformation of view rather than a cure. It involves recognizing your intrinsic wholeness and, simultaneously, your connectedness to everything else. Above all it involves coming to feel at peace within yourself. As we have seen and will see even more in further sections, this can lead to dramatic improvements in symptoms and a renewed ability to move toward greater health and well-being.

14

Doctors, Patients, and People: Moving Toward a Unified Perspective on Health and Illness

This is an exciting time in the history of medicine and the medical sciences. More is known about the details of the structure and functioning of living organisms on every level than ever before. Biological research is being carried out at a feverish pace, and more is being learned every day. Since 1944, the year that DNA was shown to be the genetic material, molecular biology has completely revolutionized the practice of medicine, providing it with a comprehensive scientific foundation that has proved to be enormously successful in many areas and continues to hold great promise for future breakthroughs.

We now know something about the genetic and molecular basis of a number of diseases. We also have an elaborate and continually growing array of drugs for controlling many infectious diseases and for regulating many of the physiological responses of the body when they get out of control. We know that our cells harbor certain genes—known as proto-oncogenes—that control normal functions within cells but when altered by a mutational event can lead to tumor growth. We know a great deal more about the prevention and treatment of heart disease than was known even ten years ago. If caught in time, a person having a heart attack, or who has just had one, can now have a specific enzyme (TPA or streptokinase) injected into the bloodstream that will dissolve the culprit blood clot in one of the coronary arteries and greatly reduce damage to the heart muscle.

185

The past twenty years have seen the development of sophisticated computer-controlled diagnostic technology, including sonography, CAT scanning, PET scanning, and MRI scans, which allows doctors to look inside the body in various ways and determine how it is functioning under various circumstances.

Comparable advances have been made in surgical procedures. Lasers are routinely used to do fine repair on detached retinas and to preserve vision; artificial hip and knee joints have been developed that can restore the ability to walk without pain to many people suffering from severe arthritis; cardiac bypass surgery, even organ transplants, have become common occurrences.

However, while more is known about disease than ever before and while we have improved ways of diagnosing and treating many diseases, far more still remains unknown. Modern medicine is nowhere near putting itself out of business by eradicating or even controlling disease. In spite of the rapid progress in genetics, molecular and cell biology, and neurophysiology, our understanding of the biology of living organisms, even the simplest ones, is still rudimentary. And when it comes down to medicine's ability to treat certain diseases and the people who have them, we discover very real limits and major areas of ignorance.

We naturally put enormous faith in modern medicine because of its spectacular successes. But at the same time we are often surprisingly uninformed of what medicine does not know and what it cannot do. Sometimes we don't discover the very real limits of medicine until it is our own body that is in pain or diseased, or that of someone we love. Then we can become severely disillusioned, frustrated, and even angry at the discrepancy between our expectations of what medicine can do and the reality.

It is hardly fair to fault an individual doctor for the limits of medical knowledge. When you come right down to it, there are few medical cures at present or on the horizon for the chronic diseases and other chronic conditions (such as many forms of pain), although they are a major cause of suffering, disability, and death in our society. It is far better to prevent them in the first place if possible than to have to be treated for them.

There are many diseases whose origins are completely mysterious or that are intimately linked to social factors such as poverty and social exploitation, dangerous working conditions, stressful and poisonous environmental conditions, and culturally entrenched habits, all of which are outside the direct influence of medicine and science as they are presently organized.

Although a great deal is known about the molecular biology of certain cancers and there are effective treatments for some forms of cancer, many cancers are presently only very poorly understood and effective treatments do not exist. Yet even in such cases there are always some people who survive much longer than expected. In some instances tumors have been known to regress or disappear altogether, even without medical treatment. Medicine knows almost nothing about why this happens or how. Yet it is known to happen. This in itself can be a source of some hope for people when they have exhausted the options available in traditional medicine.

Most doctors acknowledge the role of the mind and social factors in healing. Often they refer to it as "the will to live." Many have observed it firsthand in their patients. Yet no one understands it. It tends to be invoked in a hand-waving, mystical sort of way, usually only after all the medical options have been exhausted. It is a way of saying, "There is nothing more we can do, but I know that it is still possible for miracles to happen, miracles that traditional medicine just doesn't have explanations for or know how to conjure up for people."

If a person believes she or he is going to die and loses hope, this emotional capitulation can itself tilt the system against recovery. Personal motivations to live are known to sometimes influence survival. Emotional disposition and support from family and friends can make a big difference in how people do in the face of serious illness.

Yet until recently doctors did not receive much, if any, training in how to help patients make use of their own inner resources for healing, or even how to recognize when they themselves might be unwittingly undermining those very resources that are the patient's best allies in the healing process.

Too often the scientific and technological sophistication of the traditional medical approach to disease leads in its practice to an impersonal approach to the patient, as if medicine's knowledge is so powerful that the patient's understanding, cooperation, and collaboration in treatment are of minor value. When this attitude is displayed by a physician in his or her relationship to a patient, when the patient is made to feel, either through omission or commission, inadequate or ignorant or in some way to blame, either for his condition or for his lack of response to the treatment, or when the person's feelings are simply ignored, these are instances of inadequate medical care.

A cardinal aphorism of traditional medicine has always been

that "care of the patient requires caring for the patient." This aphorism needs to be more actively kept in mind by health professionals. In an optimal encounter between patient and physician, each has a vital area of expertise, and both areas are important to the healing process, which starts in the initial encounter, even before diagnosis. The dignity of the patient needs to be honored and preserved throughout the entire sequence of medical encounters, whether they lead to a "successful" outcome or not.

It is not uncommon for doctors who become ill to discover for the first time in their lives the little and not-so-little insensitivities in the health care system that rob people of their dignity and sense of control. At such times they may be more likely to see, as they make the transition from "doctor" to "patient," that the latter role puts you at immediate risk for shame, loss of control, and reduced dignity, even though you are the same person you were before the role change. If this is true for physicians, who understand the process much better than most people, it is not hard to understand how alienating the health care system can be for people who have no background or understanding to help them sort out what they are going through.

When we become ill and seek medical care and take on the role of "patient," we are usually in a particularly vulnerable psychological state because we are naturally concerned about the larger implications of our illness. We are also for the most part in a position of substantial ignorance and little authority compared with our doctors, even though it is our body that is the subject of all the attention. In this situation we may be unusually sensitive to the messages, both verbal and nonverbal, that we get from our doctors. These messages can either augment the healing process in us or subvert it altogether if our doctor is insensitive to his or her own behaviors and the effects they can have on his or her patients.

A story told by Bernard Lown, a renowned cardiologist, about an incident he observed while he was in training, illustrates this powerfully:

The experience still provokes in me a shudder of disbelief. Some thirty years ago I had a postdoctorate fellowship with Dr. S. A. Levine, professor of cardiology at the Harvard Medical School and at the Peter Bent Brigham Hospital. He was a keen observer of the human scene, had an awesome presence, was precise in formulation, and was blessed with a prodigious memory. He was, in effect, the consummate clinician at the bedside. Dr.

Levine conducted a weekly outpatient cardiac clinic at the hospital. After we young trainees examined the patient, he would drop in briefly to assess our findings and suggest further diagnostic workup or changes in the therapeutic program. With patients, he was invariably reassuring and convincing, and they venerated his every word. In one of my first clinics, I had as a patient Mrs. S., a well-preserved middle-aged librarian who had a narrowing of one of the valves on the right side of her heart, the tricuspid valve. She had been in low-grade congestive heart failure with modest edema [swelling] of the ankles, but was able to maintain her job and attend efficiently to household chores. She was receiving digitalis and weekly injections of a mercurial diuretic. Dr. Levine, who had followed her in the clinic for more than a decade, greeted Mrs. S. warmly and then turned to the large entourage of visiting physicians and said, "This women has TS," and abruptly left.

No sooner was Dr. Levine out of the door than Mrs. S.'s demeanor abruptly changed. She appeared anxious and frightened and was now breathing rapidly, clearly hyperventilating. Her skin was drenched with perspiration, and her pulse had accelerated to more than 150 a minute. In reexamining her, I found it astonishing that the lungs, which a few minutes earlier had been quite clear, now had moist crackles at the bases. This was extraordinary, for with obstruction of the right heart valve, the lungs are spared the accumulation of excess fluid.

I questioned Mrs. S. as to the reasons for her sudden upset. Her response was that Dr. Levine had said that she had TS, which she knew meant "terminal situation." I was initially amused at this misinterpretation of the medical acronym for "tricuspid stenosis." My amusement, however, rapidly yielded to apprehension, as my words failed to reassure and as her congestion continued to worsen. Shortly thereafter she was in massive pulmonary edema. Heroic measures did not reverse the frothing congestion. I tried to reach Dr. Levine, but he was nowhere to be located. Later that same day she died from intractable heart failure. To this day the recollection of this tragic happening causes me to tremble at the awesome power of the physician's word.

In this story we get to see the microanatomy of a dramatic and very rapid mind-body interaction resulting, almost unbelievably, directly in death. We witness through Dr. Lown's eyes the appearance of a particular thought in the mind of the patient, triggered by the unexplained use of a technical term by her doctor, for whom she had the highest regard. The thought that her situation was terminal, although completely untrue, *was believed by her to be true*. It set off an immediate psychophysiological reaction. Her belief in that thought was so firmly entrenched that she was completely closed off even to authoritative reassurances from another doctor that it was in fact a misunderstanding. By that point her mind was in a state of turbulence, clearly overwhelmed by anxiety and fear. Apparently her emotional state overwhelmed her body's regulatory mechanisms that normally maintain physiological balance. As a result her body went into a severe stress reaction from which neither she nor her doctors were able to extricate her. Not even the heroic life-support and rescue measures of one of the best hospitals in the world could save her once this chain of events was unleashed, even though it had been triggered by a seemingly innocent, if insensitively delivered remark.

Dr. Lown's story graphically illustrates the enormous power that strongly held beliefs, which are in actuality just thoughts, can have on our health. Had this woman been a little less reactive, a little more willing to look at this suddenly acquired belief as a thought that might require some clarification or that might be inaccurate, had she been able to let go of her thought at least enough to entertain the notion that what Dr. Lown was telling her might be true, she might have lived. Unfortunately she did not have that flexibility of mind at the time. Perhaps she believed too strongly in her doctor and not enough in herself. In any event we can clearly see, through Dr. Lown's account, that an emotional reaction to a misunderstood comment by her doctor was the direct cause of her death.

Had her doctor left her bedside a little less abruptly and had he observed the effect of his words on her, as Dr. Lown had no trouble doing, he would have noticed that she was distressed. Had he noted and inquired into her immediate anxiety reaction, he might have been able to allay her fears on the spot and prevent this entire sequence of events.

Although death under such circumstances is a rare occurrence in medical practice, the pain and humiliation that patients experience at the hands of the health care system, sadly, is not. Much of it could be easily avoided if physicians were trained to value making observations of a psychological and social nature in addition to attending to the physical aspects of patient care.

Dr. George Engel, professor emeritus at the University of Rochester Medical School, has long advocated training doctors to value observing their patients with the same scientific care and rigor that they bring to their consideration of their patients' lab reports and X rays. Dr. Engel is a major voice articulating an expanded model for the practice of medicine, a model that takes into account the importance of psychological and social factors in health and disease and that takes a systems perspective (see Chapter 12) on health and illness and the patient as a whole person. Dr. Engel's model is known as the *biopsychosocial model*. Elaborated over ten years ago, it is influencing a whole generation of young doctors, who are being trained to go beyond the limits of the traditional medical model in the way they practice medicine.

Until Dr. Engel's model was put forth, the effect of psychological factors on physical illness was not addressed in a major way in the curriculum of modern medical education, although it had been recognized since the days of Hippocrates that the mind plays a major and sometimes primary role in disease and health. The virtual exclusion of the domain of the mind from the major currents in medical education was due mainly to the fact that, since the time of Descartes in the seventeenth century, Western scientific thinking has divided the intrinsic wholeness of being into separate, essentially noninteracting domains of *soma* (body) and *psyche* (mind). While these are convenient categories for facilitating understanding on one level, the tendency has been to forget that mind and body are separate in thought only. This dualistic way of thinking and seeing has so permeated Western culture that it had closed off the entire realm of mind-body interactions in health as a legitimate domain of scientific inquiry. Only very recently has this begun to change, as the major weaknesses of this dualistic paradigm have become apparent.

One notable weakness was the failure of the standard medical model to explain why some people get sick and others do not, given the same exposure to disease agents and environmental conditions. While genetic variability might account for some differences in resistance to illness, other factors seemed to play a role as well. The biopsychosocial model proposed that psychological and social factors could either protect a person from illness or increase his or her susceptibility to it. Such factors include a person's beliefs and attitudes, how supported and loved a person feels by family and friends, the psychological and environmental stresses to which one is exposed, and personal health behaviors. The discovery that the immune system can be influenced by psychological factors bolstered the biopsychosocial model by providing one plausible biological pathway for explaining such mind-body interactions.

Another important element pointing toward the need to include a role for the mind in a more accurate model of health and illness was the *placebo effect*, a very well known phenomenon for which the standard biomedical model has no explanation. Numerous studies have shown that when people believe that they are taking a drug of a particular potency, they show significant clinical effects typical of the drug in question, even when they did not actually get the drug but only a sugar pill, known as a *placebo*. Sometimes the magnitude of the placebo effect comes close to the magnitude of the drug itself. This phenomenon can only be explained by assuming that the *suggestion* that you are taking a powerful drug in some way influences the nervous system to create conditions in the body similar to those produced on a molecular level by the presence of the drug. It suggests that, by whatever mechanism, a person's beliefs can either change his or her biochemistry or functionally mimic a change in biochemistry. The power of suggestion lies at the root of the phenomenon of hypnosis, which has long been known to be able to dramatically affect many different human activities, including pain perception and memory. Of course the standard medical model has no place for hypnotic phenomena either.

Another influence in the movement toward an expanded perspective on health and illness came through the acceptance of acupuncture in the West. The most dramatic moment came when James Reston of *The New York Times*, while in China, suffered a ruptured appendix and underwent an operation with only acupuncture for anesthesia. Since acupuncture is based on a five-thousand-year-old classical Chinese model of health and disease, and treatment consists of stimulating energy pathways, called *meridians*, that have no anatomical basis in Western medical thought, the mind-set in the West was expanded to at least entertain the notion that a different way of looking at the body might lead to effective diagnostic and treatment methods.

Studies by Dr. Herbert Benson of the Harvard Medical School in the early 1970s on people practicing a form of meditation known as Transcendental Meditation, or TM, demonstrated that meditation can produce a pattern of significant physiological changes, which he termed *the relaxation response*. These include a lowering of blood pressure, a reduced oxygen consumption, and an overall decrease in arousal. Dr. Benson proposed that the relaxation response was the physiological opposite of *hyperarousal*, the state we experience when we are stressed or threatened. He hypothesized that if the relaxation response were elicited regularly, it could have a positive influence on health and protect us from some of the more damaging effects of stress. Dr. Benson pointed out that all religious traditions have ways of eliciting this response and that there is a kind of wisdom associated with prayer and meditation that is relevant to the health of the body and deserving of further study.

In the late 1960s and the 1970s, a great deal of research in the field of biofeedback and self-regulation showed that human beings could learn to control many physiological functions that had previously been considered involuntary, such as heart rate, skin temperature, skin conductance, blood pressure, and brainwaves, when they were given feedback from a machine that told them how they were doing. This research was pioneered by Drs. Elmer and Alyce Green at the Menninger Foundation, Drs. David Shapiro and Gary Schwartz who were at Harvard at the time, Dr. Chandra Patel in England, and many others. Many of these biofeedback studies actually made use of relaxation, meditation, or yoga to help people to learn to control these bodily responses.

In 1977 a book appeared that brought together many of these various strands for the first time and made them accessible to the general public. Entitled *Mind as Healer, Mind as Slayer,* by Dr. Kenneth Pelletier, the book presented a wide range of compelling evidence that the mind was a major participant in illness and could be a major factor in health as well. It inspired widespread interest in mind-body interactions, giving voice to the many compelling reasons for taking responsibilty for one's own health rather than waiting for it to break down under stress and then counting on medical care to make things better. This book has since become a classic in the field.

Norman Cousins's writings have also contributed substantially to broad public interest in taking charge of one's own health, especially when it breaks down. Cousins's books recounting his own experiences with illness and his determination to take the primary responsibility for healing out of the hands of his doctors and into his own created much controversy and debate within the medical establishment. In *Anatomy of an Illness as Perceived by the Patient,* Cousins detailed his successful efforts to overcome a degenerative collagen disease using, among other things, large doses of self-prescribed laughter therapy. Laughter appears to be a profoundly healthful state of momentary body-mind integration and harmony. In Cousins's view cultivating strong positive emotional states through humor and not taking oneself so seriously, even in the face of life-threatening circumstances, are of major therapeutic value in the healing process. Certainly this is very much in the spirit of Zorba, who dances and sings in the face of the full catastrophe.

In *The Healing Heart* Cousins describes his experiences following a heart attack that occurred some years after his experience with the collagen disease. In both books he recounts how he approached these illnesses by analyzing current medical knowledge and its limits in terms of his particular problems and circumstances and then describes how he went on to chart his own intelligent and idiosyncratic course toward recovery, in close collaboration with his sometimes bemused doctors.

Because of his fame as the editor of the *Saturday Review* and his sophistication about medical matters, Cousins received very special treatment from his doctors. On the whole they were extraordinarily tolerant of his ideas and of his desire to be a full participant in all aspects of the decision-making process involving his medical treatment.

Not just Norman Cousins but *anybody* who wants to participate in the process of recovery from an illness in this way deserves this kind of "treatment partnership" with his or her doctors and with the health care system. To make this happen requires that we ask for information and explanations from our doctors and insist on being actively involved in the decisions concerning us. Many physicians welcome and encourage this kind of interaction with their patients. Cousins has inspired many people with illnesses, as well as many of those treating them, to view the patient's role as a participant as essential to the healing process. However, a lot of people tend to be intimidated by the authority of physicians. This is especially so when they are feeling vulnerable about their health and they themselves have little knowledge of medicine. If you feel this way, you may have to work extra hard at asserting yourself and at maintaining your own balance of mind and self-confidence when you find yourself in such situations. Directing mindfulness to your interactions with your doctors, both before you see them and during your encounters with them, can help you to formulate and ask the questions you want answers to and to advocate more effectively for yourself.

Another influence pushing medicine toward a new paradigm, if only indirectly, stems from the revolution in the science of physics that started around the turn of the century and is still continuing. The most rigorous of the physical sciences has had to come to terms with some fundamental discoveries that showed that, at the deepest and most fundamental level, the natural world is neither describable nor understandable in conventional terms. Our basic notions that things are *what* they are, that they are *where* they are, and that one set of conditions always causes the same thing to happen had to be completely revised to understand the world of the very small and the very fast. For instance it is now known that the subatomic particles (such as electrons, protons, and neutrons) that make up the atoms of which all substances, including our bodies, are composed have properties that appear sometimes wavelike and sometimes particlelike; furthermore, they cannot be said to have a particular energy at a particular time with complete certainty; and the connections between events on this level of physical reality are only describable by probability.

Physicists had to drastically expand their view of reality in order to describe what they found inside the atom. They coined the term *complementarity* to convey the idea that one "thing" (say, an electron) can have two totally different and seemingly contradictory sets of physical properties (i.e., appear as either a wave or a particle), depending on what method you use to look at it. They were obliged to invoke a principle of *uncertainty* as a fundamental law of nature to explain that one can know either the position of a subatomic particle or its momentum, but not both at the same time. And they had to develop the idea of a *quantum field*, which posits that matter cannot be separated from the space surrounding it, that is, that particles are simply "condensations" of a continuous field that exists everywhere. In this world description it may not be meaningful to ask what "causes" the appearance or disappearance of matter out of the void, although this is known to occur. These new descriptions of reality, of the internal structure of the very atoms that make up our own bodies and the world, are so far from our ordinary mode of thinking that they require a major shift in our thinking.

These revolutionary concepts, which physicists have been grappling with for the past ninety years, have gradually filtered down in the intellectual culture, prompting people to think more in terms of complementary ways of knowing in general. This means that it is now more acceptable to posit, for instance, that while science and medicine have a *particular description* of health, *this description may not be the only possible valid one*. The notion of complementarity reminds us that all systems of knowledge may be incomplete and need to be seen as aspects of a larger whole that lies beyond all the models and theories that attempt to describe it. Far from invalidating knowledge in a particular realm, complementarity merely points to the fact that knowledge is limited and needs to be used within the domains where its descriptions are valid and relevant.

One doctor's ideas about the implications that this new way of thinking in physics might have on medicine are presented in *Space, Time and Medicine,* by Larry Dossey. Dr. Dossey takes the position that "our ordinary view of life, death, health and disease rests solidly on seventeeth-century physics, and if this physics has been scuttled in favor of a more accurate description of nature, an inescapable question occurs: must not our definitions of life, death, health, and disease themselves change?" Dr. Dossey believes that "we face the extraordinary possibility of fashioning a [health care] system that emphasizes life instead of death, and unity and oneness instead of fragmentation, darkness, and isolation."

◆

As we have seen, the need to conceptualize health and illness in a larger framework than the traditional one has led to the formulation of a new paradigm, still in its infancy, but already having substantial repercussions in the practice of medicine. One of those repercussions has been the development of a new field within medicine known as *behavioral medicine*, which is devoted to a deeper understanding of what we mean by health and to exploring how we can best promote health and prevent disease and how we can best treat and heal the diseases and disabilities we do experience.

Behavioral medicine was formally established in 1977. It explicitly recognizes that mind and body are intimately interconnected and that an appreciation of these interconnections and their scientific study is vital to a fuller understanding of health and disease. It is an interdisciplinary field, uniting the behavioral sciences with the biomedical sciences in the hope that the cross-fertilization will yield a more comprehensive picture of health and illness than either could alone. Behavioral medicine recognizes that our thought patterns and emotions may play a significant role in health and disease. It recognizes that what people believe about their bodies and their illnesses may be important for healing and that how we live our lives, what we think, and what we do may all influence our health in important ways.

The field of behavioral medicine offers new hope for people who ordinarily tend to fall through the cracks of the health care system and come away unhelped, frustrated, and bitter. In clinical programs such as the stress clinic, people are presented with the opportunity to try to do something for themselves as a *complement* to more traditional medical approaches. People are now being encouraged by their doctors to pursue such programs and to learn meditation and other methods as aids in coping with stress, illness, and pain. In these programs people learn to face their life problems and develop personalized strategies for working with them rather than giving themselves over solely to "experts" who are supposed to just "fix them" or make their problems magically disappear. Such programs are vehicles in which people can work to become healthier and more resilient, in which they can change their beliefs about what they are capable of doing and learn to relax and cope more effectively with life stress. At the same time they can work at changing their life-styles in key ways that might directly affect their health and physical well-being. Perhaps the most important step they can take in such programs is to expand the way they see themselves and their relationship to their life and to the world.

Behavioral medicine expands the traditional model of medical care so that it addresses mind as well as body, behavior and beliefs and feelings as well as signs and symptoms and procedures. By involving people in this expanded definition of medicine and health care in a *participatory* way, behavioral medicine helps people to shift the balance of responsibility for their well-being away from an exclusive dependency on their doctors and closer to their own personal efforts, which they have more direct control over than they do over hospitals, medical procedures, and doctors.

Coming to the stress clinic at the suggestion of their doctors is one way in which people with medical problems can take personal responsibility for participating in and contributing to the process of healing themselves. A small but important element of their experience in the clinic involves learning about some of the research findings in behavioral medicine that illustrate the importance of paying attention to mind-body interactions. Knowing something of the evidence for the connections between mind and health can give people a better idea about why health professionals make the recommendations for life-style change that they do. It demystifies medical knowledge by showing people where what health professionals know comes from and how statements of "fact" are arrived at. In the stress clinic we encourage people to think for themselves about the implications and limits of such knowledge, as well as to ask questions about its relevance to their own case. The results of studies investigating the relationship of psychological factors to health and illness can stimulate people to examine their own often very limiting beliefs about themselves and their illnesses and about what might be possible.

In this way, our patients come to see that science is confirming what has long been known, namely that each one of us has an important role to play in our own well-being. This role can be more effectively played if we can become conscious of and modify certain aspects of the way we live which can affect our health. These include our attitudes, thoughts, and beliefs; our emotions; our stance in relationship to society; and our behaviors. All can influence our health in different ways; all are related to stress and our attempts to cope with it; and all are directly influenced by the practice of mindfulness. In the next chapter we will examine a range of evidence that supports a new, unified mind-body perspective on health and illness and highlights the importance of becoming mindful of our own patterns of thinking, feeling, and behaving.

15

Mind *and* Body: Evidence That Beliefs, Attitudes, Thoughts, and Emotions Can Harm or Heal

THE ROLE OF PERCEPTIONS AND THOUGHT PATTERNS IN HEALTH

In the last chapter we saw a dramatic example of how a thought, triggered by a misunderstood remark, led to an overwhelming mind-body crisis that resulted in a woman's death. Although we are often unaware of our thoughts as thoughts, they have a profound effect on everything we do and they can have a profound effect on our health as well, which can be for better or for worse.

Our thought patterns dictate the ways we perceive and explain reality, including our relationship to ourself and to the world. We all have particular ways in which we think about and explain to ourselves why things happen to us. Our thought patterns underlie our motives for doing things and for making choices. They influence the degree of confidence we have in our ability to make things happen. They are at the core of our beliefs about the world, how it works, and what our place in it is. Thought patterns can be grouped into categories and studied systematically by scientists to determine how people with a particular pattern compare with those with a different pattern.

Optimism and Pessimism—Basic Filters on the World

Dr. Martin Seligman and his colleagues at the University of Pennsylvania have been studying health differences between people who can be identified as being basically optimistic or basically pessimistic in their thinking about why things happen to them. These two groups of people have very different ways of explaining the causes of what Dr. Seligman calls the "bad" events that happen to them in their lives. ("Bad" events include natural disasters, such as floods or earthquakes; personal defeats or setbacks, such as loss of a job or rejection by someone you care about; an illness, injury, or other stressful occurrence.)

Some people tend to be pessimistic in the ways they explain to themselves the causes of a bad event. This pattern involves blaming themselves for the bad things that happen to them, thinking that the effects of whatever happened will last a long time and that the bad event will affect many different aspects of their lives. Dr. Seligman refers to this *attributional style*, as it is technically called, as the "It's me, it's going to last forever, it's going to affect everything I do" pattern. In the extreme this pattern reflects a person who is highly depressed, hopeless, and very self-preoccupied. Some people call this mode of thinking *catastrophizing*. An example of this style might be the reaction "I always knew I was stupid and this proves it; I can never do anything right" when you experience a failure of some kind.

An optimist experiencing the same event would see it quite differently. People who are optimists tend not to blame themselves for bad events or, if they do, they see them more as momentary events which will become resolved. They tend to see bad events as limited in time and in how pervasive the damage they cause will be. In other words they focus on the *specific consequences* of what happened and do not make sweeping global statements and projections that blow the event out of proportion. An example of this style might be "Well, I really blew it that time, but I'll figure out something, make some adjustments and next time it will fly."

Dr. Seligman and his colleagues have shown that people who have a highly pessimistic attributional style are at significantly higher risk for becoming depressed when they encounter a bad event than are people who have the optimistic way of thinking. Pessimists are also more likely to come down with physical symptoms and show hormonal and immune-system changes characteristic of increased susceptibility to disease following a bad event than are optimists. In a study of cancer patients these researchers showed that the worse the attributional style, the earlier the patient died of the disease. In another study they showed that baseball players in the Hall of Fame who had a pessimistic attributional style when they were young and healthy were more likely to die young than those who had an optimistic attributional style.

Dr. Seligman's overall conclusion from these and other studies is that it is not the world per se that puts us at increased risk of illness so much as how we see and think about what is happening to us. A highly pessimistic pattern of explaining the causes of bad or stressful events when they occur seems to have particularly toxic consequences. Dr. Seligman's work suggests that this way of thinking puts people at risk for illness and may explain why some people are more susceptible to illness and premature death than others when other factors such as age, sex, smoking habits, diet have been taken into account. A pattern of optimistic thinking in response to stressful events, on the other hand, appears to have a protective effect against depression, illness, and premature death.

Self-efficacy—Your Confidence in Your Ability to Grow Influences Your Ability to Grow

One thought pattern that appears to be extremely powerful for improving health status is what is called *self-efficacy*. Self-efficacy is a belief in your ability to exercise control over specific events in your life. It reflects confidence in your ability to actually do things, a belief in your ability to make things happen, even when you might have to face new, unpredictable, and stressful occurrences. Dr. Albert Bandura and his colleagues at Stanford University Medical School have shown that a strong sense of self-efficacy is the best and most consistent predictor of positive health outcomes in many different medical situations, including who will recover most successfully from a heart attack, who will be able to cope well with the pain of arthritis, and who will be able to make life-style changes (such as quitting smoking). A strong belief in your ability to succeed at whatever you decide to do can influence the kinds of activities in which you will engage in the first place, how much effort you will put into something new and different before giving up, and how stressful your efforts to achieve control in important areas of your life will be.

Self-efficacy increases when you have experiences of succeeding at something you feel is important. For example, if you are practicing the body scan and, as a result, feel more in touch with your body and more relaxed, then that taste of success will lead you to feel more confident in your ability to relax when you want to. At the same time, such an experience will make it more likely that you will keep practicing the body scan.

Your self-efficacy can also increase if you are inspired by the examples of what other people are able to do. In the stress clinic classes, when one person reports a positive experience with the body scan, in controlling pain for instance, it usually has a dramatic positive effect on other people in the class who have not yet had such an experience. They are likely to say to themselves, "If that person can do it with his problems, then I can do it with mine." So seeing one person with a problem succeed can boost the confidence of others, both in their own ability and in the techniques they are using.

Dr. Bandura and his colleagues studied self-efficacy in a group of men who had had heart attacks and were undergoing cardiac rehabilitation. They were able to show that those men who had a strong conviction that their heart was very robust and could recover fully were much less likely to be derailed from their exercise programs than were those who were less confident, even though the severity of heart disease in the two groups was the same. Those with high self-efficacy were able to exercise on the treadmill without worrying or feeling defeated by the normal feelings of discomfort, shortness of breath, and fatigue that are a natural part of any exercise program. They were able to accept their discomfort without worrying that it was a "bad sign" and could focus instead on the positive benefits of their exercise program, such as feeling stronger and being able to do more. On the other hand, the men who did not have this kind of positive conviction tended to stop exercising, mistaking normal discomfort, shortness of breath, and fatigue as signs of an ailing heart. Further studies showed that when people who have low self-efficacy undergo training to develop mastery experiences, their confidence in their ability to function successfully and to control areas of their life that once felt out of their control grows and flourishes.

◆

One interesting line of research on the effects of thoughts and feelings on health involves studying people who seem to thrive on stress or who have survived extremely stressful situations. Here the goal is to see whether certain people have particular personality characteristics that may account for their apparent "immunity" to stress and to stress-related illnesses. Dr. Suzanne Kobasa of the City

University of New York and her colleagues, and Dr. Aaron Antonovsky, a medical sociologist in Israel, have both conducted studies in this area.

Hardiness

Dr. Kobasa has studied business executives, lawyers, bus drivers, telephone company employees, and other groups of people who lead high-stress lives. In every group, as you might expect, she found some people who were much healthier than others experiencing the same amount of stress. She wondered whether the healthier people had some personality characteristic in common that might be protecting them from the negative effects of high stress. She found that a particular psychological characteristic differentiated those who got sick often from those who stayed healthy. She called this characteristic *psychological hardiness*. Sometimes it is also referred to as *stress hardiness*.

As with the other psychological factors we have looked at, hardiness, too, involves a particular way of seeing oneself and the world. According to Dr. Kobasa, stress-hardy individuals show high levels of three psychological characteristics: *control*, *commitment*, and *challenge*. People who are high in *control* have a strong belief that they can exert an influence on their surroundings, that they can make things happen. This sounds similar to Dr. Bandura's notion of self-efficacy. People who are high in *commitment* tend to feel fully engaged in what they are doing from day to day and are committed to giving these activities their best effort. People who are high in *challenge* see change as a natural part of life that affords at least some chance for further development. This view allows stress-hardy individuals to see new situations more as opportunities and less as threats than might other people who do not share this orientation toward life as an ongoing challenge.

Dr. Kobasa emphasizes that there are many things a person can do to increase his or her level of stress hardiness. She suggests that the best way to develop greater hardiness is to come to grips with your own life by being willing to ask yourself hard questions about where your life is going and how it might be enriched by specific choices and changes you could make in the areas of control, commitment, and challenge. She also emphasizes that hardiness could be improved in high-stress work settings by restructuring roles and relationships within organizations to promote greater control, commitment, and sense of challenge among individual employees.

Sense of Coherence

Dr. Aaron Antonovsky's research has focused on people who have survived extreme stress, such as the Nazi concentration camps. In Dr. Antonovsky's view, being healthy involves an ability to continuously restore balance in response to its continual disruption. He wondered what allowed some people to resist very high levels of stress even as their resources for coping with the stress and tension were constantly being disrupted or threatened with disruption, as they were in the Nazi concentration camps. Dr. Antonovsky found that people who survive extreme stress have what he terms an inherent *sense of coherence* about the world and themselves. This sense of coherence is characterized by three components, which he calls *comprehensibility, manageability,* and *meaningfulness.* People who have a high sense of coherence have a strong feeling of confidence that they can make sense of their internal and external experience (that it is basically *comprehensible*), that they have the resources available to meet and manage the demands they encounter (*manageability*), and that these demands are challenges in which they can find meaning and to which they can commit themselves (*meaningfulness*).

THE ROLE OF EMOTIONS IN HEALTH—CANCER

The studies we have looked at so far have had a predominantly cognitive focus, that is, they have looked primarily at thought patterns and beliefs and their effects on health and illness. A parallel line of research has concerned itself with the role of emotions in health and illness. Obviously our thought patterns and our emotions shape and influence each other. It is often difficult to determine in a particular situation whether one is more fundamental than the other. We will now take a look at some research findings from studies focusing primarily on the relationship between emotional patterns and health.

For some time now there has been considerable debate about whether certain personality types are more prone to certain diseases. For instance, some studies suggest that there may be a "cancer-prone" personality, others that there may be a "coronary-heart-disease-prone" personality. The cancer-prone pattern is frequently described as someone who tends to conceal his or her feelings and is very other-oriented while actually feeling deeply alienated from others and feeling unloved and unlovable. Feeling a lack of closeness with one's parents when young is strongly associated with this pattern.

Much of the evidence in support of this link comes from a forty-year study conducted by Dr. Caroline Bedell Thomas of Johns Hopkins Medical School. Dr. Thomas collected large amounts of information on the psychological status of the incoming medical students at Johns Hopkins starting in the 1940s and then followed these individuals periodically over the years as they got older and, in some cases, got sick and died. In this way she was able to correlate particular psychological characteristics and early family-life experiences that these doctors reported when they were young and healthy (around age twenty-one) with a range of different diseases that some of them experienced over the next forty years. The results demonstrated, among other things, that *there was a particular constellation of features in early life that was associated with an increased likelihood of having cancer later in life*. Prominent among these characteristics were a lack of close relationship to parents and an ambivalent attitude toward life and human relationships. The conclusion, of course, is that our emotional experiences early in life may play a strong role in shaping our health later in life.

Dr. Bernie Siegel, a surgeon associated with Yale University and well-known author of *Love, Medicine and Miracles* and *Peace, Love and Healing*, sees a strong relationship between surviving cancer and the degree to which you can love yourself and be open to receiving love. His books recount numerous case histories of people with cancer who used the experience of having cancer to learn to find new love for themselves. Based on his widespread experience working with people with cancer, and highly conscious of his role as healer as well as his role as a surgeon who removes tumors from people's bodies, Dr. Siegel emphasizes the crucial importance of examining one's emotional life if one chooses to work *with* one's cancer to enhance the healing process. He strongly advocates meditation for cancer patients, saying in *Love, Medicine and Miracles*, "I know of no other single activity that by itself can produce such great improvement in the quality of life."

◆

As we examine research relating thought patterns and emotional factors to health, it is important for us to keep firmly in mind that it is always dangerous and almost always wrong to assume that because a connection has been found between certain personality traits or behaviors and a disease, this means that being a certain way or thinking a certain way *causes* you to get a particular disease. It is more accurate to say that it *may* increase to some extent (that extent depending on the strength of the correlation and a lot of other factors) your risk of getting the disease. This is because research studies always result in statistical relationships, not in a one-to-one correspondence. Not all people who have a particular personality trait that has been shown to be associated with cancer always get cancer. In fact not all people who smoke cigarettes die from lung cancer, emphysema, or heart disease, even though smoking has been proven beyond all doubt to be a strong risk factor for all of these diseases. The relationship is a statistical one, having to do with probabilities.

Therefore it is wrong to conclude from any of the evidence pointing to a possible relationship between emotions and cancer that certain personality traits directly "cause" the disease. Nevertheless, there is mounting evidence that certain psychological and behavioral patterns may *predispose* a person to at least some forms of cancer, while other personality attributes may protect a person from cancer or increase the chances of surviving it. In this regard the feelings you experience toward yourself and other people and how you express or don't express them seem to be particularly important.

For example, Dr. David Kissen and his collaborators at the University of Glasgow in Scotland, conducted a series of studies on male patients with lung cancer starting in the late 1950s. In one study they analyzed the personal histories of several hundred patients taken at the time they entered the hospital with chest complaints, but before any diagnosis was made. Those men who were later found to have lung cancer reported significantly more adversities in childhood, such as an unhappy home or the death of a parent, than had those who turned out to have other diagnoses. This finding is consistent with Dr. Thomas's more recent results from the Johns Hopkins medical-student study, in which, as we saw, she found that cancer later in life was associated with a lack of closeness to parents and ambivalent feelings toward relationships reported forty years earlier. In the Kissen study those men who were found to have lung cancer had also reported more adversities as adults, including disturbed interpersonal relationships. The researchers observed that, as a group, those with lung cancer showed particular difficulty in expressing their emotions. They did not express their feelings about bad events, especially those that involved bonds with other people (such as marital problems or the death of somebody close to them), although, to the researchers, these were obviously sources of current emotional upset in their lives. Instead they tended to deny that they were feeling emotional pain and talked of their difficulties during the interviews in matter-of-fact tones that seemed inappropriate to the interviewers under the circumstances. This was in marked contrast to the patients in the control group (who were later found to have diseases other than lung cancer), who described similar situations with appropriate expressions of emotion.

The inability to express emotions was strongly linked to mortality among the lung cancer patients in this study. *Those people who had the poorest ability to express emotions had more than four and a half times the yearly death rate than those lung cancer patients with the highest ability for emotional discharge.* This finding held true regardless of whether or how much they smoked cigarettes, although, as you might expect, the heavy smokers had ten times the incidence of cancer as those who had never smoked.

More evidence relating emotional factors to cancer came from researchers at King's College Hospital in London, who conducted a similar study on women with breast cancer. Drs. S. Greer and Tina Morris conducted in-depth psychological interviews with 160 women as they were admitted to the hospital for a lump in the breast before it was known whether or not it was cancerous. At the time of the interview all the women were under the equal stress of not knowing whether they had cancer or not. The interviews with the women and with their husbands and other relatives were used as a means of measuring the degree to which the women concealed or expressed their feelings.

The majority of women who were later found not to have breast cancer had what these researchers termed a "normal" pattern of emotional expression. However, the majority of women who were later found to have breast cancer had either a lifelong pattern of extreme suppression of their feelings (for the most part, anger) or of "exploding" with emotion. Both extremes were associated with a higher risk of cancer. However, it was much more common for these women to suppress their feelings than to be "exploders."

In a five-year follow-up of fifty women with breast cancer, all of whom had been treated surgically, the researchers found that those women who were judged to be facing their situation three months after surgery with what they called a "fighting spirit," that is, a highly optimistic attitude and a belief in their own ability to survive, were much more likely to be alive than those who at three months had adopted either an attitude of stoic acceptance toward their disease or who were completely overwhelmed by it and felt helpless, hopeless, and defeated. Women who denied altogether that they had cancer and refused to discuss the subject and who showed no emotional distress about their situation also were much more likely to survive to five years. The results of this study suggest that emotions may play some role in cancer survival, with strong positive emotions (a fighting spirit, total denial) appearing protective and blocked emotional expression (stoicism or helplessness) decreasing survival. However, as these researchers themselves pointed out, their study was of a relatively small number of people and thus their findings can only be considered suggestive.

For unequivocal links to be established between a psychological characteristic and an illness, very large (and often extremely expensive) studies known as clinical trials need to be conducted. The results of one such study which looked into the relationship of depression to cancer in over 6,000 men and women in the United States were recently reported. Although many smaller and less well-designed studies had reported an association between depression and cancer, no link was found in this larger study. The group of people with symptoms of depression and the group that did not both had cancer rates of around ten percent. Yet many well-designed studies do show an unequivocal link between a behavioral pattern related to depression, known as helplessness, reduced immunological functions including natural killer cell levels, and increased tumor growth in animals. The relationship of these findings and of the work on helplessness in human beings, which has also shown a relationship to reductions in immune function, to this negative outcome of the clinical trial on depression and cancer remains to be seen as more research is conducted. This is an area of continued controversy.

◆

Cancer is a condition in which cells within the body lose the biochemical mechanisms that keep their growth in check. Consequently, they multiply wildly, in many cases forming large masses called tumors. Many scientists believe that the production of cancerous cells in the body is happening at a low level all the time as a "normal" process and that the immune system, when healthy, recognizes them and destroys them before they can do any damage. According to this model it is when the immune system is weakened, either through direct physical damage or through the psychological effects of stress, and it can no longer effectively identify and destroy these small numbers of cancerous cells that the cancer cells multiply out of control. Then, depending on the type of cancer, either they develop a blood supply of their own and eventually form a solid tumor or they overwhelm the system with large numbers of circulating cancer cells, as in leukemia.

Of course it is possible for a person to be exposed to such massive levels of carcinogenic substances that even a healthy immune system would be overwhelmed. This happened to people living in areas where there has been toxic dumping, such as the infamous Love Canal. Similarly, exposure to high doses of radiation, as occurred following the bombings of Hiroshima and Nagasaki and following the nuclear accident at Chernobyl, can cause the formation of cancerous cells and at the same time weaken the immune system's ability to recognize and neutralize them. In short, the development of any kind of cancer is a multistage, complex occurrence involving our genes and our cellular processes, the environment, and our individual behavior and actions.

◆

Even if it turns out that there is a statistically important relationship between negative emotions and cancer, to suggest to a person with cancer that his or her disease was caused by psychological stress, unresolved conflict, or unexpressed emotions would be totally unjustifiable. It amounts to subtly or not so subtly blaming the person for his or her disease. People often do this unwittingly, perhaps in an attempt to rationalize a painful reality and to cope with it better themselves. Whenever we can come up with an explanation for something, it makes us feel a little better because we can reassure ourselves, however wrongly, that we "understand" why that person "got" cancer. But doing this amounts to a violation of the other person's psychic integrity, based on ignorance and surmise. It also robs people of the present by directing their attention to the past when they most need to focus their energies and face the reality of having a life-threatening disease. Unfortunately, this kind of thinking, which seeks to attribute a subtle psychological deficiency as the "cause" of the cancer, has become fashionable in certain circles. This attitude is far more likely to result in increased suffering than in healing. From everything we know about the emotions and health, acceptance and forgiveness are what we need to cultivate to enhance healing, not self-condemnation and self-blame.

If a person who has cancer believes that emotional factors may have been important in his or her illness, that is his or her prerogative. It may be very helpful to explore this question, and it may not be, depending on the person's life and on how the subject is approached. Some people are empowered by the realization that there may have been ways in which they contributed to their illness by the way they handled emotions and feelings in the past. For them, it means that by becoming more aware of these particular issues and areas now and by making changes, they might be able to enhance their healing and recovery. But this perspective should not be *imposed* by others. Explorations in this domain need to be undertaken with great compassion and caring, whether by the person or with the help of a physician or therapist. Inquiry into possible factors that might have contributed to one's illness can only help if they come out of non-judging, out of generosity and compassion and acceptance of oneself and of one's past, not out of condemnation.

Whether psychological factors played a causal or exacerbating role in a particular disease in a particular person will never be known with certainty. Since mind and body are not really separate in the first place, one's state of physical health will always be affected to some extent by psychological factors. But by the time a person has been diagnosed with a particular illness, the issue of causal psychological factors can be at best of secondary importance. At that juncture it becomes much more important to take responsibility for what needs doing in the present. Since there is evidence that positive emotional factors can enhance healing, a diagnosis of cancer can be a particularly important turning point in a person's life, a time for mobilizing an optimistic, coherent, self-efficacious, and engaged perspective and for working at being less susceptible to the pull of pessimistic, helpless, and ambivalent mind states. Purposefully directing gentleness, acceptance, and love toward oneself is a very good place to begin.

HIGH BLOOD PRESSURE AND ANGER

There is evidence that suppressing emotional expression may play a role in hypertension as well as cancer. In this area the focus has been primarily on anger. People who habitually express anger when provoked by others have lower average blood pressures than people who habitually suppress such feelings. In a study of 431 adult men living in Detroit, Margaret Chesney, Doyle Gentry, and their collaborators found that blood pressure was highest in men reporting high job or family stress *and* a tendency to suppress feelings of anger. It seems that in high-stress situations, an ability to vent one's angry feelings is protective against high blood pressure. Other studies suggest that high blood pressure may be associated with both extremes of emotional behavior, either always suppressing anger or always expressing it overtly, as was also noted with the women in the breast cancer study, who either had trouble expressing their feelings or tended to "explode" with them.

CORONARY HEART DISEASE, HOSTILITY, AND CYNICISM

Perhaps the greatest scientific scrutiny of personality factors in relationship to chronic disease has focused on the question of whether or not there is a heart-disease-prone personality. For some time it was thought that there was conclusive evidence that there was indeed a particular behavior pattern associated with increased risk of coronary heart disease, known as *Type-A behavior.* But recent research has shown that in all likelihood, it is not the entire Type-A pattern as originally described but only one aspect of it that is related to heart disease.

Type A's are described as driven by a sense of time urgency and competitiveness. They are characteristically impatient, hostile, and aggressive. Their gestures and speech tend to be hurried and abrupt. In this terminology people who do not show the Type-A pattern are referred to as Type B's. According to Dr. Meyer Friedman, one of the originators of the Type-A concept, Type B's are more easygoing than Type A's. They are not driven by time urgency and are free from a generalized irritability, hostility, and aggressiveness. They are also more inclined toward periods of contemplation. Yet there is no evidence that Type B's are any less productive or less successful than Type A's.

The original evidence relating Type-A behavior to coronary heart disease came from a large research project known as the Western Collaborative Group Study. This study characterized 3,500 men as either Type A or Type B when they were healthy and had no signs of disease. Eight years later they looked again to see who had developed heart disease and who had not. It turned out that the Type A's developed coronary heart disease at two to four times the rate (depending on age, the younger men having the greater risk) of the Type B's.

Many other studies confirmed the connection between the Type-A behavior pattern and coronary heart disease and demonstrated that it was true for women as well as for men. But recently other studies, particularly those by Dr. Redford Williams of Duke University Medical School and his collaborators, have looked at just the hostility component of the Type-A behavior pattern and have found it to be a stronger predictor of heart disease all by itself than the full Type-A pattern. In other words, the evidence suggests that you are at less risk of heart disease as a Type A if you are low in hostility, even if you feel a strong time urgency and are competitive. What is more, *high hostility scores predicted not just myocardial infarction and death from heart disease, they also predicted increased risk of death from cancer and all other causes as well!*

In one fascinating study, Dr. Williams and his collaborators did a follow-up study on male physicians whose level of hostility on a particular psychological test had been measured when they were medical students twenty-five years earlier. They found that those men with low hostility scores when they were in medical school had about one-fourth the risk of having heart disease twenty-five years later than those with high hostility scores. When they looked at death from all causes, the results were also dramatic. Since they had graduated from medical school, only 2 percent of the men who were in the low-hostility group had died, whereas 13 percent of those in the high-hostility group had died in the same time period. In other words those who showed high hostility on a psychological test they took twenty-five years ago are now dying at a rate that is six and a half times the rate of those whose hostility was low at that time.

Williams describes hostility as "an absence of trust in the basic goodness of others," grounded in "the belief that others are generally mean, selfish and undependable." He emphasizes that this attitude is usually acquired early in life from caregivers such as our parents or others and that it probably reflects an arrested development of "basic trust." He points out that this attitude has a strong element of cynicism in it as well as hostility, as exemplified by two typical items on the questionnaire they used to measure hostility: "Most people make friends because friends are likely to be useful to them" and "I have frequently worked under people who seem to have things arranged so that they get credit for good work but are able to pass off mistakes onto those under them." Anyone who strongly believes these two statements probably has a very cynical view of people in general. With such a view of the world and other people, hostile and cynical people can be expected to feel and either suppress or display anger and aggression much more frequently than others.

The study of these doctors provides strong evidence that a hostile and cynical outlook on the world may, in and of itself, put one at much greater risk for illness and premature death than a more trusting view of people. It seems an ingrained cynical and hostile attitude is highly toxic to well-being. These and other findings are detailed in Dr. Williams's book, *The Trusting Heart,* in which he also points out that all the major religious traditions of the world emphasize the value of developing the qualities that science now seems to be showing are good for your health.

OTHER PERSONALITY TRAITS AND HEALTH

Dr. David McClelland, a renowned psychologist formerly at Harvard and now at Boston University, has been conducting research into the relationship between motivation and health for over twenty years. Motivational factors underlie not only our actions but also the ways we organize our experience into a worldview. Dr. McClelland has identified a particular motivational type that is more susceptible to disease than others. He calls it *the stressed power-motivation syndrome.* People who are high in this characteristic have a strong need for power in their relationships with people. Their need for power outweighs any need they might have for affiliation with people. They tend to be aggressive, argumentative, competitive, and join organizations to increase their personal status and prestige. But they also get very frustrated and feel blocked and threatened whenever stressful events occur that may challenge their sense of power. People with this particular motivational pattern get sick when under such stress much more readily than others who do not share this drive.

Dr. McClelland has also identified an opposite motivational pattern which seems to confer hardiness or resistance to illness. He calls it *unstressed affiliation motivation.* People high in unstressed affiliation have a strong need for affiliation. They are drawn to being with people and want to be friendly and liked by others, not as a means to an end (as with the cynical Type A's) but as an end in its own right. They are also free to express their need for affiliation since it is not blocked or threatened by stressful events. In a study of college students, those scoring above the average in stressed power motivation had more reported illness than other students, while those who were above average in the unstressed affiliation syndrome reported the least illness.

Once again we find evidence that there is a certain way of looking at the world that predisposes a person to illness and another way that seems to enhance a high degree of health.

PERSONALITY STUDIES ON PEOPLE IN THE STRESS CLINIC

We are presently collaborating with Dr. McClelland and his colleagues, Dr. Joel Weinberger and Carolyn McCleod, studying how motivational patterns change in the patients undergoing mindfulness training in the stress clinic. In one study we found that most people showed major increases in *affiliative trust* (a motivational pattern associated with increased immune function and reduced likelihood of illness) while they were in the program. By contrast a group of patients who were waiting to get into the program and who were tested over the same period of time did not show any change in affiliative trust.

In related studies we found that the people in the stress clinic also showed significant improvements on Dr. Kobasa's *hardiness* scale and on Dr. Antonovsky's *sense of coherence* scale over the eight weeks they were in the program. Those with the largest improvements in sense of coherence also showed the largest improvements in their physical and psychological symptoms.

Preliminary analyses of these ongoing studies show that the people in the stress clinic appear to be undergoing a profound change not only in their symptoms and in their ability to relax but also in the very patterns of their thinking and feeling. These motivational characteristics have traditionally been seen as associated with deep and stable personality structures and are not usually thought to be amenable to change, particularly in a short time period. The changes we are seeing in these personality variables in the people who go through the stress clinic suggest that *training in mindfulness meditation can have a profound positive influence on one's view of oneself and of the world, including an ability to be more trusting of oneself and others.*

SOCIAL INFLUENCES ON HEALTH

We have reviewed some of the evidence from studies in behavioral medicine suggesting that our thought patterns, our beliefs, our emotions, in short our very personality, may affect our health in major ways. There is also considerable evidence that suggests that social factors, which of course are related to psychological factors, also play an important role in health and illness. It has long been known, for instance, that, statistically speaking, people who are socially isolated tend to be less healthy, psychologically and physically, and more likely to die prematurely than people who have extensive social relationships. Death rates from all causes are higher in unmarried people than in married people at all ages. There seems to be something about having ties to others that is basic to health. Of course this is intuitively understandable. We all have a strong need to belong and to feel a part of something and a need to associate with other people. Dr. McClelland's studies on affiliative trust suggest that these kinds of ties are extremely important for people's health.

Evidence supporting the importance of social connections for health has been bolstered by several major studies of very large populations in this country and abroad over the past twenty years. All show a relationship between ties to others and health. People who have a very low degree of social interaction in their lives, as measured by marital status, contacts with extended family and friends, church membership, and other group involvements, are between two and four times as likely to die in the succeeding ten-year period as are people who have a very high level of social interaction, when all other factors such as age, prior illness, income, health habits such as smoking, alcohol consumption, physical activity, race, and the like are taken into account.

There are a number of studies that suggest why this might be so. Dr. James Lynch, of the University of Maryland and author of *The Broken Heart: The Medical Consequences of Loneliness*, has shown that physical contact with or even the presence of another person can have a calming effect on cardiac physiology and reactivity in a stressful intensive care unit. In other studies Dr. Lynch showed that people live longer after a myocardial infarction if they have a pet than if they don't. He also showed that just the presence of a friendly animal can decrease one's blood pressure.

Human-animal contact seems to benefit not only the humans but the pets as well. According to Dr. Lynch, petting reduces cardiovascular reactivity in stressful situations among dogs, cats, horses, and rabbits. One remarkable study of human-animal inter-action came about after researchers at the University of Ohio noticed that rabbits on a high-fat, high-cholesterol diet designed to give them heart disease had much less severe heart disease if they were in lower cages in the room rather than higher ones. This finding didn't make any sense at all. Why should the position of their cages make a difference in the degree of heart disease when the rabbits were all genetically identical, were on the same diet, and were being treated the same way. Then one researcher observed that they were *not* being treated in exactly the same way. It turned out that one of the members of the team was taking out the rabbits in the lower cages from time to time, stroking them, and talking to them.

This led the researchers to perform a carefully controlled experiment, petting some rabbits and not others while keeping them all on the same high-fat, high-cholesterol diet. The results demonstrated conclusively that affectionate stroking of rabbits made them much more resistant to heart disease than their unpetted kin. The petted rabbits had 60 percent less severe disease than the unpetted ones. They repeated the whole experiment a second time to make sure it wasn't a fluke and got exactly the same result.

♦

To summarize, all the studies we have discussed and many others support the notion that our physical health is intimately connected with our patterns of thinking and feeling about ourselves and also with the quality of our relationships with other people and the world. The evidence suggests that certain patterns of thinking and certain ways of relating to our feelings can predispose us to illness. *Thoughts and beliefs that foster hopeless and helpless feelings; a sense of loss of control; hostility and cynicism toward others; a lack of commitment and enthusiasm about life's challenges; an inability to express feelings; and social isolation appear to be particularly toxic.*

On the other hand, other patterns of thinking, feeling, and relating appear to be associated with robustness and health. People who have a basically optimistic perspective, who have the ability to "let go" of a bad event, who can see that it is impermanent and that their situation will change, tend to be healthier than their pessimistic counterparts. Optimists know intuitively that there are always choices that can be made in life, that there is always the possibility of exercising some control. They also tend to be able to laugh at themselves, to have a positive sense of humor.

Other health-related psychological traits include a strong sense of coherence, the conviction that life can be comprehensible, manageable, and meaningful; a spirit of engagement in life, taking on obstacles as challenges; and confidence in one's ability to make changes that one decides are important.

Healthy social traits include valuing relationships, honoring them, and feeling a sense of goodness and basic trust in people.

Since all the evidence we have looked at is only statistically valid, we cannot say that a particular belief or attitude causes disease, only that more people get sick or die prematurely if they have strong patterns of thinking that way, for whatever reasons. As we will see in the next chapter, it makes more sense to think of health and illness as opposite poles on a continuum than to think that you are *either* "healthy" *or* "sick." There will always be a flux of different forces at work in our lives at any given time; some may be driving us toward illness, others shifting the balance toward greater health. Some of these forces are under our control, or might be if we put our resources to work for us, whereas others lie beyond what any individual can control. The ultimate limits beyond which the system breaks down completely are not precisely known and are probably different for different people and even at different times for the same person. But this dynamic interplay of multiple forces that influence our health is happening wherever we are on the health-illness continuum at any particular time, and it goes on changing throughout our lives.

HOW WE CAN USE THIS KNOWLEDGE IN OUR PRACTICE

The relevance of the evidence presented here to us as individuals lies primarily in our ability to bring awareness to our own thoughts and feelings and their physical, psychological, and social consequences *as we observe them*. If we can observe *in ourselves* the toxicity of certain beliefs, thought patterns, and behaviors as they arise in the moment, then we can work to lessen their hold on us. Knowing something of the evidence, we might be motivated to look a little more closely at those moments when we find ourselves thinking pessimistically, or suppressing our feelings of anger, or thinking cynically about other people. We might bring mindfulness to the consequences of these very thoughts, feelings, and attitudes as they arise in us.

For instance, you might observe how your body feels when you hold in your anger. What happens when you let it out? What are its effects on other people? Can you see the immediate consequences of your own hostility and distrust of others when these feelings surface? Do they cause you to jump to unwarranted conclusions or to think the worst of people and to say things you later regret? Can you see how such attitudes cause pain to others in the moment that they are happening? Can you see how these attitudes create unnecessary trouble and pain *for you* at the time that these feelings surface?

On the other hand, you might also be mindful of positive thoughts and feelings as they occur. How does your body feel when you see obstacles as challenges? How does it feel when you are experiencing joy? When you are trusting others? When you are generous and showing kindness? When you are loving? What are the effects of these inner experiences of yours on others? Can you see the immediate consequences of your positive emotional states and of your optimistic perspective at those times? Do these influence other people's anxiety and pain? Is there a sense of greater peace within yourself at these times?

If we can be aware, *in our own personal experience* as well as from the evidence from scientific studies that certain attitudes and ways of seeing ourselves and others are health-enhancing, that affiliative trust and seeing the basic goodness in others and in ourselves has intrinsic healing power, as does seeing crises and even threats as challenges and opportunities, then we can work mindfully to consciously develop these qualities in ourselves from moment to moment and from day to day. They become new options for us to cultivate, new ways of seeing and being in the world.

16
Connectedness
—

Imagine the following experiment, which was actually carried out by Drs. Judith Rodin and Ellen Langer, two social psychologists now at Yale and Harvard. They studied elderly residents in a nursing home. With the cooperation of the nursing-home staff, Drs. Rodin and Langer divided the participants in the study into two groups that were the same in terms of age, sex, severity of illness, and kinds of illnesses. Then one group of people was explicitly encouraged to make more decisions for themselves about life in the nursing home, such as where to receive visitors and when to see movies, while the other group was explicitly encouraged to let the staff help them with these kinds of decisions.

As part of the study each person was also given a plant for his or her room. However, the two groups of patients were told quite different things about the plant they were being given. People in the first group, who were being encouraged to make more decisions for themselves, were told something like "This plant is to brighten up your room. It is your plant now and whether it lives or dies is your responsibility. You decide when to water it, where it will do best." The people in the other group, who were encouraged to let the staff make decisions for them, were told something like "This plant is to brighten up your room a little. But don't worry, you don't have to water it or take care of it. The housekeeper will do that for you."

What Drs. Rodin and Langer found was that by the end of a year and a half, a certain number of people in both groups had died, as would have been predicted for these nursing-home residents. But the remarkable finding was that the two groups differed dramatically in *how many* people had died over the same period of time. It turned out that the people who were encouraged to let the staff help them with their decisions about visitors and other details of their lives and who were told that the staff would take care of the plant they had been given died at the same rate as was usually seen in that nursing home. But *the people who were encouraged to make decisions for themselves and who were told that the plant was their responsibility died at about half the usual rate!*

Dr. Rodin and Dr. Langer interpreted these findings to mean that enabling these nursing-home residents to take more control in their lives, even over "little" decisions, such as when to water the plant, protected them from an earlier death in some way. Anybody who is familiar with nursing homes knows that there are few things in that environment that really are under a person's control. (This interpretation is consistent with Dr. Kobasa's work on hardiness, which identified control as one important factor in resistance to illness.)

There is a complementary interpretation that I find myself drawn to, one that places the emphasis slightly differently. One might equally say that those people who were told that the plant was their responsibility to take care of were given an opportunity to bond to the plant, to feel needed in some small way. In fact they may have come to feel that the plant depended on them for its well-being. This way of looking at the experiment emphasizes the connectedness between the person and the plant rather than the exercise of control. Even when making decisions about where to meet visitors and when to go to the movies, it is at least plausible that the encouragement to make decisions for themselves led to their feeling as if they were participating more, were connected more with the nursing home, belonged there more than the group that was not encouraged in this way.

When you feel connected to something, that connection immediately gives you a purpose for living. Relationship itself gives meaning to life. We have already seen that relationships, even relationships with pets, are protective of health. We have also seen that affiliation, meaning and a sense of coherence are attributes of well-being.

Meaning and relationship are strands of connectedness. They weave your life as an individual into a larger tapestry, a larger whole, which, you might say, actually gives your life its individuality. In the case of the plant experiment in the nursing home, we might suppose that those people who were given the plant but were not told that they were to be responsible for it would be less likely to develop this kind of relationship, a connectedness with the plant. It is more likely that they saw the plant as just another neutral item in

the room, like the furniture, rather than as something that depended on them for its well-being.

To my mind, connectedness may be what is most fundamental
about the relationship of mind to physical and emotional health.
The studies of social involvements and health certainly suggest that
this is so. They show that just the *number* of relationships and
connections one has through marriage, family, churches and other
organizations is a strong predictor of mortality. This is a very crude
measure of relationship, since it does not take into account the
quality of those relationships and their meaningfulness to the individuals studied.

It would not be hard to imagine that a happy hermit, living in
isolation, might feel connected to everything in nature and all
people on the planet and not be at all affected by a dearth of human
neighbors. We might speculate that such a person probably would
not suffer ill health or premature death from such voluntary isolation. On the other hand, people who are married might have very
rocky and tenuous connections, which might make for very high
stress and a susceptibility to illness and premature death. The fact
that studies could show a relationship between the sheer *number* of
social connections and the death rate in a large population implies
that our connections play very powerful roles in our lives. It suggests that even negative or stressful connections with people may be
better for our health than isolation, unless we know how to be
happy alone, which few of us do.

Many studies with animals also support the idea that connectedness is important for health. As we have seen, stroking
and petting appear to be health enhancing for both people and
animals. Animals raised in isolation when they are young never
function as normal adults and tend to die sooner than animals raised
among littermates. Four-day-old monkeys will cling to a terrycloth
surrogate "mother" if separated from their real mother. They will
spend more time in physical contact with the soft terrycloth
"mother" than with a wire-mesh surrogate, *even when the wire one
provides milk and the soft one doesn't!* Dr. Harry Harlow of the
University of Wisconsin performed such experiments in the late
1950s and clearly demonstrated the importance of warm physical
contact between mother and infant in monkeys. Harlow's baby
monkeys chose soft touch with an inanimate object over physical
nourishment.

The renowned anthropologist Ashley Montagu documented

the profound importance of touch and its relationship to physical and psychological well-being in a remarkable book called *Touching: The Human Significance of the Skin*. Physical touch is one of humanity's most basic ways of connecting. For instance, shaking hands and hugging are symbolic rituals that communicate an openness to connecting. They are formalized acknowledgments of relationship. And they become much more, tapping a deeper domain of connectedness, a channel for the expression of feelings, when they are engaged in with awareness.

While physical touch is a wonderful way in which to communicate our feelings, it is hardly the only one. We have many other channels for touching besides the skin. We make contact with each other and connect through all our senses, with our eyes, our ears, our noses, our tongues, our bodies, and our minds. These are our doors of connection to each other and to the world. They can hold extraordinary meaning when the contact is made with awareness rather than out of habit.

When touching is perfunctory or habitual, the meaning "embodied" in it rapidly changes from connectedness to disconnectedness and from there to feelings of frustration or annoyance. No one likes to be treated mechanically, and we certainly do not like to be touched mechanically. If we think for a moment about making love, one of the most intimate expressions of human connectedness through touching, we might recognize and admit to ourselves that lovemaking suffers when the touching is automatic and mechanical. It is almost always felt as lacking in affection and bonding, a sign that the other person is not fully present. This distance can be felt in all aspects of the touching: in body language, timing, movement and speech. Perhaps one person's mind is somewhere else in a particular moment. This can lead to a break in the energy flow between the two people. When this happens, it seriously erodes positive feelings. If it becomes a chronic pattern, it can easily lead to resentment, resignation, and alienation. But usually an inability to bring awareness to making love and to experiencing full connectedness with the other person is only symptomatic of a larger pattern of disconnectedness, one likely to manifest itself in various ways in the relationship, not just in bed.

We might say that the degree to which a person's mind and body are connected and in harmony reflects the degree of awareness that person brings to present-moment experience. If you are not in touch with yourself, it is very unlikely that your connections with others will be satisfactory in the long run. The more centered you are yourself, the easier it will be for you to be centered in your relationships, to appreciate connectedness with others, and to be able to fine-tune it. This is a very fruitful area of application of the meditation practice, as you will see in Part IV.

◆

In the last chapter we saw that a lack of closeness to one's parents during childhood was associated with an increased risk of cancer in Dr. Caroline Bedell Thomas's study of doctors. We might speculate that this has something to do with the extreme importance of early experiences of connectedness to later health as an adult. Perhaps it is in childhood that all the positive attitudes, beliefs, and emotional competencies that we looked at in the last chapter, and in particular basic human trust and the need for affiliation, take root. If we were denied such experiences in childhood, for whatever reasons, it is likely that special attention to the cultivation of those qualities will be particularly important if we are to experience ourselves as whole when we are adults.

The fact is that everybody's original experiences of life were, literally, even biologically, experiences of connectedness and oneness. Each of us came into the world through the body of another being. We were once part of our mother, connected to her body, contained within it. We all bear the sign of that connectedness. Surgeons know not to excise the belly button if they have to make a midline incision; nobody wants to lose their belly button, "useless" though it is. It's a sign of where we came from, our membership card in the human race.

After babies are born, they immediately seek another channel for connecting to their mother's body. They find it through nursing if their mothers are aware of this channel and value it. Nursing is reconnecting, a merging again into oneness, this time in a different way. Now the baby is on the outside, her body separate yet drawing life from the mother's body through the breast while touching her, being warmed by her body, enveloped in her gaze and sounds. These are early moments of connectedness, moments that cement and deepen the bond between mother and child even as the baby gradually learns about being separate.

Without parents or others to care for them, human babies are completely helpless. Yet protected and cared for within the web of connectedness that the family represents, they thrive and grow, complete and perfect in themselves yet completely dependent on others for their basic needs. Each one of us was at one time this complete and also this helpless.

As we grew older, we found out more and more about our separateness and individuality, about having a body, about "me," "my," and "mine," about having feelings, about being able to manipulate objects. As children learn to separate and to feel themselves as separate selves with increasing age, they also need to continue to feel connected in order to feel secure and in order to be psychologically healthy. *They need to feel that they belong*. It is not a matter of being dependent or independent, but of being *interdependent*. They can no longer be one with their mothers in the old ways, but they do need to experience ongoing emotional connections with them and with their fathers and others in order ultimately to feel whole themselves.

The energy that feeds this ongoing connectedness, of course, is love. But love *itself* needs nurturing to flower fully, even between children and parents. It's not that it isn't "always there" so much as that it can easily be taken for granted and remain underdeveloped in its expression. It means little if you love your children or your parents deep in your heart but the expression of it is constantly being subverted or inhibited by strong feelings of anger or resentment or alienation. Love means little if the major way you have to express it is to pressure others to conform to your views of how they should be or what they should do. It is particularly unfortunate if you have no awareness of what you are doing at such times and no sense of how it is being perceived by others.

The path to developing our capacity to express love more fully is to bring awareness to our actual feelings, to observe them mindfully, to work at being non-judgmental and more patient and accepting. If we ignore our own feelings and behavior and just coast in the belief that the love is there and that it is strong and good, sooner or later our connections with our children may become strained or badly frayed, even broken. This is especially so if we are unable to see and accept them for who they actually are. This is an area in which regular practice of lovingkindness meditation (see Chapter 13) even for brief moments, can provide strong nourishment for the outward expression of our unconditional loving feelings.

◆

The majority of pediatricians and child psychologists used to believe that babies were senseless when they were born, that they couldn't feel pain the way adults do or that it wouldn't affect them if they did because they wouldn't remember it later, and that therefore it didn't matter how you treated children when they were babies. What the mothers felt was probably quite different, but even a mother's instinctive responses to her baby are strongly influenced by cultural norms and especially by the authoritative pronouncements of her pediatrician.

Studies of newborn babies in the past twenty years have dispelled the viewpoint that they are insensitive to pain and unaware of the outside world at birth. They show that babies are alert and aware even in the womb. From the time they are born and even before, their "view" of the world and their feelings are being shaped by the messages they received from the surrounding environment. Some studies suggest that if a newborn baby and its mother are separated at birth for a prolonged period, usually due to medical circumstances totally beyond the control of the mother, and if consequently the normal infant-maternal bonding process is unable to occur within that time, the future emotional relationship between the child and the mother may be more emotionally disturbed and distanced. The mother may never feel the strong attachment toward that child that mothers usually do. There may be a lack of feelings of deep connectedness. No one can say with certainty how this might translate into specific emotional or health problems for this child twenty or thirty years later, but there appears to be some connection.

Early childhood experiences of isolation, cruelty, violence, and abuse can lead to severe emotional disabilities in later life. They strongly shape a person's view of the world as meaningful or meaningless, benevolent or uncaring, controllable or uncontrollable, and of the person as worthy or unworthy of love and esteem. While some children are true survivors and find ways of growing and healing from such experiences no matter what, countless others never recover from the early rupture of their connections with warmth and acceptance and love. They carry around scars that have never healed and that are seldom even understood or defined. Dr. Alice Miller, a Swiss psychiatrist, has made a fascinating study of this process in her book, *For Your Own Good*. Children of alcoholics, drug addicts, and young victims of physical or sexual abuse often suffer grievously in this way, but others who were less overtly abused also carry deep emotional scars and wounds from childhood.

A lack of closeness with your parents when you were a child can leave a deep wound, whether you are conscious of it or not. It is a healable wound, but it needs to be recognized as a wound, as a broken connection, for deep psychological healing to occur. It may well express itself in feelings of alienation, even from your own body. This, too, is healable. The woundedness of our connection to our own body at times cries out for healing. Yet too often these cries go unheeded or unrecognized, even unheard.

What would it take to initiate the healing of such wounds? First, an acknowledgment that they are there. Second, a systematic way of listening to and reestablishing a sense of connectedness with your own body and with your positive feelings toward it and toward yourself.

We see such wounds and the scarring they produce every day in the stress clinic. Many people come to the clinic with much more pain than only that caused by their physical problems and by the stress in their lives. Many find it difficult to feel much, if any, love and compassion for themselves. Many feel unworthy of love and unable to express warmth toward members of their own family, even when they want to. Many feel disconnected from their bodies. Their lives are devoid of feelings of coherence or connectedness. Many got messages from their parents or from school or from church or sometimes all three when they were children that they were bad or stupid or ugly or unworthy or selfish. And those messages were internalized, became part of their self-image and of their view of the world, and were carried into adulthood deep in their own psyches.

Of course for the most part adults, whether they be parents, teachers or clergy, don't *mean* to give children such messages. It is just that without paying attention to this domain of our relationships, we tend to hardly ever be aware of what we are really doing or saying. We have elaborate psychological defenses that allow us to believe unquestioningly that we know what is best for children, that we know exactly what we are doing and why. Most of us would be shocked if a neutral third party were to suddenly stop the action at certain times and point things out from the perspective of the child, or to highlight the likely consequences to the child of what we were saying or doing.

To take a simple example, when a parent calls a child a "bad boy" or a "bad girl," in all likelihood what is really meant is that the parent does not like what the child is doing. But that is not what is actually being communicated. What is being communicated is that the child is "bad." When a child hears this, the tendency is to take it literally. You are being told that you are unworthy of love. This message is all too easily internalized by the child. It is all too easy to think that there really is something wrong with you. Sometimes parents even say outright, "I don't know what is the matter with you!"

It is likely that the level of subtle psychological violence perpetrated on children by parents, teachers, and other adults who are unconscious of their actions and the effects of these actions on the self-esteem of children far exceeds the epidemic proportions of outright physical and psychological abuse of children in our society and influences generation after generation of people in terms of how they feel about themselves and what they conceive of as possible in their lives. We carry around the scars of such treatment in the form of a lot of missed connections. We try to compensate in many ways in order to feel good deep in our hearts. But until the wounds are healed rather than covered over and denied, our efforts are not likely to result in wholeness or health. They are more likely to result in disease. We have already seen quite a few examples of this.

A MODEL OF CONNECTEDNESS AND HEALTH

Dr. Gary Schwartz, a psychologist formerly at Yale University and now at the University of Arizona, has proposed a model that attributes the ultimate origin of disease to disconnectedness and of health to connectedness. His model is based on a systems perspective, which, as we have seen in Chapter 12, considers complex systems of any kind as "wholes" rather than reducing the whole to its component parts and only considering the parts in isolation. Dr. Schwartz's model is an example of how the new paradigm in science is finding expression within medicine.

We saw in Chapter 12 that living systems maintain inner balance, harmony, and order through their capacity to self-regulate via feedback loops between particular functions and systems. We saw that heart rate varies with the degree of muscle exertion, and our eating as a function of hunger. Self-regulation is the process whereby a system maintains *stability* of functioning and at the same time, *adaptability* to new circumstances. It includes regulating the flow of energy in and out of the system and the use of that energy to maintain the living system's organization and integrity in a complex and ever-changing dynamic state as it interacts with the environment. In order to achieve and maintain a condition of self-regulation, the individual parts of the system need to relay information about their status to the other parts of the system with which they interact. That information can be used to regulate, in other words selectively control, the functioning of the network of individual parts to maintain overall balance of energy flow within the system as a whole.

Dr. Schwartz uses the term *disregulation* to describe what happens when a normally integrated self-regulating system, such as a human being, becomes imbalanced with regard to its feedback loops. Disregulation follows as a consequence of a disruption or *disconnection* of essential feedback loops. A disregulated system loses its dynamic stability, in other words its inner balance. It tends to become less rhythmic and more *disordered* and is then less able to use whatever feedback loops are still intact to restore itself. This disorder can be seen in the behavior of the system as a whole and by observing its component parts in interaction. The disordered behavior of a living system such as a person is usually described medically as a *disease*. The specific disease will depend on which particular subsystems are most disregulated.

Dr. Schwartz's model emphasizes that one major cause of disconnection in people is *disattention*, that is, not attending to the relevant feedback messages of our body and our mind that are necessary for their harmonious functioning. In his model, disattention leads to disconnection; disconnection to disregulation; disregulation to disorder; and disorder to disease.

Conversely, and very importantly from the point of view of healing, the process can work in the other direction as well. *Attention leads to connection; connection to regulation; regulation to order; and order to ease* (as opposed to dis-ease), *or more colloquially, to health.* So, without going into all the physiological details of our feedback loops, we can simply say that the quality of the connections within us and between us and the outside world determine our capacity for self-regulation and healing. And the quality of those connections is maintained and can be restored by paying attention to relevant feedback.

So it becomes important to ask, what does relevant feedback mean? What does it look like? Where should we be putting our attention in order to move from disease toward "ease," from disorder toward order, from disregulation toward self-regulation, from disconnectedness toward connectedness? Some concrete examples may help you to grasp the simplicity and power of this model in practical terms and relate it to the meditation practice.

When your whole organism, your body and your mind to-
gether, is in a relatively healthy state, it takes care of itself without
too much attention. For one thing almost all of our self-regulatory
functions are under the control of the brain and the nervous system
and are ordinarily occurring without our conscious awareness. And
we would hardly want to control them consciously for any length of
time, even if it were possible. It would leave us no time for anything
else.

The beauty of the body is that ordinarily our biology takes care
of itself. Our brain is continually making adjustments in all of our
organ systems in response to the feedback it gets from the outside
world and from the organs themselves. But some vital functions do
reach our consciousness and can be attended to with awareness.
Our basic drives are one example. We eat when we are hungry. The
message in the "hungry" feeling is feedback from the organism. We
eat, and then we stop eating when we are full. The message in the
"full" feeling is feedback from the body that it has had enough.
This is an example of self-regulation.

If you eat for other reasons than because your body is producing a "hungry" message, perhaps because you are feeling anxious or
depressed, emotionally empty or unfulfilled, and you seek to fill
yourself in any way you can, a lack of attention to what you are
doing and the consequences of it may throw your system out of
regulation, especially if it becomes a chronic behavior pattern. You
might wind up eating compulsively, overriding the feedback messages from the body telling you that it has had enough. The simple
process of eating when hungry and stopping when full can become
highly disregulated in this way and lead to disease, the so-called
"eating disorders" now so common in postindustrial societies.

Pain and feeling sick are also messages that should cause us to
pay attention, since they connect us to important needs of the
organism. For example, if our response to stomach pain from
repeatedly eating certain foods, from stress or from too much
alcohol or smoking is simply to take antacids and continue to live in
the same old way, we are not heeding this highly relevant message
from our own body. Instead, we are unknowingly disconnecting
from the body, overriding its efforts to restore balance and order.
On the other hand, when we attend to such a message, we are likely
to modify our behavior in some way or other in order to seek relief
and restore regulation and order to the system. We will return to the
whole question of paying appropriate attention to our body's messages in Chapter 21.

When we seek help from doctors, they become part of our feedback system. They pay attention to our complaints and to what they can detect in our bodies using their diagnostic tools. Then they prescribe whatever treatments they believe appropriate to reconnect the feedback loops within the organism so that it can self-regulate once again. And what we tell them about the effects of their treatment gives *them* feedback that might cause them to modify their approach, since we are usually closer to what is happening within our body than they are.

We function relatively well without awareness because so many of our connections and feedback loops within the body take care of themselves when we are relatively healthy. But when the system goes out of balance, *the restoring of health requires some attention to reestablish connectedness.* We must be aware of the feedback to know whether the responses we are making are moving us in a direction of health. And even when we are relatively healthy, the more we tune in and establish sensitive connections with our body, our mind, and the world, the more likely we will be able to move the system as a whole to even greater levels of balance and stability. *Since the processes of healing and "diseasing" can be thought of as happening all the time within us, their relative balance at any point in our lives may hinge on the quality of attention we bring to the experience of our body and mind and the degree to which we can establish a comfortable level of connectedness and acceptance.*

◆

Most of us are not particularly sensitive to either our body or our thought processes. This becomes all too clear when we begin to practice mindfulness. We can be surprised at how difficult it is just to listen to the body or attend to our thoughts as events. When we work systematically to bring our undivided attention to the body, as we do when we practice the body scan or the sitting or the yoga, we are literally increasing our connectedness with it. We know our body better as a result. We trust it more, we read its signals more accurately, and we know how good it can feel to be completely at one with our body in a state of deep relaxation. We also learn to regulate its level of tension intentionally, in ways that are not possible without awareness.

The same is true for our thoughts and feelings and for our relationship to the environment. When we are mindful of the process of thought itself, we can more readily catch our own lapses of mind, the inaccuracies in our thinking, and the self-subverting behaviors that often follow from them. As we have seen, the great delusion of separateness that we indulge in, coupled with our deeply conditioned habits of mind, the scars we carry, and our general level of unawareness, can result in particularly toxic and dis-regulating consequences for both our body and our mind. The overall result is that we may feel deeply inadequate when it comes to facing and living within and changing the full catastrophe of our lives.

On the other hand, the more conscious we are of the intercon-nectedness of our thoughts and feelings, our choices and our actions in the world, the more we can see with eyes of wholeness, the more effective we will be when faced with obstacles and challenges and stress.

If we wish to mobilize our most powerful inner resources to help us to move toward greater levels of health and well-being, we will have to learn how to tap into them in the face of the sometimes blistering levels of stress that we live immersed in. Toward this end, in the following section we will examine what we mean by stress in the first place. We will look at the common ways we react to it, how stress can disregulate our bodies and our very lives, and how we might make use of it to grow, to heal and to come to peace within ourselves.

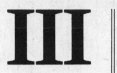

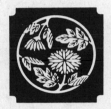

STRESS

17

Stress

The popular name for the full catastrophe nowadays is *stress*. Any concept that covers such a broad scope of life circumstances as does this particular term is bound to be somewhat complex. Yet at its heart the notion of stress is also very simple. It unifies a vast array of human responses into a single concept with which people strongly identify. As soon as I say to someone that my job is in stress reduction, the response is invariably, "Oh, I could really use that." People know exactly what it means, at least to them.

But stress occurs on a multiplicity of levels and originates from many different sources. We all have our own version of it, one which may be continually changing in its details while its overall pattern remains the same. In order to understand what stress is in its broadest formulation and to know how to work with it effectively under many different circumstances, it makes sense to think about it from a systems perspective. In this chapter we will look at the origin of the concept of stress, various ways of defining it, and at a unifying principle that will help us to handle it more effectively in our own lives.

Stress can be thought of as acting on different levels, including the physiological level, the psychological level, and the social level. As you might expect, all these levels interact with each other. These multiple interactions influence the actual state of your body and mind under specific circumstances. They also influence the range of options you have for facing and coping with stressful events. For simplicity we will consider these various levels separately while keeping in mind that they are interconnected and are different aspects of one phenomenon.

Dr. Hans Selye first popularized the term *stress* in the 1950s based on his extensive physiological studies of what happens when animals are injured or placed under unusual or extreme conditions.

In its popular usage the word has become an umbrella term connoting all the various pressures we experience in life. Unfortunately, this way of using the word confuses whether stress is the *cause* of the pressures we feel or the *effect* of those pressures, or in more scientific terms, whether stress is the stimulus or the response. We often say things like "I feel stressed," which implies that stress is what we are experiencing in response to whatever is making us feel that way, and on the other hand, "I've got a lot of stress in my life," which implies that stress is an outside stimulus that causes us to feel a certain way.

Selye opted to define stress as a response, and he coined another word, *stressor,* to describe the stimulus or event that produced the stress response. He defined stress as *"the nonspecific response of the organism to any pressure or demand."* In his terminology stress is the total response of your organism (mind *and* body) to whatever stressors you experience. But the picture is further complicated by the fact that a stressor can be an internal as well as an external occurrence or event. For instance, a thought or a feeling can cause stress and therefore can be a stressor. Or, under other circumstances, that same thought or feeling might be a response to some outside stimulus and therefore be the stress itself.

The interplay of external and internal factors in identifying the ultimate cause of disease was very much in Selye's mind when he developed his theory of stress and the notion that diseases could originate from failed attempts to adapt to stressful conditions. Thirty years before the emergence of the field of psychoneuroimmunology, Selye was well aware that stress could compromise immunity and therefore resistance to infectious organisms:

> Significantly, an overwhelming stress (caused by prolonged starvation, worry, fatigue, or cold) can break down the body's protective mechanisms. This is true both of adaptation which depends on chemical immunity and of that due to inflammatory barricades. It is for this reason that so many maladies tend to become rampant during wars and famines. If a microbe is in or around us all the time and yet causes no disease until we are exposed to stress, what is the "cause" of our illness, the microbe or the stress? I think both are—and equally so. In most instances, disease is due neither to the germ as such, nor to our adaptive reactions as such, but to the inadequacy of our reactions against the germ.

The genius of Selye's insight was in emphasizing the non-specificity of the stress response. He claimed that the most interesting and fundamental aspect of stress was that the organism undergoes a generalized physiological response in its efforts to adapt to the demands and pressures it experiences, whatever they might be. Selye called this response the *General Adaptation Syndrome* and saw it as a pathway by which organisms are able to maintain fitness, even life itself, in the face of threat, trauma, and change. He emphasized that stress is a natural part of life and cannot be avoided. Yet at the same time, stress ultimately requires adaptation for the organism to survive.

Selye saw that, under certain circumstances, stress might lead to what he called *diseases of adaptation*. In other words, our actual attempts to respond to change and to pressure, no matter what their particular source, might *in themselves* lead to breakdown and disease if they are inadequate or disregulated. From this it follows that the more we can bring attention to the *effectiveness* of our efforts to cope with the stressors we experience, the more we will be able to guard against disregulation and perhaps avoid making ourselves sick or sicker.

As we saw when we discussed Dr. Seligman's studies on optimism and health, *it is not the potential stressor itself but how you perceive it and then how you handle it that will determine whether or not it will lead to stress.* We all know this from personal experience. Sometimes the slightest little thing can trigger an emotional overreaction in us, completely out of proportion to the offending event itself. This is more likely to happen at times when we are under pressure and we feel anxious and vulnerable. At other times we might be able to handle not just little annoyances but major emergencies with almost no sense of effort. At such moments you may not even realize that you are under stress. It may only be later, after the event is over, that you feel the effects of what you went through, perhaps in the form of feeling emotionally drained or physically exhausted.

To some extent our ability to cope with stressors depends on how virulent they are. At one end of the spectrum are stressors that, if not avoided, will destroy life regardless of the way we perceive them. Among these are exposure to high levels of toxic chemicals or radiation or being hit by bullets that destroy vital organs. Absorption of high enough levels of energy of any kind into the body will kill or severely damage any living thing.

At the other end of the spectrum, there are many forces that impinge on us that almost nobody finds particularly stressful. For instance, we are all continuously subjected to the gravitational pull of the earth, just as we are all continually exposed to the changing seasons and to the weather. Since gravity is always affecting us, we tend not to notice it. We are hardly aware of how we adapt to it by shifting the body from one leg to the other in the standing posture or by propping ourself up against a wall. But if you work for eight hours at a time standing in one place on a concrete floor, you will be very aware of gravity as a stressor.

Of course, unless you are an iron worker, a steeple painter, a trapeze artist, or a ski jumper, gravity is usually the least of your stress problems. But it illustrates the point that some stressors are unavoidable and that we are continually adapting to the demands they place on our body. As Selye pointed out, such stressors are a natural part of living. The example of gravity reminds us that, in and of itself, stress is neither good nor bad, it's just the way things are.

In the vast middle range of stressors, where exposure is neither immediately lethal, like bullets or high-level radiation or poison, nor basically benign, like gravity, the general rule for those causing psychological stress is that *how you see things and how you handle them makes all the difference in terms of how much stress you will experience*. You have the power to affect the balance point between your internal resources for coping with stress and the stressors that are an unavoidable part of living. By exercising this capacity consciously and intelligently, you can control the degree of stress you experience. Moreover, rather than having to invent a new way of dealing with every individual stressor that comes up in your life, you can develop a way of dealing with change *in general*, with problems *in general*, with pressures *in general*. The first step, of course, is recognizing when you are under stress in the first place.

Much of the early research on the physiological effects of stress was carried out on animals and did not distinguish between a psychological component of the stress reaction and a physiological component. For example, Selye's critics point out that the physiological damage seen in an animal forced to swim in freezing water might be due more to the animal's terror than to purely physiological reactions to either cold or water as stressors. So Selye might have been measuring the effects of a psychological response to a harmful experience rather than a purely physiological response, as he thought. With this in mind, researchers set about to investigate the role of psychological factors in the stress response in animals as well as in people. These efforts led to the demonstration that psychological factors are an important part of an animal's response to physical stressors. In particular it has now been shown conclusively that the extent to which an animal is given options to respond effectively to a particular stressor strongly influences how much physiological disregulation and breakdown will occur as a result of exposure to a stressor. *Control,* a psychological factor, is a key factor in protecting an animal from stress-induced disease.

From everything we know about stress in human beings, the same relationship holds. (Recall that control was a major factor in the study of nursing home residents—the plant experiment described in Chapter 16, and in Dr. Kobasa's work on psychological hardiness, described in Chapter 15.) And since people usually have many more psychological options than do animals in laboratory experiments, it stands to reason that by becoming conscious of our options in stressful situations and by being mindful of the relevance and effectiveness of our responses in those situations, we may be able to exert considerable control over our experience of the stress and thereby influence whether or not it will lead to disease.

Stress studies with animals demonstrated the extreme toxicity of *learned helplessness,* a term describing a condition in which we discover that nothing we do matters. But if helplessness can be learned, it can also be unlearned, at least by people. Even if there is no actual course of *external* action we can take that will have a meaningful effect under certain extremely stressful circumstances, human beings still have profound *internal* psychological resources that can give us a sense of being engaged and in control to some degree and thereby protect us from helplessness and despair. Certainly this is suggested by Dr. Antonovsky's studies of the survivors of concentration camps.

Dr. Richard Lazarus, a prominent stress researcher, and his colleagues at the University of California at Berkeley emphasize that perhaps the most fruitful way to look at stress from a psychological point of view is to consider it as a *transaction* between a person and his or her environment. Dr. Lazarus defines psychological stress as *"a particular relationship between the person and the environment that is appraised by the person as taxing or exceeding his or her resources and endangering his or her well-being."* This means, as we have already discussed, that an event can be more stressful for one person, who for one reason or another has fewer resources for dealing with it, than for another person, who has greater coping resources. It also implies that the meaning of the transaction will determine whether a situation is labeled as stressful or not. If you appraise or interpret an event as threatening your well-being, then it will be taxing to you. But if you see it differently, then the same event might not be stressful at all, or a good deal less stressful to you.

This is good news because, given a particular situation, there are usually many ways of seeing it and many potential ways of handling it. It means that the way we see, appraise, and evaluate our problems will determine how we respond to them and how much distress we will experience. It also implies that we may have much more control over things that may potentially cause us stress than we might ordinarily think. While there will always be many potential stressors in our environment over which we cannot have immediate control, *by changing the way we see ourselves in relationship to them, we can actually change our experience of the relationship and therefore modify the extent to which it taxes or exceeds our resources or endangers our well-being.*

The transactional view of psychological stress also implies that you can be more resistant to stress if you build up your resources and enhance your physical and psychological well-being in general (via exercise and meditation, for example) during times when you are not particularly taxed or overwhelmed. The word *resources* really means that combination of inner and outer supports and strengths that helps us to cope with a changing field of experiences. Supportive family members, friends, and membership in groups that you care about are examples of external resources that could help buffer your experiences of stress. Inner resources might include your beliefs about your ability to handle adversity, your view of yourself as a person, your views on change, your religious beliefs, and your levels of stress hardiness, sense of coherence, and affiliative trust. All these can be strengthened, as we have seen, by practicing mindfulness.

Stress-hardy individuals have greater coping resources than other people under similar circumstances because they view life as a challenge and assume an active role in attempting to exert meaningful control. The same is true of people with a high sense of coherence. Strong internal convictions about the comprehensibility, manageability, and meaningfulness of life experiences are powerful internal resources. People who cultivate such strengths are less likely to feel taxed or threatened by events than someone with fewer resources of this kind. This is also true for all the other health-enhancing cognitive and emotional patterns that we looked at in Chapter 15.

If, on the other hand, our reactions to things are usually clouded by emotions of fear, hopelessness, or anger, or by underlying motives of greed and distrust, then our actions will more than likely create additional problems and dig us deeper into a hole, to the point where it may be hard for us to see our way out of what seems more and more overwhelming. We bog down and get stuck. This can lead to feelings of vulnerability and helplessness.

But Dr. Lazarus's definition also implies that for something to be psychologically stressful, it has to be appraised in some way as a threat. Yet we know from experience that there are many times when we are *unaware* of the degree to which our relationships with our inner or outer environment are taxing our resources even though they are. For example, much of our life-style may be undermining our health, exhausting us physically and mentally without our conscious acknowledgment of it. Moreover, our negative attitudes and beliefs about ourselves and others and about what is possible may also be major factors preventing us from growing or healing or taking control in times of difficulty. These, too, may be below our level of conscious awareness.

Precisely because perception and appraisal or the lack of them play such a major role in our ability to adapt and respond appropriately to change and to pain and to threats to our well-being, the major avenue available to us *as individuals* for handling stress effectively is to *understand* what we are going through. We can best do this by cultivating our ability to perceive our experience in its full context, as we did with the puzzle of the nine dots in Chapter 12. In this way, we can discern relationships and feedback that we may not have been aware of before. This allows us to see our life situation more clearly and thereby influence the level of stress associated with our habitual reactions in difficult situations. It also frees us from the tight grip of our many unconscious beliefs that ultimately inhibit our growth. So it can be particularly helpful to keep in mind from moment to moment that it is not so much the stressors in our lives but how we see them and what we do with them that determines how much we are at their mercy. If we can change the way we see, we can change the way we respond.

18

Change: One Thing You Can Be Sure Of

The concept of stress suggests that, in one way or another, we are continually faced with the necessity of adapting to all the various pressures we experience in life. Basically this means adapting to *change*. If we can learn to see change as an integral part of life and not as a threat to our well-being, we will be in a much better position to cope effectively with stress. The meditation practice itself brings us face-to-face with the undeniable experience of continual change within our own minds and bodies as we watch our constantly changing thoughts, feelings, sensations, perceptions, and impulses. This alone should be enough to demonstrate to us that we live immersed in a sea of change, that whatever we choose to focus on changes from one moment to the next, it comes and it goes.

Even inanimate material is subject to continual change: continents, mountains, rocks, beaches, the oceans, the atmosphere, the earth itself, even stars and galaxies all change over time, all evolve, and are spoken of as being born and dying. We humans live for such a brief time, relatively speaking, that we tend to think of these things as permanent and unchanging. But they are not. Nothing is.

If we consider the major forces that impinge on our lives, the first thing we will have to acknowledge is that nothing is absolutely stable, even when our lives seem to be on "an even keel." Just being alive means being in a continual state of flux. We, too, evolve. We go through a series of changes and transformations to which it is difficult to affix an exact beginning or an exact end. We emerge as discrete individuals out of a stream of preceding beings of whom our parents are only the most recent representatives. And at a certain point, usually unknown to us, our life as a discrete individual comes to an end. But unlike inanimate matter and most living things, we know the inevitability of change and of our own death. We are able to think about the changes we experience and wonder about them and even fear them.

Consider just the physical changes we go through. During our lives, the body is constantly changing. A discrete human life begins its journey as a single cell, the fertilized human egg. This microscopic entity contains all the information necessary to become a new human being. As it descends through a fallopian tube and becomes implanted in the wall of the uterus, it begins dividing: from this one cell come two; then those two divide to make four; then those four divide to make eight; and so on. As the cells continue to divide, they gradually develop from a clump into a hollow sphere. The cells at the top differentiate slightly from those at the bottom of this tiny sphere that is to become the body. The sphere grows as the cells continue to divide. As it does, it also changes its shape. It folds in upon itself, creating different layers and regions that ultimately differentiate into specialized tissues and organs with different functions: bones and nerves, muscles and skin, all the inner organs and organ systems, the eyes, ears, nose, tongue, hair, teeth.

Yet even in the body's earliest stages, death is part of the process. Some of the cells that are originally laid down to form the structures of the hands and feet die selectively to give rise to the spaces between the fingers and toes so that we don't wind up with paddles at the ends of our arms and legs. And many cells within the developing nervous system die before we are born if they don't find other cells to connect up with. Even on the cellular level, connectedness to the whole appears to be of vital importance.

By the time we are born, our body consists of over ten trillion cells, all doing their jobs, all more or less in the right place. If they are, then we come out whole, ready for the ongoing transformations we will experience during infancy, toddlerhood, preadolescence, adolescence, and young adulthood; and, if we are receptive to the idea, growth and development and learning need not stop at young adulthood. In fact there is no need for us ever to stop growing and learning.

At the far end of this seamless process, if we make it that far, our bodies grow old and die. Death is part of their nature. The life in individuals always comes to an end, even as the potential for life continues on in the flow of the genes and the emergence of new members of the family and the species.

The point is that life is constant change from the word go. Our bodies change in countless ways as we grow and develop over the course of a lifetime. So do our views of the world and of ourselves. Meanwhile the external environment in which we live is also in continual flux. In fact, nothing at all is permanent and eternal, although some things appear that way since they are changing so slowly.

◆

Living organisms have developed impressive ways of protecting themselves from all the unpredictable fluctuations in the environment and of preserving the basic internal conditions for life against too much change. The concept of inner biochemical stability was first articulated by the French physiologist Claude Bernard in the nineteenth century. He hypothesized that the body has evolved finely tuned regulatory mechanisms that are controlled by the brain and mediated by the nervous system and the secretion of hormone messenger molecules into the bloodstream to ensure that the conditions throughout the body that are necessary for the optimal functioning of its cells are maintained in spite of large fluctuations in the environment. These fluctuations may involve temperature changes, lack of food for long stretches of time, and of course threats from predators and competitors. The regulatory responses, all accomplished via feedback loops, preserve the dynamic internal balance, called *homeostasis*, by keeping the corresponding fluctuations of the organism within certain limits. Body temperature is regulated in this way, as are the concentrations of oxygen and glucose in the blood.

We have evolved drives and instincts that support homeostasis by directing our behavior to satisfy our body's needs. In this category are instincts such as thirst when the body needs water and hunger when the body needs food. Of course we can also regulate our physiological state to some extent through our own conscious actions, such as putting on or taking off clothes depending on the outside temperature or opening a window to cool things off.

So while constant change is the hallmark of the world outside the individual organism, including both the natural and the social environment, to a large extent our bodies are protected and buffered from outside changes. We have built-in mechanisms for stabilizing our "inner chemistry" in order to increase our chances of survival under changing conditions. We also have built-in repair mechanisms that allow biological mistakes to be recognized and corrected, cancer cells to be detected and neutralized, broken bones to mend, blood to clot over a wound, and wounds to seal over and heal.

These regulatory pathways function in response to specific signals within the organism, our body's inner chemical language. We never have to think about our liver chemistry. Fortunately for us it self-regulates. We never have to think about taking the next inbreath; it takes care of itself. We don't have to remind the pituitary to secrete growth hormone on a certain schedule so that we grow to be the right size in adulthood. And when we are cut or injured, we don't have to think about making the blood clot to form a scab or making the skin heal underneath.

On the other hand, if we abuse the system too much, say by drinking more alcohol than the body can tolerate, then later on we may wind up having to give some thought to our liver. But by that point it may be disregulated beyond repair. The same goes for smoking and the lungs. Even with elaborate repair capabilities and built-in protective and purifying systems, the body can take only so much abuse before it is overwhelmed.

◆

We may find it comforting to know that our bodies have very robust and resilient built-in mechanisms, developed over millions of years of evolution, for maintaining stability and vitality in the face of constant change. This biological resilience and stability is a major ally when it comes to facing stress and change in our lives. It helps us to remember that we have every reason to trust our bodies and to work in harmony with them and not against them.

As we have seen, Hans Selye emphasized that a stress-free life is impossible, that the very process of being alive means that there will be wear and tear associated with the need to adapt to a changing outer and inner environment. The question that concerns us is, How much wear and tear does there have to be?

In the 1960s researchers began to investigate whether there was a relationship between how much change a person goes through in a year and what happens to his or her health at later times. Drs. Thomas Holmes and Richard Rahe of the University of Washington Medical School listed a number of life changes, including the death of a spouse, divorce, imprisonment, personal injury or illness, getting married, getting fired from work, retirement, pregnancy, sexual problems, death of a family member or close friend, change in line of work or work responsibilities, taking out a mortgage, outstanding personal achievement, change in living conditions, change of personal habits, going on vacation, and getting a traffic ticket. They ordered these "life events" in terms of what they thought was the degree of adjustment they would require and gave them arbitrary numerical values, starting with 100 for death of a spouse and going down to 11 for a minor violation of the law. They found that a high score on their life-change index was associated with a higher probability of illness in the following year than a low score. This suggested that change itself could predispose a person to illness.

Many of the life changes on their list, such as getting married, getting promoted, or having an outstanding personal achievement, are usually considered "happy" occasions. They are included because even events that may appear "positive" are nevertheless profound life changes that require adaptation and are therefore stressful. In Selye's terminology they are examples of *eustress,* or "good stress." Whether they later lead to *distress* depends in large measure on how you adapt to them, which hinges on what they really mean to you and whether that meaning changes over time. If you adjust easily, then the eustress is relatively harmless and benign; it does not threaten to tax or overwhelm your ability to handle the changes. But it is all too easy to see how a positive life change might turn from eustress to distress if you have a hard time adjusting to your new circumstances.

For instance, you may have been looking forward to retirement for years and be happy at first when it comes and you can finally stop getting up early and going to work. But after a while you may not know what to do with all the time you have. You may come to miss the connectedness you felt when you were working. Unless you are forming new connections and finding new opportunities for meaning in your life, you may be failing to *adapt* to this major life change and it could wind up being a source of stress for you even though you couldn't wait for it to happen.

The high divorce rate in our society attests to the fact that the happy occasion of marriage can also lead to major distress and suffering. This is particularly so if the initial match was less than compatible or if the individuals are unable to adjust to the changes associated with living together, including, of course, allowing for your own and the other person's growth and change. The stress on a marriage is compounded if the couple is unable to adjust to the enormous demands of parenthood and the changes in roles and life-style that it brings. The eustress of having children can easily turn to distress and worse. The same is true of job promotions, graduating from school, aging, and all other positive life changes. They require adapting to the change itself.

The meaning that life changes have for you will strongly depend on their total context. If your spouse has been suffering from a long, wasting illness or if your relationship to that person has been one of extended misery or exploitation or alienation, then the meaning of his or her death may be very different and the difficulty of adjusting to it also very different than if the death occurred suddenly and the relationship was extremely close. Assigning "death of a spouse" a score of 100 in all cases, as Drs. Holmes and Rahe did, does not take into account the *meaning* of the experience for the surviving spouse and the degree of adjustment or adaptation that he or she will have to make as a result.

It is not only the major turning points in our lives that require us to adapt. Every day we face a range of moderately important to trivial obstacles and occurrences with which we have to deal, whether we want to or not, and which we may turn into much larger problems than they need to be if we lose our perspective and balance of mind.

◆

The ultimate effect on our health of the total psychological stress we experience depends in large measure on how we come to perceive change itself, in all its various forms, and how skillful we are in adapting to continual change while maintaining our own inner balance and sense of coherence. This in turn depends on the meaning we attribute to events, on our beliefs about life and ourselves, and particularly on how much awareness we can bring to our usually mindless and automatic reactions when our "buttons" are pushed. It is here, in our mind-body reactions to the occurrences in our lives that we find stressful, that mindfulness most needs to be applied and where its power to transform the quality of our lives can best be put to work.

19

Stuck in Stress Reactivity

Human beings are actually remarkably resilient to stress. One way or another we manage to persevere, to survive, and to have our moments of pleasure, peace, and fulfillment. We are expert copers and problem solvers. We cope through prayer and religious beliefs, through involvements and diversions that feed our needs for joy and belonging and for stepping outside of ourselves. We cope and are buoyed up by sharing love and by receiving encouragement and support from family and friends.

At the same time, however, our physiological/psychological balance, stable though it is, can be pushed over the edge into disregulation and disorder if it is taxed beyond its limits to respond and adapt. Health can be undermined by a lifetime of ingrained behavior patterns that compound and exacerbate the pressures of living we continually face. Ultimately our automatic reactions to the stressors we encounter determine in large measure how much stress we experience. Automatic reactions, triggered out of unawareness, usually compound and exacerbate stress, making what might have remained basically simple problems into worse ones. They prevent us from seeing clearly, from solving problems creatively, from expressing our emotions effectively when we need to communicate with other people, and ultimately they prevent us from attaining peace of mind. Instead, each time we react, we stress our intrinsic balance even more. A lifetime of unconscious reactivity is likely to increase our risk of eventual breakdown and illness significantly.

Consider yourself for a moment to be the person depicted in the center of Figure 9. External stressors (small arrows on top of the figure) in the form of all the forces—biological, physical, social, economic, and political—that bear on us and that generate changes

FIGURE 9

THE STRESS-REACTION CYCLE

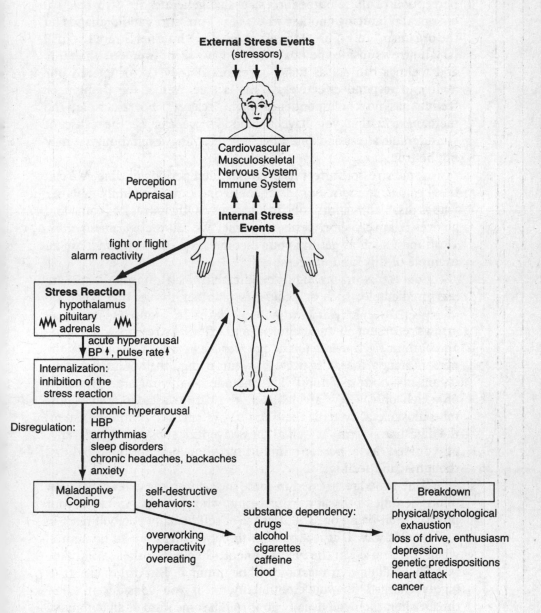

in our bodies, our lives, and our social status all impinge upon us from the outside.

From the inside our mind not only changes in response to our perception of these outer forces; it also generates its own reactive energies, producing another whole set of pressures and demands on the organism. In Figure 9 these are labeled "Internal Stress Events" (small arrows inside the box). As we have seen, even our thoughts and feelings can act as major stressors if they tax or exceed our ability to respond effectively. This is true even if the thought or feeling has no correspondence with "reality." For example, the mere *thought* that you have a fatal disease can be the cause of considerable stress and could become disabling, even though it may not be true.

Some stressors affect us over extended periods of time. We call these *chronic stressors*. For instance, taking care of a family member who is disabled is a form of chronic stress. Other stressors come and go over relatively short periods of time. We call these *acute stressors*. Deadlines, such as getting your income taxes done on time, are an example of this kind of pressure.

Some stressors are highly predictable, such as taxes. Others are less predictable, such as accidents or other things that come up unexpectedly that you have to deal with. In Figure 9, the small arrows represent all these internal and external stressors, both acute and chronic, as they are felt *at any moment in time*. The figure of the person stands for all aspects of your being, the totality of your organism—body *and* mind. This includes all of your organ systems, of which only a few are labeled, the cardiovascular system, the musculoskeletal system, the nervous system, the immune system, the digestive system, as well as the conventional psychological sense of yourself as a person, including your perceptions, beliefs, thoughts, and feelings.

When you are stressed in some moment to the extent that your mind identifies a threat to your being, whether it is a threat to your physical well-being or to your sense of self, usually you will react in a particular way. If it is a passing threat or turns out to be neutral when reappraised in the next moment, then either there will be no reaction at all or your reaction will be minimal. But if the stressor is highly charged for you emotionally, or if you consider it to be threatening, then you usually go through some kind of an automatic *alarm reaction*.

The alarm reaction is our body's way of clearing the decks for defensive or aggressive action. It can help us in threatening situations to protect ourselves and to maintain or regain control. Our nervous systems are "wired" up to perform in this way under certain circumstances. The alarm reaction enables us to call on the full power of all our internal resources in life-threatening situations.

Walter B. Cannon, the great American physiologist who worked at the Harvard Medical School in the early part of this century and who coined the term *homeostasis* to describe the internal stability of our physiology, studied the physiology of this alarm reaction in a number of experimental systems. In one he studied what a cat goes through when threatened by a barking dog. Cannon termed the cat's reaction the *fight-or-flight reaction* because the physiological changes the threatened animal goes through are those that mobilize the body for fighting or fleeing.

People go through the same physiological reaction that animals do. When we feel threatened, the fight-or-flight reaction occurs almost instantly. The result is a state of physiological and psychological *hyperarousal*, characterized by a great deal of muscle tension and strong emotions, which may vary from terror, fright, or anxiety to rage and anger. The fight-or-flight reaction involves a very rapid cascade of nervous-system firings and release of stress hormones, the most well known of which is *epinephrine (adrenaline)*, which are unleashed in response to an immediate acute threat. This leads to heightened sense perceptions so that we can take in as much relevant information as possible as quickly as possible: the pupils of our eyes dilate to let in more light, the hair on our body stands erect so that we are more sensitive to vibrations. We become very alert and attentive. The output of the heart jumps by a factor of four or five by increasing the heart rate and the strength of the heart-muscle contractions (and thereby the blood pressure) so that more blood and therefore more energy can be delivered to the large muscles of the arms and legs, which will be called upon if we are to fight or run.

At the same time the blood flow to the digestive system shuts down, as does digestion itself. After all, if you are about to be eaten by a tiger, there is no point in continuing to digest food in your stomach. It will get digested in the tiger's stomach just as well if you are caught. Both fighting and running require that your muscles get as much blood as possible. You may feel this rerouting of your blood flow in times of stress as "butterflies in your stomach."

All these changes in your body and in your emotions come about because of the activation of a particular branch of what is called the *autonomic nervous system* (ANS). The autonomic nervous system is that part of your nervous system that regulates the internal states of your body such as your heart rate, blood pressure, and the digestive process. The particular branch of the ANS that is stimulated in the fight-or-flight reaction is known as the *sympathetic branch*. Its function is to speed things up. The other branch, known as the *parasympathetic branch*, acts as a brake. Its function is to slow and calm things down.

The *hypothalamus* controls the activity of both of these branches. It is the master control switch of the autonomic nervous system. The hypothalamus is a gland that is itself part of what is called the *limbic system*, a region located deep within the brain. The limbic system can be thought of as the "seat of our emotions." It has connections, through the hypothalamus, not only to the autonomic nervous system but also to the endocrine system of glands and to our musculoskeletal system. These interconnected pathways allow our emotions and our organ systems to respond in a coordinated and integrated fashion to external events.

The limbic system is responsible for, among other things, the regulation of our internal body states as well as of our emotions and drives. It is one of the major control centers of our biological regulatory mechanisms. When it triggers the sympathetic nervous system via stimulation of specific areas in the hypothalamus, the result is a massive discharge of nervous signals that influence the functioning of every organ system in our body. This is accomplished in two ways; one by direct hard-wire neuron (nerve cell) connections to all the internal organs; the other by the secretion of hormones and neuropeptides into the bloodstream. Some hormones are secreted by glands, others by nerve cells (these are called neuropeptides), others by both. These hormones and neuropeptides are chemical messengers that travel far and wide in the body to transmit information and trigger specific responses from different cell groups and tissues. When they arrive at their targets, they bind to specific receptor molecules and transmit their message. You might think of them as chemical keys, turning on or off specific control switches in the body. It may well be that all of our emotions and feeling states are dependent on the secretion of specific neuropeptide hormones under different conditions.

Some of these hormone messengers are released as part of the fight-or-flight reaction. For example, epinephrine and norepinephrine are released into the bloodstream by the *adrenal medulla* (part of the adrenal glands located on top of your kidneys) when the adrenal glands are stimulated by signals from the hypo-thalamus via sympathetic nerve pathways. These hormones give you the "rush" and sense of extra power in emergency situations that we have labeled the "Stress Reaction" in Figure 9. In addition, the pituitary gland in the brain is also stimulated when we are stressed. It triggers the release of other hormones (some from a region of the adrenal glands called the *adrenal cortex*) that are also part of the stress reaction.

◆

The story of Arnold Lemerand illustrates the remarkable power inherent in the stress reaction. A news item from the *Boston Globe,* November 1, 1980, read as follows:

> Arnold Lemerand, of Southgate, Mich., is 56 years old and had a heart attack six years ago. As a result, he doesn't like to lift heavy objects. But this week, when Philip Toth, age 5, became trapped under a cast iron pipe near a playground, Lemerand easily lifted the pipe and saved the child's life. As he lifted it, Lemerand thought to himself that the pipe must weigh 300 to 400 pounds. It actually weighed 1800 pounds, almost a ton. Afterward, Lemerand, his grown sons, reporters and police tried to lift the pipe but couldn't.

This anecdote illustrates the power of the fight-or-flight reaction and the surge of energy it provides in life-threatening situations. It also demonstrates that in an emergency you really don't stop to think. If Mr. Lemerand had thought about the weight of the pipe before he tried to lift it, or about his own heart condition, he probably would not have been able to lift it. But the necessity of action in the face of a life-threatening situation triggered an immediate state of hyperarousal in which his thinking shut down for a moment and sheer action took over. But when the threat was over, he was unable to perform the same feat, even with lots of help.

It is easy to see how the fight-or-flight reaction would increase an animal's chances of survival in a dangerous and unpredictable environment. It works the same way for us. The fight-or-flight reaction helps us to survive when we find ourselves in life-threatening situations. So it is not at all bad that we have this vital capacity. What is bad is when we can't control it or use it constructively and it starts to control us.

The fight-or-flight reaction can be triggered in animals when they encounter members of another species. It also comes into play when animals are defending their social standing within their own species and when they are challenging the social status of another animal in their group. When an animal's social position is challenged, the fight-or-flight reaction is unleashed and the two animals in question fight until one either submits or runs away. Once an animal submits to another, it "knows its place" and doesn't keep going through the same reaction every time it is challenged. It readily submits.

People have many more choices in situations of social stress and conflict, but often we get stuck in these same patterns of submission, fleeing, or fighting all the same. Our reactions in social situations are often not that different from those of animals. Yet animals of the same species seldom kill each other in social conflicts the way humans do.

Much of our stress comes from threats, real or imagined, to our social status, not to our lives. *But the fight-or-flight reaction kicks in even when there is no life-threatening situation facing us. It is sufficient for us just to feel threatened.*

By causing us to react so quickly and so automatically, the fight-or-flight reaction often creates problems for us in the social domain rather than giving us additional energy for resolving our problems. Anything that threatens our sense of well-being can trigger it to some degree. If our social status is threatened, or our ego, or our strongly held beliefs, or our desire to control things or to have them be a certain way ("my" way, for instance), then the sympathetic nervous system lets loose. We can be catapulted into a state of hyperarousal and fight-or-flight whether we like it or not.

◆

Unfortunately, hyperarousal can become a permanent way of life. Many of our patients start out describing themselves as tense and anxious "all the time." They suffer from chronic muscle tension, usually in the shoulders, the face, the forehead, the jaw, and the hands. Everybody seems to have his or her own special areas that store muscle tension. Heart rate is also frequently elevated in a state of chronic hyperarousal. You can feel shaky inside, feel "butterflies" in your stomach, feel skipped heartbeats or palpitations, or have chronically sweaty palms. The urge to flee may surface frequently, as can impulses to lash out in anger or to get into arguments and fights.

Certainly these are common responses to everyday stressful situations, not just to life-threatening ones. They come about because our body and mind react automatically to perceived threat or danger. Since the capacity to trigger a fight-or-flight reaction is part of our nature even though we do not usually run into tigers in our daily lives, and since it is liable to have major unhealthy consequences psychologically, socially, and physically if it runs out of control, it is important for us to be aware of this inner tendency and how easily it can be triggered if we hope to reverse a lifelong pattern of automatic stress reactivity. As you will see shortly, *awareness* is the critical element in learning how to free yourself from your stress reactions at those moments when your first impulse is to feel threatened and to run or take some other kind of evasive action or to fight.

♦

So what *do* we usually do in all those situations when the fight-or-flight reaction is building up inside of us but we feel unable to fight or run because both are socially unacceptable and, besides, we know neither will solve our problems? We still feel threatened, hurt, fearful, angry, resentful. We still have the stress hormones and neurotransmitters clearing the decks for fight or flight. Our blood pressure is rising, our heart is pounding, our muscles are tense, our stomach is churning.

One common way we deal with it in social situations is to suppress these feelings as best we can. We wall them off. We pretend we are not aroused. We dissimulate, hiding our feelings from others and sometimes even from ourselves. To do so, we put the arousal the only place we can think of, deep inside us. We internalize it. We inhibit the outward signs of the stress reaction and carry on as usual, holding it all inside.

The nice thing about fighting or running is that at least these activities exhaust you, so that ultimately, after the stressful situation is encountered, you rest. Your blood pressure and heart rate return to baseline, your blood flow readjusts, your muscles relax, and you move toward a state of recovery and recuperation.

When you internalize the stress reaction, you don't get the resolution that fighting or running brings. You don't peak, and you don't get the physical release and recovery afterward. Instead, you just carry the arousal around inside you, both in the form of stress hormones, which are playing havoc with your body, and in the form of your agitated thoughts and feelings.

We encounter a lot of different situations from day to day, many of which tax our resources to one degree or another. If each time we run into some aspect of the full catastrophe, our automatic response is a mini or not so mini fight-or-flight reaction, and if most of the time we inhibit its expression outwardly and just absorb its energy, by the end of the day we will be incredibly tense. If this becomes a way of life, and if we have no healthy way of releasing the built-up tension, then over a period of weeks and months and years we will more than likely drift into a perpetual state of chronic hyperarousal from which we rarely get any break and that we might even come to think of as "normal."

There is mounting evidence that chronic stimulation of the sympathetic nervous system can lead to long-term physiological disregulation, resulting in problems such as increased blood pressure, cardiac arrhythmias, digestive problems, chronic headaches, backaches, and sleep disorders, as well as to psychological distress in the form of chronic anxiety. Of course, having any of these problems creates even more stress. They all become additional stressors that just feed back on us, compounding our problems. This is shown in Figure 9 by the arrow going from these symptoms of chronic hyperarousal back to the person.

We see the results of this way of living every day in the stress clinic. People come to us when they have had enough, when they get desperate enough, when they decide that there just has to be a better way to live and to handle their problems. In the first class everybody gets to say what they are like when they are their most relaxed selves. Many say, "I can't remember, it's been so long," Or "I don't think I have ever felt relaxed!" They instantly recognize the hyperarousal syndrome sketched out in Figure 9. Many say, "This describes me to a tee."

We all use various coping strategies to keep on an even keel and to deal with the pressures in our lives. Many people cope remarkably well with extremely trying personal circumstances and have developed their own strategies for doing so. They know when to stop and take time out, they have hobbies and other interests to take their mind off of things, they give themselves advice, reminding themselves to look at things differently and not to lose perspective. People who do this tend to be the stress-hardy ones.

But many people cope with stress in ways that are actually self-destructive. These attempts at control are labeled "Maladaptive Coping" in Figure 9 because, although they do help us to tolerate stress and give us some sense of control, in the long run they wind up compounding the stress that we experience. You can think of maladaptive as meaning unhealthy, causing more stress.

One favorite maladaptive coping strategy is to deny that there is any problem at all. "Who me, tense? I'm not tense." says the denier, all the while radiating body language that speaks of stored muscle tension and unresolved emotions. For some people it takes a long time to come close to admitting to themselves that they are carrying around a lot of body armor or that they feel hurt and angry inside. It's very hard to release tension if you won't even admit it's there. And if you are challenged about your denial, strong emotions can surface that can take many forms, including anger and resentment. These are sure signs that you are resisting looking at something deeper within yourself.

However, denial doesn't have to be maladaptive. It is sometimes a good temporary way of coping with relatively unimportant problems until you can't deny them anymore. Then you have to do something else to deal with them. Sometimes denial is, sadly, the only thing that a person believes he or she can do in a very harmful situation, such as the child who is being abused and threatened with death if she divulges anything. Some of the patients we see who had such experiences as children had no other options when they were young, especially if their tormentor was a parent or someone whom they were supposed to love—and often did. This was the case for Mary, whose dilemma we discussed in Chapter 5. Denial allowed her to keep her sanity in a world of madness. But sooner or later, denial stops working and you have to come up with something else. And in the end, even if it was the best you could do at the time, there is usually a serious price to be paid for it.

There are many other unhealthy ways we try to control our stress besides denial. They are unhealthy precisely because, in one way or another, they avoid perceiving and dealing with the real problems. *Workaholism* is a classic example. If you feel stressed and dissatisfied by family life, for instance, then work can be used as a wonderful excuse for never being home. If your work gives you pleasure and you get positive feedback from colleagues, if you feel in control when you are there and you have power and status and feel productive and creative, it is easy to immerse yourself in work. It can be intoxicating and addicting, just like alcohol. And it provides a socially acceptable alibi for not being available for the family, since there is always more work to do than you can possibly get done. Some people drown themselves in their jobs. Most do it unconsciously, with all the best intentions in the world, because deep down they are reluctant to face other aspects of their lives and the need to strike a healthy balance.

Filling up your time with *busyness* is another self-destructive avoidance behavior. Instead of facing up to your problems, you can run around like crazy doing good things until your life is overflowing with commitments and obligations and you can't possibly make time for yourself. For all the running around, you may not really know what you are doing. This kind of hyperactivity sometimes functions as an attempt to hold on to the feeling of control when it seems to be slipping away.

We also love to look outside ourselves for quick fixes when we feel stressed or uncomfortable. One popular way of handling stress is to use *chemicals* to change our body-mind state when we don't like how we are feeling, or just to make our moments "more interesting." To cope with the stress and distress in our lives, we use alcohol, nicotine, caffeine, sugar, and all sorts of over-the-counter and prescription drugs. The impulse to go in this direction usually comes from a strong desire to feel different at a low moment. And we have lots of low moments. The level of substance dependency in our culture is dramatic testimony to our individual pain and our yearning for moments of inner peace.

Many people do not feel that they can get through the day, even the morning, without a cup of coffee (or two or three). Having a cup of coffee becomes a way of taking care of yourself, a way of stopping, of connecting with others or with yourself. People use coffee breaks to pace themselves as they face the demands of the day. Others use cigarettes in the same way. Cigarettes are commonly if unconsciously used to get through moments of stress and anxiety. You light up, take a deep breath, the world stops for a moment, there is a momentary sense of peace, of satisfaction, of relaxation, then you move on. Until the next stressful moment. Alcohol is another chemical means of coping with stress and with emotional pain. It offers the added elements of muscle relaxation and escape from the weight of your problems. With a few drinks inside you, life can seem more tolerable. Many people only feel optimistic, social, self-confident, and hopeful when they have been drinking. The people you drink with are likely to provide emotional and social comfort and to reinforce the idea that drinking can help you to feel in control.

Food can also be used to cope with stress and emotional discomfort in a similar way, almost as if it were a drug. Many people eat whenever they feel anxious or depressed. Food becomes a crutch for getting through uncomfortable moments and a reward for afterward. If you have a feeling of emptiness inside, it's only natural to try to fill it. Eating is an easy way to do it. At least you are literally filling yourself. The fact that it doesn't really make you feel better does not prevent people from continuing to do it. Using food for comfort can be a powerful addiction. As with any addiction it is very hard to break out of, even when you are aware of it, unless you have a strategy for doing so and the strong determination to stick with it.

People are also accustomed to using *drugs* to regulate their levels of psychological well-being. Tranquilizers are the most widely prescribed medication in the United States. They are most often prescribed for women. The message is, If you are feeling some discomfort or having trouble sleeping, or are anxious, or yelling at the kids all the time, or overreacting to little things at home or at work, "take one of these" to take the edge off things, to be your old self, to get things under control. This attitude toward the validity of using drugs as the first line of defense to regulate anxiety reactions and symptoms of stress is very prevalent in medicine. Drugs are convenient and they work. Why not use them? Why not give someone a convenient and effective way of feeling in control?

For the most part this perspective goes unquestioned in medicine. It is a tacit framework within which the daily work of medicine is conducted. Doctors are bombarded with drug advertisements in medical journals and with drug salespeople, who are always dropping off free samples of the latest drugs to try out on their patients as well as notepads, coffee cups, calendars, pens—all covered with drug names. The pharmaceutical companies make sure that medicine is practiced within a sea of highly visible drug messages.

There is nothing wrong with drugs per se. In fact, as we all know, medications play an extremely important role in medicine. But the climate that is created by aggressive advertising and sales tactics can have strong subconscious influences on the practitioners of the art, leading them to think first and foremost about *which* drug they should be prescribing rather than *whether* they should be prescribing any drug at all as the first approach to the problem.

Of course, this attitude toward drugs pervades the entire society, not just medicine. We are a drug-ingesting culture. Patients often come to the doctor with the *expectation* that they will be "given something" to help them. If they don't leave with a prescription, they might feel the doctor is not really trying to help. The over-the-counter products for pain relief, for controlling cold symptoms, and for speeding up or slowing down movement through the colon alone constitutes a multibillion-dollar industry in this country. We are inundated with messages telling us that if our body or mind is not feeling the way we would like it to feel, we should just take "X" and things will come back to "normal" and we will be in control once again.

Who could resist? Why would anyone go through the discomfort of a headache when you could take an aspirin or a Tylenol? The fact that we take drugs on many occasions just to suppress symptoms of disregulation usually goes unnoticed. We use them to avoid paying attention to the headache or the cold instead of asking ourselves whether there is a deeper pattern underneath our immediate symptoms and discomfort that might be worth attending to.

Given the prevalence of this attitude toward drugs, it is little wonder that there is an epidemic of illegal drug use in our country. The driving force among the consumers of illegal drugs is ultimately the same mind-set, namely, if you don't like things as they are, take something that will put you in a better state. When people feel alienated from the dominant social institutions and norms, they are likely to explore ways of relieving those feelings of alienation through the most convenient and immediately powerful means available. Drugs are convenient and they have very immediate effects. Illegal drug use is presently occurring at all levels of society, from the widespread use of drugs and alcohol among teenagers to the use of so-called recreational drugs, such as cocaine, among the successful strata of society to the rampant epidemics of crack and heroin in the inner cities.

Many of the ways people use chemicals, legal and illegal, for attaining a sense of control, peace of mind, relaxation, and good feelings inside themselves are, in essence, examples of maladaptive coping attempts. They are particularly unhealthy when they become habitual and when they become the only or the dominant means we employ for controlling our reactions to stress. They are maladaptive because they compound stress in the long run, even if they provide some relief in the short run. They do not help us to adapt effectively to the stressors we live with nor to the world as it is.

The fact that they ultimately add to the stress and pressure on us is indicated in Figure 9 by the arrow going from substance dependency back to the person. Reliance on chemicals easily leads to distortions in perceptions, clouding our ability to see clearly, and undermining our motivation to find healthier ways to live. In these ways, they prevent us from growing and healing.

These substances we seek out to relieve stress are also stressors on the body in their own right. Caffeine has been implicated in disregulation of blood pressure and heart rate; nicotine and the other chemicals in smoke in heart disease, cancer, and lung disease; alcohol in liver, heart and brain disease; and cocaine in cardiac arrhythmias and sudden cardiac death. All are psychologically addicting; nicotine, alcohol, and cocaine are physiologically addicting as well.

◆

A person can live for many years cycling through episodes of stress and stress reactivity followed by maladaptive attempts to keep body and mind under control, followed by more stress, followed by more maladaptive coping, as shown in Figure 9. The habits of overworking, overeating, hyperactivity, and substance dependency can keep you going for a long time. If you choose to look, it is usually evident that things are getting worse, not better. If you are in this situation, the people closest to you are probably trying to get you to see it and to admit it and seek professional help. But it is very easy to discount what other people are telling you and even to deny what your own body or mind is trying to tell you when your habits have become a way of life. They provide a certain comfort and security that you don't want to give up, even if they are killing you. Ultimately, all maladaptive coping is addictive.

As Figure 9 suggests, sooner or later the accumulated effects of stress reactivity, compounded by inadequate ways of dealing with it, lead to breakdown in one form or another. Mostly it will happen sooner rather than later because our internal resources for maintaining homeostasis can take only so much overload and abuse before they break down.

What gives out first will depend to a large extent on your

genes, on your environment, and on the particulars of your mal-adaptive life-style. The weakest link is what goes first. If you have a strong family history of heart disease, you might have a heart attack, especially if other factors that increase the risk of heart disease—such as smoking, a high-fat diet, high blood pressure, and cynical and hostile behavior toward others—are prominent features of your life.

Alternatively, you may reach a state of disregulation of immune functioning, which may make cancer of some kind the more likely outcome. Here, too, your genes, your exposure to carcinogens during your lifetime, your diet, and your relationship to your emotions might make this pathway either more or less likely. A stress-provoked drop in immune function could also lead to greater susceptibility to infectious diseases.

Any organ system could be the ultimate weak link that leads to disease. For some it might be the skin, for others the lungs, for others the cerebral vasculature leading to a stroke, for others the digestive tract or the kidneys. For others it might be an injury, such as a disk problem in the neck or lower back, made worse by an unhealthy life-style.

Whatever the actual form of the breakdown, if it does not result in death, then it is just one more major stressor that you now have to face and work with on top of all the others you already had in your life. In Figure 9, breakdown itself becomes the source of one more arrow feeding back on the person and requiring even greater adaptation.

There is another branch of the stress reaction pathway, one not depicted in Figure 9, that becomes important when a person is faced with unavoidable stress sustained over long periods of time. Examples might be caring for an elderly parent who is ill or who has Alzheimer's disease or caring for a disabled child. Here all the stressors of daily living are compounded by a whole other set of potentially overwhelming stressors associated with the long-term demands of the situation. If *adequate* short and long term strategies for adapting to the situation are not developed, the pressures of daily living can mount to the point where the person is constantly in a state of hyperarousal, reacting repeatedly to even insignificant stressors with tension, irritability, and anger. However, continued arousal with little ultimate control over the fundamental stressor can reach the point where feelings of helplessness and hopelessness begin to dominate. Rather than hyperarousal, chronic depression can set in, leading to a different spectrum of hormonal and immune system changes that, over time, can also undermine health and lead to breakdown.

Breakdown in the stress reaction pathway does not have to be primarily physical. Too much stress and not enough effective coping can lead to a depletion of psychological resources to the point where you might experience what is sometimes called a *nervous breakdown,* a feeling of being completely unable to function in your ordinary life anymore. This condition may reach the point of requiring hospitalization and drug treatment. Nowadays it is fashionable to use the word *burnout* to describe a similar state of near or total psychological exhaustion with an accompanying loss of drive and enthusiasm for the details of your life. What used to give you pleasure no longer does.

The person experiencing burnout feels alienated from work, family, and friends; nothing seems meaningful anymore. A deep depression can set in under these conditions and can lead to a loss of ability to function effectively. Joy and enthusiasm disappear. As with the physical examples of breakdown, if psychological breakdown occurs, it becomes one more major stressor that the person now has to deal with, one way or another.

This cycle of a stressor triggering a stress reaction of some kind, often accompanied by an internalizing of the stress reaction, leading to inadequate or maladaptive attempts to keep things under control, leading to more stressors, more stress reactions, and ultimately to an acute breakdown in health, perhaps even to death, is a way of life for many of us. When you are caught up in this vicious cycle, it seems that it is just the way life is, that there is no other way. You might think to yourself that this is just part of getting older, a normal decline in health, a normal loss of energy or enthusiasm or feelings of control.

But getting stuck in the stress-reaction cycle is neither normal nor inevitable. As we have already seen, we have far more options and resources for facing our problems than we usually know we have. The healthy alternative to being caught up in this self-destructive pattern is to stop *reacting* to stress and to start *responding* to it. This is the path of mindfulness in daily life.

20

Responding to Stress Instead of Reacting

And so we come back to the key importance of mindfulness. The very first and most important step in breaking free from a lifetime of stress reactivity is to be mindful of what is actually happening while it is happening. In this chapter we will look at how we do this.

Let's consider once again the situation of the person in Figure 9 that we analyzed in the last chapter. As we have seen, at any moment in time this person may be encountering a combination of internal and external stressors that can trigger a cascade of feelings and behaviors we have been calling the *stress reaction*. Figure 10 shows the same stress-reaction cycle as in Figure 9, but now includes an alternative pathway, which we call the *stress response*, to distinguish it from the automatic stress reaction. The stress response is the healthy alternative to the stress reaction. It represents collectively what we call *adaptive*, or healthy, coping strategies as opposed to maladaptive attempts to cope with stress.

You do not have to go the route of the fight-or-flight reaction nor the route of helplessness every time you are stressed. You can actually choose not to. This is where mindfulness comes in. Moment-to-moment awareness allows you to exert control and to influence the flow of events at those very moments when you are most likely to react automatically and plunge into hyperarousal and maladaptive attempts to cope.

By definition, stress reactions happen automatically and unconsciously. As soon as you bring awareness to what is going on in a stressful situation, you have already changed that situation dramatically, just by virtue of not being unconscious and on automatic pilot anymore. You are now fully present while the stressful event is

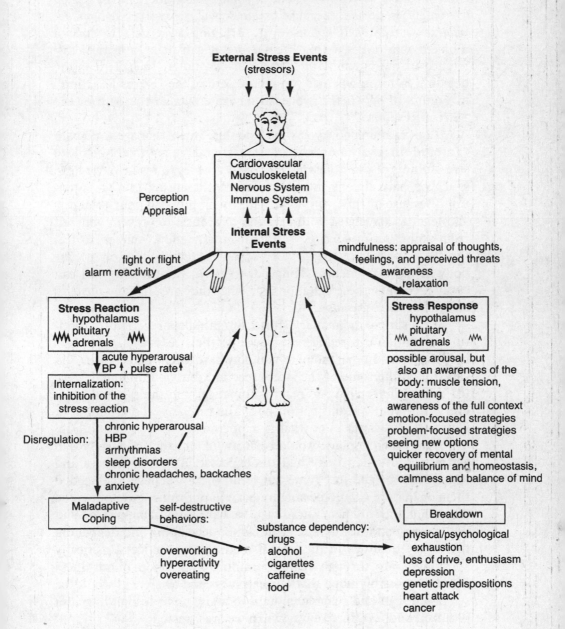

FIGURE 10

**COPING WITH STRESS:
RESPONDING VS. REACTING**

unfolding. And since *you* are an integral part of the *whole* situation, *by increasing your level of awareness, you are actually changing the entire situation, even before you do anything.* This inner change can be extremely important because *it gives you a range of options for influencing what will happen next.* Bringing awareness to such a moment only takes a split second but it can make a critical difference in the outcome of a stressful encounter. In fact, it is the deciding factor in whether you go the path of the "Stress Reaction" in Figure 10 or whether you can navigate over to the path of the "Stress Response."

Let's examine how you would do this. If you manage to remain centered in that moment of stress and recognize both the stressfulness of the situation *and* your impulses to react, as we have said, you have already introduced a new dimension into the situation. Because of this, you don't have to suppress all your thoughts and feelings associated with heightened arousal to prevent yourself from going out of control. You can actually allow yourself to feel threatened or fearful or angry or hurt and to feel the tension in your body in these moments. Being conscious in the present, you can easily recognize these agitations for what they are, namely *thoughts and feelings and sensations.*

This simple momentary shift from mindless reaction to mindful recognition can reduce the power of the stress reaction and its hold over you. In that moment you now have a very real choice. You can still go the route of the stress reaction, but you no longer have to. You no longer have to react automatically in the same old way every time your buttons get pushed. You can *respond* instead out of your greater awareness of what is happening.

This inner response would be an awful lot to ask of ourselves in a stressful situation if we had the expectation that awareness and centeredness could just come out of nowhere whenever we needed them or that we should be able to just *will* our mind and body to be calm when they are not. But in fact, we have been training mind and body to respond in this way right along, developing and deepening these very qualities in the formal meditation practice. Practically speaking, only through regular training to develop mindfulness could we possibly hope that our calmness and awareness would be strong enough and reliable enough to assist us in responding in a balanced and imaginative way when we are stressed.

The capacity to respond mindfully develops each time we experience discomfort or pain or strong feelings during meditation and we just observe them and work at letting them be there as they are, without reacting. As we have seen, the practice itself grounds us in alternative ways of seeing and responding to reactive states within ourselves, moment by moment. It introduces us to an entirely different kind of control. We come to see from our own experience that effective control can come out of inner calmness, acceptance, and openness; that we don't have to struggle with our thoughts and feelings or force things to be as we want them to be.

One thing is certain. We know where the fight-or-flight reaction will lead if it is left to play itself out automatically. We have been on that route most of our lives. The challenge now is for us to realize that at any moment we are in a position to actually decide to do things differently.

Choosing to go the route of the stress response obviously does not mean that you will never feel threatened or fearful or angry or that you will never do anything silly or self-destructive. What it does mean is that you might be more aware of those feelings and impulses more of the time when they are present. Your awareness may or may not temper the intensity of the arousal you feel. That will depend on the circumstances. But in general, awareness either reduces arousal at the time or it helps you to recover from it more quickly afterward. This is indicated in Figure 10 by the smaller "squiggles" in the box labeled "Stress Response" as compared with the box labeled "Stress Reaction."

In many situations, emotional arousal and physical tension are totally appropriate. At other times they may be inappropriate. In either case, how you handle them will depend on your degree of awareness.

In some situations, your feeling threatened may have more to do with your state of mind than with the triggering event itself. When you bring awareness to stressful moments, you might see more clearly how your own unbalanced view could be contributing to an inappropriate overreaction on your part, one that is out of proportion to what the actual circumstances warrant. Then you might remind yourself to try letting go of your own self-limited view, right in that moment, just to see what would happen. You might try trusting that things will become more harmonious if you make the effort to meet the situation with calmness and clarity. Why not test this possibility for yourself once or twice? What do you have to lose?

When you experiment in this way, you may be surprised at how many things that used to "push your buttons" no longer get you aroused. They may no longer even seem stressful to you, not because you have given up and have become helpless and defeated or resigned but because you have become more relaxed and trusting of yourself. Responding in this way under pressure is an empowering experience. You are maintaining your own balance of mind and of body, what is sometimes called maintaining your *center*.

◆

How do we consciously cultivate the stress response in daily life? The same way we cultivate mindfulness in the formal meditation practice: moment by moment, grounding ourselves in our body and in our breathing. When your buttons are pushed or you find yourself feeling stressed, when feelings of fight or flight come up, you might try bringing your awareness to your face and shoulders as they tense up, to your heart beginning to pound, to your stomach beginning to feel funny, to whatever you might notice about how your body feels at that moment. See if you can be aware of your feelings of anger or fear or hurt as you feel them rising inside of you. You might even try saying to yourself, "This is it" or "Here is a stressful situation" or "Now is a time to tune in to my breathing and center myself." Mindfulness sets the stage for you to respond appropriately right here in the moment. If you are quick enough, you can sometimes catch the stress reaction before it develops completely and turn it into a response instead.

It takes practice to catch stress reactions as they are happening. But don't worry. If you are like most of us, you will have plenty of opportunities to practice. When you are willing to bring awareness to them, each situation you encounter becomes another occasion for you to practice responding instead of reacting. You can be certain that you won't be able to respond to *every* situation. It is unrealistic to expect that of yourself. But just by *trying* to bring a larger view to each one of these moments, you are transforming the stressors into challenges and passageways for growth. The stressors now become like the wind, here for you to use to propel you where you want to go. As with any wind, you may not be able to "control" the entire situation, but you will be in a good position either to work with it creatively and put its energies to work for you or to protect yourself better from it.

◆

The place to start, of course, is with your breathing. If you can manage to bring your attention to your breathing for even the briefest moment, it will set the stage for facing that moment and the next one mindfully. The breath itself is calming, especially when we can tune in to it at the belly. It's like an old friend; it anchors us, gives us stability, like the bridge piling anchored in bedrock as the river flows around it. Or, alternatively, it can remind us that ten or twenty feet below the agitated surface of the ocean there is calmness.

The breath reconnects you with calmness and awareness when you lose touch momentarily. It brings you to an awareness of your body in that moment, including any increase in muscle tension. It can also remind you to check your thoughts and feelings. Perhaps you will see how reactive they are. Perhaps you will question their accuracy.

In maintaining your own center in the face of stress, it is much more likely that, right in that moment, you will have an awareness of the full context of the situation, whatever it is. Your impulses to run or fight, to struggle or protect yourself or perhaps to fall apart will be seen within this larger picture along with all other relevant factors in that moment. Perceiving things in this way allows you to remain more calm from the start or to recover your inner balance more quickly if it is thrown off initially by your reaction. One executive who completed the stress clinic put the nine dot puzzle (see Chapter 12) in a prominent place on the wall in her office to remind her to remember to look for the whole context when she feels stressed at work.

When you are grounded in calmness and moment-to-moment awareness, you are more likely to be creative and to see new options, new solutions to problems. You are more likely to be aware of your emotions and less likely to be carried away by them. It will be easier for you to maintain your balance and sense of perspective in trying circumstances.

If the original cause of your stress has already passed, you will be more likely to see that, at that moment, whatever has happened has *already* happened. It is already in the past. This perception frees you to put your energies into facing the present and dealing with whatever problems require your immediate attention.

When you channel your energies in this way, you will experience a quicker recovery of your mental equilibrium, even in very stressful situations, and also of your physiological equilibrium (what we have been calling homeostasis) as your bodily reactions calm down. Notice in Figure 10 that, unlike the path of the stress reaction, *the stress response doesn't generate more stress*. It doesn't feed back more stress arrows onto the person. You respond and then it's finished. You move on. The next moment will have less carryover from the preceding ones because you faced them and dealt with them when they came up. Responding mindfully to stress from moment to moment will minimize the tension that we allow to build up inside of us, thereby reducing our need to cope with the discomfort that accompanies internalized tension.

Having an alternative way of handling pressure can reduce our dependence on the common maladaptive coping strategies we so often resort to and get stuck in when we feel tense. One returning graduate of the stress clinic said at the end of an all-day session that she figured out that her strongest impulses to go for a cigarette lasted about three seconds. She noticed that a few breaths took about the same time. So she thought she would try bringing awareness to her breathing and just ride the wave of her impulse, watching it crest and then fall, without taking the cigarette. She hasn't had a cigarette now in two and a half years.

As relaxation and peace of mind become more familiar to you through the formal meditation practice, it becomes easier to call upon them when you need them. When you are stressed, you can allow yourself to ride the waves of the stress. You will neither have to shut if off nor run away. True, you may be going up and down some, but much less than if you are always at the mercy of your own automatic reactivity.

◆

Each week people in the stress clinic come to class with anecdotes—sometimes inspiring, sometimes amusing—of the ways in which they found themselves handling stress differently than before. Phil reported he used the stress response to successfully control his back pain and concentrate better when he took his exams to become an insurance salesman; Joyce was able to remain calm in the hospital and deal with her anxious feelings about her surgery by reminding herself to breathe; Pat actually used it to stay collected and cope with the humiliation of the police coming to her house and taking her off in the middle of the night in front of her neighbors because, it turned out, her psychiatrist was going away for the weekend and mistakenly thought from a phone conversation that Pat was suicidal; Janet, the young doctor described in the introduction, was able to control her nausea and fear and to fly medical missions in the helicopter; Elizabeth decided to just remain silent when her sister started in on her with her usual hostility rather than being hostile in return. It surprised her sister so much that they started talking about it, which led to their first good communication in years.

Doug was involved in an automobile accident in which no one was hurt. The accident was not his fault. He said that previously, he would have been furious at the other driver for ruining his car and for the inconvenience it caused him on a very busy day. Instead he just said to himself, "No one was hurt, it has already happened, let's go from here." So he tuned in to his breathing and proceeded, with a calmness that was totally uncharacteristic of him, to deal with the details of the situation.

Marsha drove her husband's new van to the hospital for her stress class one night. The last thing her husband said to her before she left was "For God's sake, be careful with the van." And she was. She drove very carefully all the way to the hospital. And to make sure the van would be safe during the class, she thought she would park it in the garage rather than in one of the open lots. So she drove into the garage. As she did so, she heard a funny noise coming from the top of the van. Too late. The low overhang at the entrance had sheared off the skylight bubble on the top of the van, which she had forgotten about. For a second, when she realized what she had done and what her husband's reaction was going to be, she almost panicked. Then she laughed instead and said to herself, "The damage is done. I don't believe I did this, but it's already done." So she came to class and told us about it and how surprised she was that she was able to control her panic, be calm, see the humor in it, and realize that her husband would just have to accept that it had happened.

Keith reported that he discovered he could meditate at the dentist's. Usually he was terrified of going and always put it off until he just had to go because of the pain. He found himself focusing on his breathing and the feeling of his body sinking into the chair. He found he could do it even as the dentist was drilling in his mouth. Instead of being white-knuckled, he was calm and centered. He was astonished at how well this worked for him.

♦

In Part IV we will be discussing in detail a range of applications of mindfulness practice. There you will find many more examples of people who were able to see and to cope with things differently after they learned to respond to stress instead of reacting to it.

Perhaps by this point, if you have been practicing on your own, you may be finding that you are also responding differently in some ways to the pressures and problems in your own life. This, of course, is what is most important!

Greater resilience in the face of stressors and reduced stress reactivity are characteristic of people who practice meditation regularly. This has been demonstrated in a number of studies. Drs. Daniel Goleman and Gary Schwartz showed in the early 1970s at Harvard that meditators not only had a heightened sensitivity and emotional involvement compared with nonmeditators when both were shown a very graphic film of industrial accidents; they also recovered their physical and mental equilibrium much more quickly afterward than did nonmeditators.

In a study by Dr. Dean Ornish and his colleagues, to be discussed in more detail in Chapter 31, people with documented coronary heart disease who completed a twenty-four-day intensive lifestyle-change program that involved a low-fat, low-cholesterol vegetarian diet and daily meditation and yoga practice greatly reduced their previously elevated blood pressure responses to a range of tasks inducing psychological stress—such as doing mental arithmetic under time pressure—whereas people in a control group who did not change their diet or practice these techniques did not show a lowered blood-pressure reactivity to stress when retested. While, as we have seen, it is normal for blood pressure to go up when we are stressed, it is remarkable that the people who went through the program were able to change their stress reactivity so dramatically within such a short time.

◆

As we have seen, the fact that you can learn to respond to stress with awareness does not mean that you will never react anymore or that you will not sometimes be overwhelmed by anger or grief or fear. We are not trying to suppress our emotions when we respond to stress. Rather we are learning how to work with all our reactions, emotional and physical, so that we may be less controlled by them and see more clearly what we should do and how we might respond effectively. What occurs in any particular situation will depend on the seriousness of what is happening and on its meaning to you. You cannot develop one plan in advance that will be your strategy in all stressful situations. Responding to stress requires moment-to-moment awareness, taking each moment as it comes. You will have to rely on your own imagination and you will have to trust in your ability to come up with new ways of seeing and responding in every moment. You will be charting new territory every time you encounter stress in this way. You will know that you no longer want to *react* in the old way, but you may not know what it means to *respond* in a new and different way. Each opportunity you get will be different. The range of options available to you will depend on the circumstances. But at least you will have all your resources at your disposal when you encounter the situation with awareness. You will have the freedom to be creative. When you cultivate mindfulness in your life, your ability to be fully present can come through even under the most trying of circumstances. It will cradle and embrace the full catastrophe itself. Sometimes this will reduce your pain and sometimes it may not. But awareness brings comfort of a certain kind even in the midst of suffering. We could call it the comfort of wisdom and inner trust, the comfort of being whole.

IV

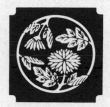

THE APPLICATIONS: TAKING ON THE FULL CATASTROPHE

21
Working with Symptoms: Listening to Your Body

The relief of symptoms of various kinds is a multibillion-dollar industry. The slightest sniffle, headache, or stomach-ache sends people scurrying to the medicine cabinet or drugstore in search of the magic something to make it go away. There are over-the-counter medications to make the digestive tract slow down, others to make it speed up, others to relieve heartburn or neutralize excess stomach acid. With a prescription from a physician, you can obtain drugs to reduce anxiety, such as Valium and Xanax, and drugs to relieve pain, such as Percodan. Tranquilizers, such as Valium and Xanax, and drugs that decrease the secretion of stomach acid, such as Tagamet and Zantac, are among the most prescribed medications in the country. They are used primarily to relieve symptoms of discomfort and they work very well in most instances. But the trouble with the widespread use of many such drugs is that the underlying problems that are producing the symptoms may not be getting addressed just because the symptoms are temporarily relieved.

This practice of immediately going for a drug to relieve a symptom reflects a widespread attitude that symptoms are inconvenient, useless threats to our ability to live life the way we want to live it and that they should be suppressed or eliminated whenever possible. The problem with this attitude is that what we call symptoms are often the body's way of telling us that something is out of balance. They are feedback about disregulation. If we ignore these messages or, worse, suppress them, it may only lead to more severe symptoms and more serious problems later on. What is more, the person doing this is not learning how to listen to and trust his or her body.

Before people begin the stress reduction program, they fill out a questionnaire in which they check off from a list of over a hundred common physical and emotional symptoms those they have experienced as problematic in the preceding month. They do the same thing again after completing the stress clinic program eight weeks later.

We observe some interesting things when we compare these two symptom lists. First, most people come into the program with a relatively high number of symptoms. The average number of symptoms is 22 out of about 110 possible ones. That is a lot of symptoms. When people leave, they are checking off on the average about 14 symptoms, or 36 percent fewer symptoms than when they started. This is a dramatic reduction in a short period of time, especially for people who have that many symptoms in the first place and have had them for quite a long time.

You might wonder whether this reduction in the number of symptoms is a nonspecific effect of having some attention paid to them, since it is well known that people can feel better temporarily when they receive almost any kind of professional attention in a medical setting. You might ask whether perhaps the reduction in symptoms is just due to their coming to the hospital every week and being part of a positive group setting rather than to anything special that they are doing in the stress clinic, such as practicing meditation.

While that is a credible supposition, in this case it is unlikely. The participants in the stress clinic have been receiving professional attention from the health care system right along for their problems. On the average, the chief medical complaint for which they are referred to us has been a problem for them for about seven years. It is unlikely that just coming to the hospital and being in a room full of other people with chronic medical problems and having attention paid to them would, by itself, result in these substantial reductions in their symptoms. But certainly one element contributing to their improvement might well be that they are challenged to do something for themselves for a change to enhance their own health. This facet of their experience in the stress clinic is a radical departure from the passive role most people assume or are forced into during treatment in the health care system.

Another reason to suspect that the symptom reduction we see among the participants in the stress clinic results from something that people actually *learn* in the program is that the reduction is maintained and even improves further after people leave. We know this from several follow-up studies in which we obtained information from over four hundred people at different times for up to four years after they completed the program.

We also know from these studies that over 90 percent of the people who complete the program say that they are keeping up their meditation practice in one form or another for up to four years after they graduate. Most rate their training in the stress clinic as very important to their improved health status.

◆

Although we see dramatic symptom reduction during the eight weeks, we actually focus very little on symptoms in the classes, and when we do, it is not to try to reduce them or make them go away. For one thing, the classes are a mix of people with many different medical problems. Each person has an entirely different and unique constellation of symptoms and concerns as well as a specific medical treatment plan. In a room with twenty to thirty-five people, all of whom are anxious and concerned about their symptoms and wanting to get rid of them, to focus primarily on the details of each person's situation would simply encourage self-preoccupation and illness behavior. Our minds being what they are, such a forum would in all likelihood give rise to never-ending discussions of what is "the matter" rather than on personal transformation. This avenue would be of little real benefit to the participants except for the sympathy and group support it would evoke, which, while certainly therapeutic, are unlikely to lead to profound changes in either view or behavior. By choosing to focus in stress clinic classes on what is "right" with people rather than on what is "wrong" with them, *without denying what is wrong,* we are able to go beyond self-involved preoccupations with the details of what is wrong and come to the heart of the matter, namely how people can begin to taste their own wholeness *as they are, right now.*

Instead of discussing symptoms as woes and how to get rid of them, when we do focus on symptoms of one kind or another it is to tune in to the actual *experience* of the symptoms themselves in those moments when they dominate the mind and body. We do this in a particular way, which might be called giving them *wise attention.* Wise attention involves bringing the stability and calm of mindfulness to our symptoms and to our reactions to them. We call it "wise" to distinguish it from the usual type of attention we pay to our problems and crises.

For example, when you have a serious chronic illness, it is only to be expected that you will be very concerned and preoccupied, perhaps even frightened and depressed about the ways in which your body has changed from what it once was and about what new problems you might have to face in the future. The result is that a lot of a certain kind of attention is spent on your symptoms, but it is not helpful or healing attention. It is the opposite of wise attention. More often than not, it is reactive, judgmental, fearful, and self-preoccupied.

The way of mindfulness is to accept ourselves right now, as we are, symptoms or no symptoms, pain or no pain, fear or no fear. Instead of rejecting our experience as undesirable, we ask, "What is this symptom saying, what is it telling me about my body and my mind right now?" We allow ourselves, for a moment at least, to go right into the full-blown feeling of the symptom. This takes a certain amount of courage, especially if the symptom involves pain or a chronic illness, or fear of death. But you can at least "dip your toe in" by trying it just a little, say for ten seconds, just to move in a little closer for a clearer look.

As we do this we may also become aware of our feelings *about* the symptom as they emerge. If there is anger or rejection or fear or despair or resignation, we look at that as well, as dispassionately as possible. Why? For no other reason than that *it is here now*. It is already part of our experience. To move to greater levels of health and well-being, we have to start from where we actually are today, in this moment, not from where we would like to be. Movement toward greater health is only possible because of now, because of where we are. So looking closely at our symptoms and our feelings about them and coming to accept them as they are is of utmost importance.

In this light, symptoms of illness or distress, plus your feelings about them, can be viewed as messengers coming to tell you something important about your body or about your mind. In the old days, if a king didn't like the message he was given, he would sometimes have the messenger killed. This is tantamount to suppressing your symptoms or your feelings because they are unwanted. Killing the messenger and denying the message or raging against it are not intelligent ways of approaching healing. The one thing we don't want to do is to ignore or rupture the essential connections that can complete relevant feedback loops and restore self-regulation and balance. Our real challenge when we have symptoms is to see if we can listen to their messages and really hear them and take them to heart, that is, make the connection fully.

When a patient in the stress clinic tells me that he or she had a headache during the body scan or during a sitting meditation, my response might be, "All right. Now tell us how you *worked* with it."

What I am looking for is whether, if you became aware that you had a headache during the time you were meditating, you used the occasion as an opportunity to look into this experience you are calling a headache, which is often a problem for you in your life anyway, even when you aren't meditating. Did you observe it with wise attention? Did you bring mindfulness and acceptance to feeling the sensations? Did you watch your thoughts at that moment? Or did the mind jump automatically into rejection and judging, perhaps to thinking that somehow you were failing at meditation, or that you "can't" relax, or that meditation doesn't "work," or that nothing can cure your headaches?

Anybody can have any or all of these negative thoughts and many others as well. They may come in and go out of your mind at different times in reaction to the headache. As with any other reaction, the challenge here is to shift your attention so that you can see them *as thoughts* and, in doing so, welcome the headache into the present moment because it is here anyway—like it or not. Can you decipher its message by directing careful attention to how your body feels right now? Are you aware now of a mood or emotion that may have preceded your realizing that you had a headache? Was there an event that triggered it that you can identify? What are you feeling right now emotionally? Are you feeling anxious, depressed, sad, angry, disappointed, discouraged, annoyed? Are you able to be with whatever you are feeling in this moment? Can you breathe with the sensations of the headache, the pounding feeling in the temples, or whatever it is? Can you see your reactions with wise attention? Can you just watch your feelings and thoughts and see them as just feelings and thoughts? Can you catch yourself identifying with them as *"my"* feelings, *"my"* anger, *"my"* thoughts, *"my"* headache, and let go of the *"my"* and just accept the moment as it is?

When you look into the headache, seeing the constellation of thoughts and feelings, the reacting, the judging, and the rejecting of how you are feeling, the wishing to feel differently that may be going on in your mind, perhaps you will realize at a certain point that you are not your headache unless you go along with this inner process of identification, unless you yourself make it *your* headache. Maybe it is just *a* headache, or maybe it is just a feeling in the head that doesn't need a name at all right now.

The ways we use language tell us a lot about the automatic way we personalize our symptoms and illnesses. For instance, we say "I *have* a headache" or "I *have* a cold" or "I *have* a fever," when it would be more accurate to say something like "the body is headaching" or "colding" or "fevering." When we automatically and unconsciously link each symptom we experience to *I* and *my*, the mind is already creating a certain amount of trouble for us. We have to perceive this identifying with the symptom when it occurs and purposefully let go of it in order to listen more deeply to its message, free from our exaggerated reactions. By seeing the headache or the cold *as a process*, we are acknowledging that it is dynamic and not static, that is not "ours" but is rather an unfolding process that we are experiencing.

When you look into a symptom with the full power of mindfulness, whether it is muscle tension, rapid heartbeats, shortness of breath, fever, or pain, it gives you much more of a chance to remember to honor your body and listen to the messages it is trying to give you. When we fail to honor these messages, either through denial or by an inflated and self-involved preoccupation with symptoms, we can sometimes create serious dilemmas for ourselves.

Usually your body will try desperately to get its messages through to you despite the bad connection with conscious awareness. A priest described his medical history in class one day this way: Looking at it after having been practicing the meditation for a few weeks, it seemed to him that his body had been trying to get him to slow down his fast-paced, Type-A life-style by giving him headaches at work. But he didn't listen, even though the headaches got worse. So his body gave him an ulcer. But still he didn't listen. Finally it sent him a mild heart attack, which scared him so much that he started to listen. He actually said that he felt grateful for his heart attack and took it as a gift. Because, he said, it could have killed him, but it didn't. It gave him another chance. He felt this could well be his *final* chance to start taking his body seriously, to listen to its messages and honor them.

22

Working with Physical Pain: Your Pain Is Not You

The next time you hit your thumb with a hammer or bang your shin on the car door, you can perform a little experiment in mindfulness. See if you can observe the explosion of sensations and the expanding shell of screamed epithets, groans, and violent body movements that ensue. It all takes place within a second or two. In that time, if you are quick enough to bring mindfulness to the sensations you are feeling, you may notice that you stop swearing or yelling or groaning and that your movements become less violent. As you observe the sensations in the hurt area, notice how they are changing, how sensations of stinging, throbbing, burning, cutting, rending, shooting, aching, and many others may flow in rapid succession through the region, blending into each other like a play of multicolored lights projected willy-nilly on a screen. Keep following the flow of sensations as you hold the area or put ice on it or put it under cold water or hold it above your head, or whatever you are drawn to do.

In conducting this little experiment, you may notice, if your concentration is strong, a center of calmness within yourself from which you can observe the entire episode unfold. It can feel as if you are completely detached from the sensations you are experiencing, as if it were not "your" pain so much as just pain. Perhaps you felt a sense of being calm "within" the pain or "behind" the pain. If you didn't, you can always try it again the next time you are unfortunate enough to bang some part of your body really hard.

Hitting your thumb with a hammer or banging your shin on something brings on immediate pain. We use the term *acute pain* to describe pain that comes on suddenly. Acute pain is usually very intense, but it also only lasts a short while. Either it goes away by itself, as when you bang your body, or it forces you to take action of some kind to make it go away, such as seeking medical help. If you try to bring mindfulness to exactly what you are feeling in those moments when you hurt yourself accidentally, you will probably find that how you relate to the sensations you experience makes a big difference in the degree of pain you actually feel and how much you suffer. It also affects your emotions and your behavior. It can be quite a revelation to discover that you have a range of options for dealing with physical pain, even very intense pain, aside from just being automatically overwhelmed by it.

From the standpoint of health and medicine, chronic pain is a much more intractable problem than acute pain. By *chronic pain* we mean pain that persists over time and that is not easily relieved. Chronic pain can be either constant or it can come and go. It can also vary greatly in intensity, from excruciating to dull and aching.

Medicine manages acute pain far better than it does chronic pain. The underlying cause of an acute pain can usually be identified rapidly and treated, resulting in elimination of the pain. But sometimes pain persists and does not respond well to the most common remedies for pain, namely drugs and surgery. And its cause may not be well defined. If it lasts more than six months or keeps coming back over extended periods of time, then a pain problem that started out as acute is said to have become chronic. In the rest of this chapter and in the one that follows, we will be discussing chronic pain and the specific ways in which you can use mindfulness to cope with it.

◆

It is important for the reader to keep firmly in mind the fact that all patients who are referred to the stress clinic have had a full medical work-up *before* they are permitted to pursue meditation training. This is absolutely necessary in order to rule out or confirm disease processes that may require immediate medical attention. Listening to your pain includes making intelligent decisions about obtaining proper medical attention. The work of mindfulness needs to be carried out in conjunction with all the other medical treatments that may be required to relieve pain. It is not meant to be a substitute for medical treatment, but it can be a vital complement to it.

Just as we saw earlier that stress per se is not bad, it is important to remember that pain per se is not a bad thing either. Pain is one of your body's most important messengers. If you didn't feel pain, you could do great harm to your body by touching a hot stove or radiator and not even know it. Or you could have a ruptured appendix, for example, and not know that anything was the matter internally. The acute pain we experience under these and similar circumstances tells us that something is the matter. It tells us in no uncertain terms that we need to pay immediate attention and to take action in some way to rectify the situation. In one case we quickly withdraw our hand from the stove; in the other we get to a hospital as quickly as possible. The pain literally drives our actions because it is so intense.

People born without intact pain circuitry have a terrible time learning the basic safety skills that we all take for granted. Without our knowing it our experiences with physical pain over the years have taught us a great deal about the world and about ourselves and our bodies. Pain is a very effective teacher. Yet if you were to ask, my guess is that most people would say that pain is categorically "bad."

As a society we seem to have an aversion to pain, even to the *thought* of pain or discomfort. This is why we are so quick to reach for medicine as soon as we feel a headache coming on and why we shift posture as soon as a little muscle stiffness generates some discomfort. As you will see, this aversion to pain is an obstacle to learning how to live with chronic pain.

Aversion to pain is really a misplaced aversion to suffering. Ordinarily we do not make a distinction between pain and suffering, but there are very important differences between them. Pain is a natural part of the experience of life. Suffering is one of many possible responses to pain. Suffering can come out of either physical or emotional pain. It involves our thoughts and emotions and how they frame the meaning of our experiences. Suffering, too, is perfectly natural. In fact the human condition is often spoken of as inevitable suffering. But it is important to remember that suffering is only *one* response to the experience of pain. Even a small pain can produce great suffering in us if we fear that it means we have a tumor or some other frightening condition. That same pain can be seen as nothing at all, a minor ache or inconvenience, once we are reassured that all the tests are negative and there is no chance that it is a sign of something serious. So it is not always the pain per se but the way we see it and react to it that determines the degree of suffering we will experience. And it is the suffering that we fear most, not the pain.

Of course, nobody wants to live with chronic pain. But the fact is, it is very widespread. The costs to the society as a whole from chronic pain as well as to the people who suffer with it are very high. It has been calculated that lower-back pain alone costs our society approximately $30 billion per year in treatment and lost productivity. The psychological costs in terms of emotional distress are staggering as well.

A lingering pain condition can be totally disabling. Pain can erode the quality of your life. It can grind you down bit by bit, making you irritable, depressed, and prone to self-pity and feelings of helplessness and hopelessness. You may feel that you have lost control of your body and of your ability to earn a living, to say nothing of enjoying the activities that usually give pleasure and meaning to life.

What is more, the treatments for chronic pain conditions, while infinitely better and more sophisticated than they were even twenty years ago, are all too often only partially successful. Many people are ultimately told by their doctor or by the staff of a pain clinic at the end of a long and often frustrating treatment course, sometimes involving surgery and usually numerous drug treatments, that they are going to have to "learn to live with" their pain. But too often they are not taught *how*. *Being told that you have to learn to live with pain should not be the end of the road—it should be the beginning*.

In the best of cases, which is probably still the exception rather than the rule, a person with chronic pain will receive the ongoing support of a highly trained multidisciplinary pain clinic staff. Psychological assessment and counseling will be integrated with the treatment plan, which might include everything from surgery to nerve blocks, trigger-point injections with steroids, intravenous lidocaine drips, muscle relaxants, analgesics, physical and occupational therapy, and, with luck, acupuncture and massage. The goal of counseling is to help the person work with his or her body and to organize his or her life to keep what pain there is under some degree of control, to maintain an optimistic, self-efficacious perspective, and to help the person engage in meaningful activities and work within his or her capacity.

In our hospital, the pain clinic refers many of the patients it treats to the stress clinic for meditation training. The deciding factor in who is referred is the willingness of the patient to try to do something for himself or herself to cope with some of the pain, particularly when it has not responded fully to medical treatment alone. People whose attitude is that they just want the doctor to "fix it" or to "make it go away" are not good candidates. They won't understand the need to take some responsibility themselves for improving their condition. They might also take the suggestion that the mind can play a role in the control of their pain to mean that their pain is imaginary, that it is "all in their head" in the first place. It is not uncommon for people to think that the doctor is implying that their pain is not "real" when he or she proposes a psychological approach to pain therapy. People who know they are in pain usually want to have something done *to* the body to make the pain go away.

This is only natural when the model you are working with is that your body is like a machine. When something is wrong with a machine, you find out what the problem is and you "fix" it. By the same token, when you have a pain problem, you would go to a "pain doctor," expecting to get what is wrong fixed, just as you would if something were wrong with your car.

But your body is not a machine. One problem with chronic pain conditions is that often it is not clear exactly what is causing the pain. Often doctors won't be able to say with certainty *why* a person is experiencing pain. The diagnostic tests, such as X-rays and myelograms and CAT scans, frequently don't show very much, even though the person is in a lot of pain. And even if the cause of the pain were known precisely in a particular case, surgeons rarely attempt to cut specific nerve pathways to lessen pain. This is only attempted in cases of unremitting, excruciating pain as a last resort. This kind of surgery used to be performed more frequently, but it usually failed, for the simple reason that pain messages do not travel in exclusive and specific "pain pathways" in the nervous system.

For these reasons, people with chronic pain conditions who seek medical treatment thinking of their body as being pretty much like an automobile and that all the doctor needs to do is to find out why they are in pain and then make it go away by cutting the right nerve or giving them some magic pills or injections are usually in for a rude awakening. Things are rarely that simple with chronic pain.

In the new paradigm, pain is not just a "body problem," it is a whole-systems problem. Sensory impulses originating both at the surface of your body and internally are transmitted via nerve fibers to the brain, where these messages are registered and interpreted as "pain." This has to happen before they are considered painful by the organism. But there are many well-known pathways within the brain and the central nervous system by which higher cognitive and emotional functions can modify the perception of pain. The systems perspective on pain opens the door for many different possible ways to use your mind intentionally to influence your experience of pain. This is why meditation can be of great value in learning to live with pain. So, if a doctor suggests that meditation might help you with your pain, it does not mean that your pain is not "real." It means that your body and your mind are not two separate and distinct entities and that, therefore, there is always a mental component to pain. This means that you can always influence the pain experience to some extent by mobilizing the inner resources of the mind.

PAIN OUTCOMES IN THE STRESS CLINIC

Before looking further into the ways we can use mindfulness to work with pain, we will review some of the results obtained from our studies of people with chronic pain conditions in the stress clinic. These studies have shown that there is a dramatic reduction in the average level of pain during the eight-week training period in the clinic, as measured by a pain questionnaire called the McGill-Melzack Pain Rating Index (PRI). This is a reproducible finding. We see it in every class, year after year.

In one study 72 percent of the patients with chronic pain conditions achieved at least a 33 percent reduction on the PRI, while 61 percent of the pain patients achieved at least a 50 percent reduction. This means that the majority of people who came with pain experienced clinically significant reductions in their pain levels over the eight weeks they were practicing the meditation at home and attending weekly classes at the hospital.

In addition to pain, we looked at how much these people changed in terms of their negative body image (the degree to which they rated different parts of their body as problematic). We found that by the end of the program they perceived their bodies as approximately 30 percent less problematic. This implies that negative views and feelings about one's body, which are especially strong when people are limited in what they can do because of pain, can improve markedly in a short period of time.

At the same time, these people also showed a 30 percent improvement in the degree to which pain interfered with their ability to engage in the normal activities of daily living, such as preparing food, driving, sleeping, and sex. This improvement was accompanied by a sharp drop (55 percent) in negative mood states, an increase in positive mood states, and major improvements in anxiety, depression, hostility, and the tendency to somatize, that is, to be overly preoccupied with one's bodily sensations. By the end of the program, people with chronic pain in this study were reporting taking less pain medication, being more active, and feeling better in general.

Even more encouraging, these improvements lasted. In a separate study, which looked at how people with pain conditions were coping up to four years after their experiences in the stress clinic, we found that, on the average, most of the gains they had achieved by the end of the program were either maintained or improved still further.

In addition, the follow-up study showed that the pain patients continued to keep up with their meditation practice, many to a very strong degree. Ninety-three percent said that they continued to practice the meditation in one form or another at some level. Almost everybody reported still using awareness of their breathing during the day, and other informal mindfulness practices. Some were practicing formally as well when they felt a need. About 42 percent were still practicing formally *at least* three times per week for *at least* fifteen minutes at a time three years later, although by four years this percentage dropped to 30 percent; all in all, an impressive level of discipline and commitment considering they had learned the practice years earlier.

The pain patients in the follow-up study were also asked to rate how important their training in the stress clinic was to them at the time they were being asked to respond. Forty-four percent (at three years) and 67 percent (at four years) rated the program between 8 and 10 on a 1-to-10 scale (where a rating of 10 meant "very important"), and over 50 percent rated it 10 at four years. Responses for six months, one year, and two years of follow-up fell between these values, from 67 percent rating it between 8 and 10 at six months to 52 percent giving it that rating at two years.

In terms of how much what they learned in the clinic was responsible for their pain reduction at follow-up, 43 percent said that 80 to 100 percent of their pain improvement at follow-up was due to what they had learned in the stress clinic, and another 25 percent said that 50 to 80 percent of their pain improvement was due to what they learned there. So by their own reports, the meditation training had lasting effects in terms of their pain improvements.

In another study, we compared two groups of pain patients. All 42 people in this study were being treated in our hospital's pain clinic using standard medical protocols as well as supportive therapies such as physical therapy. But one group of 21 patients was also practicing the meditation in the stress clinic in addition to their pain clinic treatments, while the other group had not yet been referred to the stress clinic. Both groups were followed over a ten-week period, the meditators between the time they started and the time they finished the stress clinic; the other group between the time they started their pain clinic treatments and ten weeks later.

We knew from previous studies that we could expect the meditators to show large reductions in pain and psychological distress on our rating scales. The question was, How would the meditators compare with other patients in the pain clinic who were not practicing meditation but who were receiving powerful medical treatments for pain?

The result was that the nonmeditators showed little change over the ten weeks that they were being treated in the pain clinic, while the meditators showed the major improvements we expected to see. For example, the meditators showed a 36 percent improvement in pain on the PRI, while the nonmeditators had no improvement; and they showed a 37 percent improvement in negative body image, while the nonmeditators had a 2 percent improvement. The meditators also showed an 87 percent improvement in mood, while the nonmeditators showed only a 22 percent improvement; and they had a 77 percent improvement in psychological distress, while the nonmeditators had an 11 percent improvement.

These results suggest that doing something for yourself, as the people in the stress clinic were doing by engaging in meditation practice *in addition* to receiving medical treatment for pain, can result in many positive changes that might not occur with medical treatment alone.

People with very different kinds of pain problems showed improvements during the program. People with low-back pain, neck pain, shoulder pain, face pain, headache, arm pain, abdominal pain, chest pain, sciatic pain, and foot pain, caused by a range of problems including arthritis, herniated disks, and sympathetic dystrophies, were all able to use the meditation practice to achieve major improvements. This suggests that many different kinds of pain respond to the mindfulness approach, which involves, above all, a willingness to open up to pain and learn from it instead of closing off from it and trying to make it go away.

USING THE MEDITATION PRACTICE TO WORK WITH PAIN

Some people have difficulty understanding why we emphasize that they try to enter *into* their pain when they simply hate it and just want it to go away. Their feeling is "Why shouldn't I just ignore it or distract myself from it and grit my teeth and just endure it when it is too great?" One reason is that there may be times when ignoring it or distracting yourself doesn't work. At such times, it is very helpful to have other tricks up your sleeve besides just trying to endure it or depending on drugs to ease it. Several laboratory experiments with acute pain have shown that *tuning in* to sensations is a more effective way of reducing the level of pain experienced when the pain is intense and prolonged than is distracting yourself. In fact, even if distraction does alleviate your pain or help you to cope with it some of the time, bringing mindfulness to it can lead to new levels of insight and understanding about yourself and your body, which distraction or escape can never do. Understanding and insight, of course, are an extremely important part of the process of coming to terms with your condition and really learning *how* to live with it, not just endure it.

So, where do you begin? If you have a chronic pain condition, hopefully by this point you already started practicing some of the mindfulness exercises suggested in Part I. Perhaps at some point in your reading or during meditation practice you found yourself thinking about your own situation from a different angle or feeling a desire to pay attention to things you may have taken for granted before. Perhaps you have also begun to practice one or more of the formal meditation techniques on the schedule outlined in Chapter 10. If you haven't, the first thing to do now is to make the commitment to yourself that you will make time to practice, starting with the body scan, for at least forty-five minutes per day, six days per week, and that you will keep it up even if you don't feel you are "getting somewhere" with it right away.

All of the suggestions in Part I will be just as relevant to you for working with pain as they are to people who do not have chronic pain. This includes cultivating the attitudes described in Chapter 2. Be aware of the tendency to identify yourself as a "chronic pain patient." Instead remind yourself on a regular basis that you are a whole person who happens to have to face and handle a chronic pain condition intelligently. Reframing your view of yourself in this way will be especially important if you have a long history of pain problems and feel overwhelmed and defeated by your situation and by your past experiences.

You will be more aware than anybody that having pain doesn't free you from all the other kinds of problems and difficulties people have. Your other life problems need to be faced too. You can work with them in the same way you will face and work with pain. It is important to remind yourself, especially if you feel discouraged and depressed at times, that you still have the ability to feel joy and pleasure in your life. If you remember to cultivate this wider view of yourself, your efforts in the meditation will have a much more fertile soil in which to produce positive results. The meditation may also wind up helping you in unsuspected ways having nothing to do with your pain.

As we saw when we discussed symptoms in the last chapter, making the pain go away is not a very useful immediate goal. Pain can disappear altogether at times, or it can subside and become more manageable. What happens depends on a great many different circumstances, only some of which are under your potential control. A lot depends on the kind of pain you have.

For instance, headaches are more likely to disappear in a short period of time and not recur than is low-back pain. In general, improving low-back pain takes more work over a longer period. But whatever your pain problem, it is best to immerse yourself in practicing the meditation regularly, keeping in mind the attitudinal factors we considered in Chapter 2, and see what happens. Your daily meditation practice will be your pain laboratory. *Your ability to control your pain or change your relationship to it will grow out of the body scan, the sitting meditation, the yoga (if it is advisable for you to be doing it), and out of the mindfulness you are bringing to daily living.*

◆

The body scan is by far the technique that works best at the beginning for people with chronic pain, especially if sitting still or moving are difficult. You can do it lying on your back or in any other convenient outstretched position. Just close your eyes, tune in to your breathing, and watch your belly expand gently on the inbreaths and recede on the outbreaths. Then, as described in Chapter 5, use your breathing to direct your attention down to the toes of your left foot. Start working from there, maintaining moment-to-moment awareness. When your mind is on one region of your body, the idea is to keep it focused on that region, feeling any and all sensations in that region (or lack of sensations if you don't feel anything), and breathing in "to" and out "from" that region. Every time you breathe out, see if you can let your whole body sink a little more deeply into the surface you are lying on as the muscles all over your body release their tension and relax. When it comes time to leave that region and move on to the next, let go of it completely in your "mind's eye" and dwell in stillness for at least a few breaths before tuning in to the next region on your journey up through your left leg, then your right leg, then through the rest of your body. The basic meditation instructions about how to work with your mind when it wanders still apply (except when you are in so much pain that you cannot concentrate on anything other than the pain itself; working with this situation is described on pages 294–296), namely, when you notice at a certain point that your mind is somewhere else, observe where it has gone, and then gently escort your attention back to the region you are focusing on. If you are using the body-scan tape, when your mind wanders off and you realize it, then bring your attention back and pick up wherever the tape is suggesting that you focus.

Move slowly, scanning in this way through your entire body. As you move through a problem region, perhaps one in which the sensations of discomfort and pain are quite intense, see if you can treat it like any other part of your body that you come to focus on, in other words gently breathing in to and out from that region, carefully observing the sensations, allowing yourself to feel them and open up to them and letting your whole body relax and soften each time you breathe out. When it comes time to let go of that region and move on (you can decide when that moment is), let go of it completely (if it helps, try saying "good-bye" in your mind silently on an outbreath), and see if you can flow *in that moment* into calmness and stillness. And even if the pain doesn't change at all or becomes more intense, just move on to the next region and direct your full attention to it.

If the painful sensations in a particular region do change in some way, see if you can note precisely what the qualities of that change are. Let them register fully in your awareness and keep going with the body scan.

It is not helpful to *expect* pain to disappear. But you may find that it changes in intensity, getting momentarily stronger or weaker, or that the sensations change, say from sharp to dull, or to tingling or burning or throbbing. It can also be helpful to be aware of any thoughts and emotional reactions that you may be having about either the pain, your body, the tape, the meditation, or anything else. Just keep up the watching and letting go, watching and letting go, breath by breath, moment by moment.

Anything you observe about your pain or about your thoughts and feelings is to be noted *non-judgmentally* as you maintain your focus in the body scan. In the stress clinic, we do this every day for weeks. It can be boring, sometimes even exasperating. But that is okay. Boredom and exasperation can also be seen as thoughts and feelings and let go of. As we have mentioned a number of times, and it is true of the body scan in particular, we tell our patients "You don't have to like it, you just have to do it." So whether you find the body scan to be very relaxing and interesting or difficult and uncomfortable or exasperating is irrelevant to whether it will serve you well. As we have seen, it is probably the best place to get started in this process. After a few weeks you can switch over to alternating it with the sitting meditation and with the yoga if you like. But even then, don't be too quick to give up on the body scan.

Also, do not be overly thrilled with "success" or overly depressed by lack of "progress" as you go along. Every day will be different. In fact every moment will be different, so don't jump to conclusions after one or two sessions. *The work of growth and healing takes time.* It requires patience and consistency in the meditation practice over a period of weeks, if not months and years. If you have had a problem with pain for a number of years, it is not exactly reasonable to expect that it will magically go away in a matter of days just because you have started to meditate. But, especially if you have tried everything else already and still have pain, what do you have to lose by practicing the meditation on a regular basis for eight weeks, or even longer? Is there something better you could be doing in those forty-five minutes per day than touching base with yourself, no matter what you think or feel at those moments, and dwelling in the domain of being? At times of discouragement, just watch the feelings of discouragement themselves and then let them come and let them go too, as you keep practicing, practicing.

When you encounter moments when the pain is so intense that it is impossible for you to direct your attention to any other part of your body, let go of the body scan, shut off the tape if you are using it, and just bring your attention to focus directly on the pain itself in that moment. There are a number of ways to approach pain besides those we have already discussed. The key to all of them is your unwavering determination to direct your attention gently, delicately, but firmly *on* and *into* the pain, no matter how bad it seems. After all, it is what you are feeling right now, so you might as well see if you can accept it a little bit at least, just because it is here.

In some moments when you go into your pain and face it openly, it may seem as if you are locked in hand-to-hand combat with it or as if you are undergoing torture. It is helpful to recognize that these are just thoughts. It helps to remind yourself that the work of mindfulness is *not* meant to be a battle between you and your pain and it won't be unless you make it into one. If you do make it a struggle, it will only make for greater tension and therefore more pain. Mindfulness involves a determined effort to observe and accept your physical discomfort and your agitated emotions, moment by moment. *Remember, you are trying to find out about your pain, to learn from it, to know it better, not to stop it or get rid of it or escape from it.* If you can assume this attitude and be calmly *with* your pain, looking at it in this way for even one breath or even half a breath, that is a step in the right direction. From there you might be able to expand it and remain calm and open while facing the pain for maybe two or three breaths or even longer.

In the clinic we like to use the expression "putting out the welcome mat" to describe how we work with pain during meditation. Since it is already present in a particular moment, we do what we can to be receptive and accepting of it. We try to relate to it in as neutral a way as possible, observing it non-judgmentally, feeling what it actually feels like in detail. This involves opening up to the raw sensations themselves, whatever they may be. We breathe with them and dwell with them from moment to moment, riding the waves of the breath, the waves of sensation.

We also ask ourselves the question, "How bad is it right now, in this very moment?" If you practice doing this, you will probably find that most of the time, even when you are feeling terrible, when you go right into the sensations and ask, "IN THIS MOMENT, is it tolerable? is it okay?" the chances are you will find that it is. The difficulty is that the next moment is coming, and the next, and you "*know*" they are all going to be filled with more pain.

The solution? Try taking each moment as it comes. Try to be one hundred percent *in* the present in one moment, then do the same for the next, right through the forty-five-minute practice period if necessary or until the intensity subsides, at which point you can go back to the body scan.

◆

There is another very important thing you can do as well as observing the bare sensations themselves. That is to be aware of any thoughts or feelings you are having about the sensations. For one thing, you may notice that you are talking about them silently in your mind as "pain." This too is a thought, a name. It is not the experience itself. Notice it if you are labeling the sensations in this way. Maybe it is not necessary to call them "pain." Perhaps it even makes them seem stronger. Why not look and see for yourself whether this is so?

There may also be all sorts of other thoughts and feelings milling about, appearing and disappearing, commenting, reacting, judging, yearning for relief. Statements such as "This is killing me," "I can't stand it any longer," "How long will this go on?" "My whole life is a mess," "There is no hope for me," "I'll never master this pain" may all move through your mind at one time or another. You may find such thoughts coming and going constantly. NONE OF THEM ARE THE PAIN ITSELF.

Can you be aware of this as you practice? It is a key realization. Not only are these thoughts not the pain itself, they are not you either! Nor, in all likelihood, are they particularly true or accurate. They are just the understandable reactions of your own mind when it is not ready to accept the pain and wants things to be different from the way they are, in other words, pain-free. When you see and feel the sensations you are experiencing *as sensations*, pure and simple, you may see that these thoughts about the sensations are useless to you *at that moment* and that they can actually make things worse than they need be. Then, in letting go of them, you come to accept the sensations simply because they are already here anyway. Why not just accept them for now?

However, you cannot reliably let go into accepting the sensations until you realize that it is your thinking that is labeling the sensations as "bad." It is your thinking that doesn't want to accept them, now or ever, because it doesn't like them and just wants them to GO AWAY. But notice, now it is not YOU that won't accept the sensations, it is just your thinking, and you already know, because you have seen it for yourself firsthand, that your thoughts are not you.

Does this shift in perspective show you another option for facing your pain? What about letting go of those thoughts on purpose, as a little experiment, when you are in a lot of pain? What about letting go of that part of your mind that wants things to be the way it wants them to be, even in the face of incontrovertible evidence that they are not that way right now? What about accepting things just as they are right now, in this very moment, even if you hate them, even if you hate the pain? What about purposefully stepping back from the hatred and the anger and not judging things at all, just accepting them?

It may also strike you at a certain point, particularly if there is a moment of calmness in the midst of the inner turmoil, that your *awareness* of sensations, thoughts, and feelings is different from the sensations, the thoughts, and the feelings themselves—the part of "you" that is aware is not itself in pain or ruled by these thoughts and feelings at all. It knows them, but it itself is free of them. When practicing the body scan or any of the other mindfulness techniques, you may come to notice that when you identify with your thoughts or feelings or with the sensations in your body or with the body itself for that matter, there is much greater turmoil and suffering than when you dwell as the non-judgmental observer of it all, identifying with the knower, with awareness itself.

We adopt this witnessing perspective throughout the meditation practice, but toward the end of the body-scan tape, there is an explicit sequence that encourages what we have called *choiceless awareness*, a disidentifying with the entire play of inner experience, whether it be the breath, sensations, perceptions, thoughts, or feelings. As the body scan comes to an end, after we have intentionally let go of it, we invite our thoughts and feelings, our likes and dislikes, our concepts about ourself and the world, our ideas and opinions, even our name, into the field of awareness and we intentionally let go of them as well.

On the tape, it then suggests that you tune in to a sense of being complete in the present moment, as you are, without having to resolve your problems or correct bad habits or pay your bills or get a college education or anything else. Can you identify with yourself as being whole and complete in this moment and at the same time part of a larger whole? Can you sense yourself as pure "being," that aspect of you that is beyond your body, beyond your name, your thoughts and feelings, your ideas, opinions, concepts, even beyond your identification of yourself as a certain age or as a male or female?

In the letting go of all of this, you may come to a point at which all concepts dissolve into stillness and there is just awareness, a knowing beyond any "thing" to be known. In this stillness, you might come to know that whatever you are, "you" are definitely not your body, although it is yours to work with and to take care of and make use of. It is a very convenient and miraculous vehicle, but it is hardly you.

If you are not your body, then you cannot possibly be your body's pain. As you learn to dwell in the domain of being, your relationship to pain in your body can undergo profound changes. These experiences can guide you in developing your own ways to come to terms with pain, to make room for it, to live with it, as so many of our patients have.

Of course regular practice is necessary, as we have been stressing all along. The domain of being is easier to talk about than to experience. To make it real in your life, to get in touch with it in any moment, takes concentrated work and determination. A certain kind of digging, a kind of inner archaeology, is required to uncover your intrinsic wholeness, covered over as it may be with layer after layer of opinions, likes and dislikes, and the heavy fog of automatic, unconscious thinking and habits, to say nothing of pain. There is nothing romantic or sentimental about the work of mindfulness, nor is your intrinsic wholeness a romantic or sentimental or imaginary construct. It is here now, as it always has been. It is part of being human, just as having a body and feeling pain are part of being human.

If you suffer from a chronic pain condition and you find that this way of looking at things resonates with you, then it may be time to test this approach for yourself. The only way to do so is to start practicing and keep practicing. Find and cultivate moments of calmness, stillness, and awareness within yourself using your pain as your teacher and guide.

It is hard work, and there will be times when you will feel like quitting, especially if you don't see quick "results" in terms of pain reduction. But in doing this work, you must also remember that it involves patience and gentleness and lovingkindness toward yourself and even toward your pain. It means working at your limits, but *gently,* not trying too hard, not exhausting yourself, not pushing too hard to break through. The breakthroughs will come by themselves in their own good time if you put in the energy in the spirit of self-discovery. Mindfulness does not bulldoze through resistance. You have to work gently at the edges, a little here and a little there, keeping your vision alive in your heart, particularly during the times of greatest pain and difficulty.

23

More on Pain

———

"Dear Jon and Peggy: I have many aches and pains but I feel great. I was able to shovel my driveway, which is *250 feet* long. Breathing, meditating, and frequent breaks for arms, legs, back, and neck exercises. I had muscle soreness but nothing to incapacitate me. In thirty years I never before attempted to shovel my driveway. Thank you, Pat." (January 15, 1982)

WORKING MINDFULLY WITH CHRONIC LOW-BACK PAIN AND BACK PROBLEMS

People who have never had a problem with chronic pain have no idea how much living with a pain condition changes your whole life and everything you do. Many people with back injuries are unable to work, especially at jobs that require lifting or driving or standing for long periods. Some spend years on workmen's compensation while trying to recover sufficiently to be able to get back to work and lead something like a normal life or to be certified as disabled so that they can receive disability payments. Often there are legal problems and battles in order to receive benefits. Living on a fixed and very reduced income, coupled with being stuck in the house in pain for days, weeks, months, sometimes even years, unable to do anything, is extremely frustrating and depressing, not just for the person in pain but for his or her entire family and circle of friends. It can make everybody feel angry, defeated, and helpless.

Whether you are disabled by your pain at all times or just have a chronic "bad back" that you have to be careful of, the effects of low-back pain on your life can be debilitating and depressing. Just bending over the sink when brushing your teeth, or picking up a pencil, or getting into the bathtub or out of a car can trigger days or

300

even weeks of intense pain that may force you onto your back in bed just to bear it. Not only pain but also the threat of pain if you make a wrong move constantly affect your ability to lead a normal life. Thousands of things have to be done slowly and carefully, taking nothing for granted. Lifting heavy objects may be out of the question. Even lifting very light objects can cause major problems. And at those times when you are not in pain, the strange feeling of instability and vulnerability in that central region of your body can still lead you to feel insecure and precarious. You may not be able to stand up straight or turn or walk in a way that feels normal. You may feel a need to brace yourself or guard yourself from people or circumstances that might throw your body off balance. It is very hard to have your body feel "right" when its central fulcrum feels unstable and vulnerable.

Sometimes your back can go out even when you are being careful. You may not have noticed anything in particular that you did, but even so, there are times when your back muscles can go into spasm, triggering a setback that may last for days or weeks. One minute you can be relatively OK, the next minute you are in trouble.

People with chronic back pain tend to have "good days" and "bad days." Often there are very few good days. It can be very discouraging to live from day to day, uncertain about how you will feel tomorrow or what you will or won't be able to do. It is hard to make definite plans, which makes it almost impossible to work at a regular job and makes it hard socially as well. And if you do have a good day now and again, you can feel so exuberant because your body feels "right" or normal for a change that you might well overdo things to compensate for all the times you were unable to do anything. Then you wind up paying for it later. This can be a vicious cycle.

A back problem almost forces you to be mindful because the results of being unaware of your body and what you are doing can be so debilitating. In order to work systematically around the edges of your limitations, in order to get stronger and healthier and to be able to do at least some of the things you want to do, mindfulness becomes absolutely essential.

The people in the stress clinic with chronic pain who are the most successful in controlling their pain cultivate a long-term perspective on rehabilitating themselves. Big improvements in mobility and pain reduction may or may not come about in eight weeks.

You are better off thinking in terms of six months, or even a year or two, and proceeding patiently and persistently, no matter how well things go at first. However, the quality of your life can begin to improve from the first time you practice the body scan, as we saw in the case of Phil (Chapter 13). This is especially true if you are willing to work with your body and your back problems slowly and systematically. Such a commitment and strategy should include a reasonable vision of what you might be able to accomplish with consistent work. It may help to imagine how your back might be in three years or five years if you were to keep up a steady, mindful physical exercise program, encouraging your whole body, not just your back, to grow stronger and more flexible. One very successful scientist I know who has severe pain "puts his body back together" for an hour every morning before he goes out to face the world. It might help if you think of yourself as in training, like an athlete.

A long-term approach to your own back rehabilitation might include mindfully working to strengthen your back by doing the physical therapy exercises prescribed for you or by practicing as much of the yoga as you are able to manage, after checking with your physical therapist to make sure that these specific exercises are appropriate in your case.

This kind of work needs to be done particularly slowly and gently when you have a back problem. A physical therapist who works with many of our patients commented that she loves to work with people after they have been through the stress clinic. She says they are noticeably more responsive, relaxed, and tuned in to their bodies during their physical-therapy sessions than people who do not know about mindfulness, who do not know how to breathe *with* their stretches and their movements and how to work *with* the body and *with* pain instead of against them. And the people themselves say the same thing, that physical therapy changes once they know how to use their breathing as they stretch and lift. We noted this already in the chapter on the yoga practice.

Taking care of your body through regular exercise is even more important for you if you have a back problem than for someone without one. Remember, "If you don't use it, you lose it." Don't let your back problem become an excuse for not taking care of the rest of your body. Maybe you could exercise by walking regularly or by using a stationary bicycle or by swimming. Perhaps you can also do some of the yoga. You don't have to do it all. Just do the exercises that you are able to do and avoid those that your doctor says are unwise for you or that you sense are not right for you now. But, in our view, if you want to rehabilitate your body, you should do something to stretch and strengthen your body every, or at least every other, day, as described in detail in Chapter 6, even if it is just for five minutes at first.

On top of working with your body in these ways as best you can, we suggest you practice the body scan daily, as described in Chapters 5 and 22, as the core of your rehabilitation strategy. Use it as a time to "rebody" yourself by getting deeply in touch with your body from moment to moment in stillness, working with pain and discomfort as they come up.

If you are out of work, you will have plenty of time for this. Time can weigh very heavily on us when we are stuck in the house. You may find yourself feeling bored and frustrated, uncomfortable and irritable, and even sorry for yourself. Anybody would. But if you intentionally make up your mind to use some of this time for healing by practicing the meditation and the yoga, you can transform a bad situation into a creative one. You obviously didn't ask for your back problem to happen, but as long as it has, you may as well decide that you will use your time to your advantage in order to rehabilitate yourself as best you possibly can. Remember, it's your body and nobody knows it as well as you do, and nobody depends on it as much as you do for your well-being.

One of the most healing things you can do for your body during the day is to use your breath periodically to penetrate the pain and help it to soften in the same way that we use it in the body scan, as described in the previous chapter. You can do this by consciously directing your breath in to the painful region, feeling it as it moves into your back and then visualizing the pain softening and dissolving as you relax and let go into each outbreath. Take a day-by-day, even moment-by-moment perspective, purposefully reminding yourself to take each day as it comes, each moment as it comes, letting go of any expectations that you should feel a certain way or that the pain should lessen, and just watching the breath do its work.

◆

Healing is truly a journey. The road has its ups and downs. So you should not be too surprised if you have setbacks and sometimes feel as if you are taking one step forward and then sliding two steps backward. This is the way it always is. If you are cultivating mindfulness and seeking ongoing advice and encouragement from your doctor and others who are supporting your efforts, you will be able to catch things as they change and be flexible enough to modify what you are doing when necessary to accommodate your changing situation. The most important thing is to believe in your own ability to persevere through the many ups and downs and to not lose sight of your wholeness and your journey toward realizing it fully.

◆

Bringing mindfulness to your daily activities is particularly valuable when you have a back condition and back pain. As we have seen, sometimes even lifting a pencil or reaching for the toilet paper the "wrong" way (isn't it amazing that there may be a "wrong" way for you to reach for the toilet paper?) or opening a window or getting out of a car can trigger an acute pain episode. So the more you are aware of what you are doing while you are doing it, the better. Doing things on automatic pilot can lead to serious setbacks. As you probably know, it is particularly important to avoid lifting and twisting simultaneously, even very light objects. First lift, always bending the knees and keeping the object close to your body, then turn. It helps to couple all your movements with awareness of your breathing and your body position. Are you twisting and standing up simultaneously when you get out of the car? Don't. Instead, do one first, then the other. Are you leaning over at the waist to push up a window? Don't. Instead, get in close to it before you attempt to lift it. Mindfulness of little things like this can make a big difference in protecting yourself from injury and pain.

Then there is the problem of getting things done around the house. There will be times that you can't do any work at all. But there may be other times, depending on the severity of your back condition, when it may be possible to do things if you do them in moderation and see them as part of your program to build up your strength and flexibility. Take vacuuming for instance. Lifting and pulling the vacuum cleaner can be dangerous if you have a back condition. But if you are going to do it, you can devise ways to do it mindfully. The movements involved in vacuuming can be very hard on the back. But with a little attention and imagination, you can make the movements of vacuuming into a kind of mindful yoga. You can do under the bed and under the couch on your hands and knees or squatting if that is possible, bending and reaching with awareness, using your breath to guide your movements, just as you would when doing the yoga exercises. If you vacuum this way, and you do it slowly and mindfully, chances are you will know when the body has had enough, and you will listen to its message. Then you might stop and do a little more in a day or two. After you stop, try doing some yoga for five or ten minutes to relax and destress your body and stretch some of the muscles that may have tensed up.

Needless to say, this is not the way most people vacuum or do anything else. But if you experiment, you are likely to find that a little awareness, coupled with the skills that come from your regular yoga and meditation practice, can go a long way toward transforming drudgery into therapy and frustrating limitations into healing opportunities. You work at the edges of what is possible, listening to your body. As you do, you might find yourself growing stronger over the weeks and months. Of course people who don't have pain might avoid back injuries by vacuuming in the same way. And if vacuuming is out of the question for you, you might try some other household chore and work with it in a similar way.

In the stress clinic, we suggest that people with back pain take a very cautious, experimental approach toward reclaiming those areas in their lives that are most compromised by their condition. Just because you have pain doesn't mean you should give up on your body. It is all the more reason to work with it to make it as strong as it can possibly be so that it can come through for you when you need it. Giving up on sex or walking or shopping or cleaning or hugging is not going to make things better.

Experiment mindfully! Find out what works for you, how to modify things so that you can do them, at least for short periods. Don't automatically deprive yourself, out of fear or self-pity, of the normal activities of life that make it meaningful and that give coherence to it. Remember, as we saw in Chapter 12, if you say "I can't," then you certainly won't. That thought or belief or statement becomes a self-fulfilling prophecy; it creates its own reality. But since it is only a thought, it is not necessarily completely accurate. Wouldn't it be better to catch yourself at those moments, see through the "I can't" or the "I could never . . ." thoughts and try instead "Maybe, somehow, it just might be possible . . . let me try it . . . mindfully."

Recall Phil, the French-Canadian truck driver who had injured his back and whose experience with the body scan in the first few weeks of the program is recounted briefly in Chapter 13. It took him several weeks to learn to do the body scan to achieve reliable pain reduction. He experienced many ups and downs in those first weeks but kept up the practice anyway. Finally, he wound up feeling much more able to control not only his back pain but other areas of his life as well.

Before he started meditating, Phil had been wearing a TENS* unit daily, which the pain clinic had prescribed for him as part of his treatment. He had felt he couldn't get along without it and wore it all day long, every day. But after a few weeks practicing the body scan, he found he could go two or three days without wearing it. He was very pleased to be able to control his pain on his own like that. To him it was a sign of his own power.

But when it came time for the class to do yoga, once again he came to a crossroads. After the program was over, he described it this way: "Ya know, I almost gave it up again in the third week when you started talking about yoga and all that stuff. I said, 'Oh my god, that's going to kill me to do that,' but then you said that if it bothers you, don't do it, so I mostly did the body scan. But I did do some yoga, too, and I did a lot during the all-day session. It bothered me at times, some of the exercises bothered me to do them, like the leg raising and the folding yourself up and rolling backward on your neck. I can't do a whole lot of that. The things I can do, that don't bother me, I do them every so often. I am definitely feeling more flexible."

In reviewing his experience at the end of the eight weeks, Phil said, "No, it [the pain] is not gone, it's still there, but you know, when I start feeling it too much, I just sit aside somewhere, take ten, fifteen, twenty minutes, do my meditation, and that seems to take over. And if I can stay at least, say fifteen or thirty minutes or better, I can walk away and not even think about it for maybe three, four, five, six hours, maybe the whole day, depending, like I say, on the weather."

He also noticed that things were different at home with his wife and children. In his own words, "We had a bit of a problem when I first came here [to the clinic]. We had problems, ya know. I had this pain problem so much on my mind and about finding another kind of a job without the education I figured I needed for most jobs or whatever . . . this stuff all built up pressure and, without realizing, I was like a madman more or less, ya know. I mean my wife was just like a slave working for me more or less, ya know, and we sat down

*Transcutaneous Electrical Nerve Stimulator: a device worn on the belt that delivers mild electric shocks to the skin that reduce the experience of pain.

one night and I got kinda frustrated and I told her, 'We gotta talk.' There wasn't much sex life going on, and that's driving me up a wall. I'm not a person who goes weeks without it, ya know, and so I says, 'Come on now, let's . . .' so she finally made me realize what was going on. She says, 'How long since you told me you love me? How long . . . ?' We sit down . . . we've got a double recliner, ya know, like a love seat, and she says, 'Let's sit down and watch TV together.' But when I'm watching TV, I'm watching TV. She'll talk and I go, 'Uh-huh, uh-huh' but it goes right through me, ya know. She'll say, 'Well, I told you . . .' and I'll say, 'Well, I'm sorry, I wasn't listening, I was watching my boxing' or whatever, ya know. Well, she finally made me realize what's going on. After I started in the stress clinic, I says, 'Wow, ya know, I *do* realize it now,' ya know. So we got away from the TV now. At night we don't sit down and watch TV no more. We go outside. We have a campfire every night when it's nice, with the neighbors. We sit down and talk, ya know, and sometimes we're with another couple, sometimes just talking or sitting watching the fire, and it just draws my attention. And the first thing ya know, they're talking, but it's just like they're a distance far away. I can find myself getting to the breathing exercise automatically, and I feel so much better after this, ya know, and it beats watching that boob tube. My relationship with my wife has improved a hundred percent, and with the kids too."

And on the subject of trying new things, Phil also observed, "One other thing I got from the program. . . . Before, I was never able to talk in public the way I did in the classes. Anytime I ever tried before, I could feel my face burning, turning as red as a tomato, because I am bashful and shy, I always was. I don't know what made me be able to talk in the classes the way I did. You see, what I did say, whenever I said something, I had a good feeling about it. It didn't come from my mouth, it came from inside, ya know, from the heart."

INTENSIVE MEDITATION AND PAIN

It is no accident that meditation practice has something to teach us about coping with pain. Over the past 2,500 years, practitioners of meditation have had a lot of experience learning from pain and developing methods to transcend it. Intensive training in meditation has traditionally been the province of monasteries and retreat centers set up for that explicit purpose. Long-term meditation practice can be very painful physically and emotionally as well as uplifting and liberating. Imagine going off somewhere and doing what we do in our all-day session (see Chapter 8) in silence for seven days or two weeks or a month or three months.

When you sit without moving, especially cross-legged on the floor, for periods of an hour or more and you do this maybe ten hours a day for days or even weeks at a time, your body can begin to hurt with excruciating intensity, primarily in the back, shoulders, and knees. The physical pain eventually diminishes by itself most of the time, but sitting through days of it can be quite challenging. You tend to learn a lot about yourself and about pain from putting yourself in this kind of situation on purpose. If you are willing to accept this pain and observe it and not run from it, it can teach you a great deal. Above all you learn that you can work with it. You learn that pain is not a static experience; it is constantly changing. You come to see that the sensations are just what they are and that your thoughts and feelings are something apart from the sensations. You come to see that your mind may play a large part in your own suffering, and it can play a large role in freeing you from suffering as well. Pain can teach you all of these things.

People who go on meditation retreats invariably have to face physical pain which comes up during long sittings. It is unavoidable in the early stages of a retreat. It comes out of sitting still in postures we are not used to. It also arises when we become aware of the accumulated physical tension we carry around with us, un-noticed, in our bodies. In many ways the qualities of this type of pain strongly resemble the spectrum of sensations that occur in many chronic pain conditions: the aching, the burning, the epi-sodes of sharp, shooting sensations in the back or the knees or the shoulders. You could stop the pain at any time by getting up and walking, but mostly, if you are a meditator, you choose to stay and be mindful of it as just another experience. In return, it teaches you how to cultivate calmness, concentration, and equanimity in the face of discomfort. But it is not an easy lesson to learn. You have to be willing to face the pain over and over again, day in and day out, and observe it, breathe with it, look into it, accept it. In this way, meditation practice can be a laboratory for exploring pain, for learning more about what it is, how to go deeply into it, and ultimately, how to come to terms with it.

ATHLETES AND PAIN

Like meditators, endurance athletes also know a certain kind of self-induced pain firsthand. They, too, know the power of the mind in working with their pain so that they are not defeated by it. Athletes are constantly putting themselves into situations that are bound to produce pain. You cannot run a marathon at your fastest pace and not face pain. In fact, few people could run a marathon at any speed and not encounter pain.

Then why do they do it in the first place? Because runners know that pain can be worked with and transcended. When the body is screaming out to stop because the metabolic pain (from the muscles not being able to get enough oxygen fast enough) toward the end of a race is so great, an endurance athlete has to reach into himself or herself and decide whether to back off the pace or to find new resources for going beyond what a normal person would consider an absolute limit.

In fact, unless a physical injury occurs (producing an acute pain-of-injury that makes you stop, and rightly so, to prevent further injury), it is invariably the mind that decides to quit first, not the body. Endurance athletes can be plagued by lapses of concentration, by fears and self-doubts as well as by the knowledge that they face certain pain during training and competition. For these reasons as well as many others, many athletes now believe that systematic mental training is every bit as necessary as systematic physical training if they hope to be able to perform at their peak. In fact, in the new paradigm, there cannot be complete physical fitness and optimal performance of any task without mental fitness. These need to be cultivated together.

In 1984, I had an opportunity to work with the United States Olympic men's rowing team, training the rowers in the same meditation techniques that the pain patients in the stress clinic use to cope with their pain. These athletes were able to use mindfulness strategies to improve their ability to face and cope with pain during training and competition just as the patients are able to use it to work with their pain, even though these two different groups of people are working at opposite ends of the physical-fitness spectrum.

Readers with chronic low-back problems might be interested to know that John Biglow, the single sculler on the 1984 U.S. Olympic rowing team, achieved his position as the best male American sculler that year in spite of a chronic back problem resulting from a herniated disk when he injured himself rowing in 1979. Following his injury, and a serious setback in 1983, when he reinjured himself, he was never able to row hard for more than five minutes at a time, after which he would have to rest for three minutes before he could row hard again. Yet he was able to rehabilitate himself by training very carefully using the knowledge of his own limits, to the point where he was able to demand of his back the enormous effort required to compete at the world-class level. In order to be the single sculler on the Olympic team, Biglow had to race against and beat all the fastest, strongest, and most competitive rowers in the country. (Races are 2,000 meters and are completed in about five minutes.) Imagine the faith and determination and bodily intelligence necessary for someone with a chronic back problem to even set out to work toward such a goal, no less to achieve it. But the goal he set for himself was meaningful enough to sustain him along the extremely arduous, painful, and lonely road he followed.

In our own way each of us, no matter what our deficit or disability, is capable of such achievements if we can define meaningful goals for ourselves and then work intelligently toward their fulfillment. Even if we don't achieve the goal completely, the effort itself can be sustaining and healing if we see meaning in the process itself and work with awareness, moment by moment and day by day.

HEADACHES

Most headaches are not signs of brain tumors or other serious pathological conditions, although such thoughts can easily enter your mind if you suffer from headaches that are constant, chronic, and severe. But if headaches persist or are extremely severe, it is always important to go through at least one full diagnostic work-up to rule out such pathology before trying to control them either with medication or meditation. In such cases, a well-trained physician will make sure this is done before referring a headache patient for stress reduction training. Most of the patients in the stress clinic who have problems with chronic headaches come with diagnoses of either tension headaches or migraines or both. All have had a full neurological work-up, which usually includes a CAT scan to rule out a brain tumor.

The majority of people who are referred to the stress clinic with chronic headaches respond well to the meditation practice. One woman came to the program with a twenty-year history of migraine headaches, for which she took cafergot every day. She had been treated at numerous headache clinics with no relief. Within two weeks of joining the stress reduction program, she had a two-day stretch with no headaches. This had not happened to her in twenty years. She remained headache-free for the duration of the course and for some time afterward.

You only need one experience of having a headache disappear that has been chronic and constant to know that it is within the realm of possibility for such a thing to happen. This can completely change the way you think about your body and your illness and can provide you with renewed faith in your ability to control what previously seemed uncontrollable.

One elderly woman told her class recently that the idea of putting out the welcome mat for her migraine struck her as particularly appropriate. So the next time she felt one coming on, she sat down to meditate and "talked" to her headache. She said things like "Come in if you want to, but you should know that I am no longer going to be ruled by you. I have a lot to do today and I just can't spend much time with you." This worked quite well for her and she seemed pleased with this discovery.

There is a place on the body-scan tape, after we have gone through the entire body, which suggests breathing out of an imaginary hole at the top of your head, much as a whale breathes through a blowhole. The idea is to feel as if your breath is actually moving in and out through this hole. Many people with headaches have used that "hole" as a release valve for their headaches. You just breathe in and out through the top of your head and let the tension or pressure or whatever the sensations are in that region flow right out of the body through the hole. Of course it is harder to do this if you have not been developing your ability to concentrate through regular meditation practice, but if you have been practicing breathing this way every day as part of your work with the body scan, when you have headachelike symptoms, they can be dispelled easily, before they build into a full-blown headache. But even then, this method can be effective in taking the edge off or even dissolving the headache.

As they get into practicing the meditation on a regular basis, whether they have a headache or not at the time they do it, most people who come to the stress clinic with headache problems report that both the *frequency* and the *severity* of their headaches decrease. The meditation practice affects both and can be used with headache problems in two different ways. It can be used to reduce the severity of a headache by breathing through the imaginary "hole" at the top of the head at the time a person has a headache. And the overall frequency of headaches can be reduced by the *relaxation* associated with regular meditation practice. Relaxation often dispels the physiological preconditions that lead to headaches in the first place.

◆

As your practice deepens, you may notice that your headaches do not come out of nowhere. There are usually identifiable preconditions that trigger their onset. The problem is that many of the physiological triggers are only poorly understood and the psychological or social triggers are often ignored or denied. Certainly, stressful situations can give rise to headaches, and many people—especially those with muscle tension headaches—are at least aware of this connection. But many other people report that they wake up with headaches or that they get them when they are not under obvious stress, when everything is going well for them, on the weekends or at other times that they feel they are not stressed.

A few weeks of mindfulness practice often generate new insights in these individuals about their headaches and why and when they get them. Sometimes people find out that they are a lot more tense and keyed up than they thought they were, even on the weekends. Sometimes they see that a particular thought or worry might precede the onset of a headache. This can even happen as you wake up in the morning and are getting out of bed. One anxious thought can make you tense before your feet touch the floor, although you may be completely unaware of the thought. All you know is that you "woke up" with a headache.

This is another way that being mindful as you go through the day can be useful. It helps to tune in to your body and your breathing from the very first moment that you know you are awake in the morning. You might even try saying to yourself as you wake up, "I am waking up now" or "I am awake now."

Over time, this kind of awareness will lead you to make connections that may have previously gone unnoticed, such as realizing the link between a thought you wake up with or a situation that occurs early in the day, perhaps even in the first few minutes that you are up, and a headache later on. This can lead you to intentionally try to short-circuit a possible headache-producing chain of events by bringing awareness right to the thought as it arises, seeing it as a thought and letting it go, or by taking action to change your relationship to a bothersome stressful situation and monitoring the results of your efforts. It may also be that you will become aware of times and places where you are more likely to get a headache and in this way identify *environmental factors* such as pollution and allergens that might be triggering some kinds of headaches.

For some people, chronic headaches may really be a metaphor for everything that is disconnected and disregulated in their lives: body, family, work, environment, the full catastrophe. They usually have so much stress in their day-to-day lives that it is difficult to know where to start in thinking about why they might be getting headaches. If this describes your present situation, it may be helpful for you to know that you do not have to *solve* any of your problems in order to get started. All that you really need to do is to start practicing and start paying more careful attention from moment to moment during your day. With time, movement toward *self-regulation* happens naturally. It may take years to work yourself out of such a situation completely, but the attempt itself, coupled with a willingness to accept where you already are and be patient, can lead to dramatic improvements in your headaches long before the rest of your problems have been resolved.

The two stories that follow are examples of ways in which chronic headaches may serve as a metaphor for a person's entire life situation at a particular point in time, and how this dilemma can be worked with and perhaps turned around to lead, ultimately, not only to relief of the headaches but, even more importantly, to some insight and resolution of the larger situation.

Fred, a thirty-eight-year-old man, was referred for anxiety associated with sleep apnea, a condition characterized by temporary cessation of breathing during sleep. The apnea was due to his obesity. At the time, Fred weighed 375 pounds and was five foot ten. In addition to his anxiety and his sleep apnea, Fred had chronic headaches. Whenever he felt stressed, he got a headache. Getting on a bus would always result in a headache. He hated buses ("they make me sick"), but he had no car and depended on them to get around. He lived with a roommate and worked managing a concession stand. His weight was so great that his neck would prevent him from breathing properly when he was lying down. This is what caused his sleep apnea. His pulmonary doctor had told him he would have to have a tracheotomy if he didn't lose weight right away. This prospect caused Fred a great deal of anxiety. He did not want to have a tracheotomy. A colleague who was counseling him for weight reduction suggested he attend the stress clinic to deal with his anxiety.

Fred came to the first class and didn't like it at all. He said to himself, "I can't wait till this is over, I won't be back." At the time he had agreed to go, it hadn't quite hit him what it would be like to be in a class with about thirty other people. He had always been uncomfortable in crowds and had never been able to talk in a group. He was shy and instinctively avoided any kind of situation that might lead to conflict. But, as he described it to me when the program was over, some "gut feeling" brought him back to the second class. He found himself saying, "If I don't do it now, I'll probably never do it" and "Everyone else has got problems or else they wouldn't be here." So, in spite of his feelings about the first class, Fred decided to keep coming. He started to use the body-scan tape that first week and by the next class he already knew that it was "going to work" for him. As he put it, "I really got into it right away." He was even able to say something in the class about how relaxing he had found it to tune in to his body.

From the time he started doing the body scan, Fred's headaches disappeared. This happened in spite of the fact that the stress in his life was increasing as it became more and more obvious that he was gaining weight, not losing it, and would have to have the tracheotomy. Yet he was able to ride on the buses without getting headaches or feeling sick by just "relaxing and going with the flow and enjoying it."

He also became more assertive. He was able to ask his roommate to leave when he stopped contributing to the rent. This was something he felt he would have never been able to do before. As he became more self-confident, Fred also started feeling more relaxed in his body. The yoga bothered him because of his weight and he didn't do much. But although he gained some weight during the program, he did not get depressed. Previously, gaining even a minuscule amount of weight would send him into a severe depression.

Fred also had high blood pressure. At one point prior to joining the stress clinic, his blood pressure was measured at 210/170, which is dangerously high. Usually it averaged around 140/95 on blood pressure medication. When he completed the stress clinic, it was averaging around 120/70, lower than it had been for fifteen years.

As a postscript, he underwent not one but two attempts at a tracheotomy in one week, but they didn't work because his neck was so thick they couldn't get the tube to stay in. Both times it fell out after a few days. So he never did get the tracheotomy.

When I saw him again a month after the course ended, he was on a diet and had lost a noticeable amount of weight. He was continuing with his meditation practice. He said he had never felt so sure of himself in his life. Losing the weight gave him a major boost in self-confidence. He said he was feeling happy for the first time in years and that his sleep apnea had diminished with his weight loss. And he had had only one headache since he finished the course.

In another class, a forty-year-old divorced woman named Laurie was referred by her neurologist for migraine headaches and work stress. She had had migraines since she was thirteen, often four times per week. These included seeing lights in front of her eyes, usually followed by nausea and vomiting. Although she was on medication, the drugs often did not help her headaches unless she took them at exactly the right time, before the headache built up. This time was always hard for her to judge. In the four months preceding her referral to the stress clinic, Laurie's headaches had gotten worse, to the point where, several times, she had sought help in the emergency room of the hospital.

In the fourth week of the program, we usually ask people to fill out Drs. Holmes and Rahe's Social Readjustment Rating Scale for homework, in addition to their meditation practice. As we saw in Chapter 18, this scale is simply a list of life events. The assignment is to check off those items that happened to you in the past year. The list includes such things as death of a spouse, change in work status, illness in the family, marriage, taking out a large mortgage, and a number of other events. Each item has a particular score, which is supposed to be related to how stressful it would be to have to adapt to such a change in one's life. In the instructions for this scale it says that a total score of over 150 means that you are under considerable stress and need to make sure you are taking steps to adapt to these situations effectively.

On the day we discussed it in class, Laurie had the highest score on the life-events scale of anyone in the class. She told us how she and her boyfriend had both tallied their scores one night. She scored 879 and he scored in the 700s. Their response was to laugh when they saw how high their scores were. They figured they must be stronger than they thought because, as she put it, looking at their scores, "It's a miracle we are not both dead." She knew they could easily have been crying rather than laughing. She said that she saw laughing as a good sign, a healthy response in itself.

Laurie's life at that time was dominated by fear that her ex-husband was trying to kill her, which, according to her, he had actually attempted to do. On top of this, her two sons had recently been injured in a car accident although not seriously, and she was going through a very stressful time at work.

She worked as a middle manager in a large corporation that was going through a major restructuring that made everybody feel insecure and under a lot of pressure. Her situation was made more complex by the fact that she, her boyfriend, and her ex-husband all worked for the same company.

In the fifth class (that is, after practicing the body scan for four weeks and the yoga for two) she said that during that week she had seen the lights that usually precede a big headache. But for the first time she had become aware of them early on. There were only a few lights, not the overwhelming array that usually meant that the headache was less than an hour away and already, as she put it, "unstoppable." She decided then and there to take one pill and get into bed and do the body scan, thinking that maybe she could avoid taking the other three pills that she was supposed to take in sequence over several hours to control the headaches with medication.

What Laurie reported with some pride was that, for the first time since she was a girl, she had been able to short-circuit a headache on her own. She never took the other three pills. She did the body scan, fell asleep toward the end, and woke up feeling completely refreshed. She attributed her success to two things: First, she felt that practicing the meditation over the preceding weeks had helped her to become more sensitive to her body and to what she was feeling. This is why, she feels, she was able to be aware of the early warning signs of the migraine (technically known as the prodrome; in Laurie's case, the lights), several hours before the full-blown headache was upon her and to take some action. Second, she now had something she could do at such a time—or at least she felt she had something she could try out as an alternative to taking a drug to control her headache. She had approached the headache in a new way, experimenting with her own inner resources for control.

Laurie continued to be headache-free over the next four weeks, even though her life was in a state of perpetual upheaval. She put the nine dots up on the wall in her office, and she tried to *respond* to the stressors in her life instead of reacting to them.

In the week following the end of the program, she had another big migraine headache. It came on the day before Thanksgiving and continued through the next day. She wouldn't let herself be taken to the emergency room, although she was in the bathroom throwing up more than she was with her family. They were begging her to let them take her to the hospital. But in her mind, her sons had come home for Thanksgiving dinner and she could only think of how awful it was that she was so sick on the one day that she was getting to see them.

When I saw her the next morning, she was pale, distraught, and tearful. She said she felt like a "failure" after all the good results she had had during the course. She had been hoping that her doctor would take her off her Inderal if she was able to remain headache-free. Now she felt she had "blown that possibility comletely." Even worse, she also felt like a failure because she had no idea why she had gotten the headache. She said that she hadn't felt stressed by the thought of Thanksgiving. On the contrary, she had been looking forward to it. But as we talked more about the days leading up to the holiday, it became clearer to her that it did have a special meaning for her that year and that she had had higher expectations than usual because her boys were coming and she had been feeling that she hadn't been seeing enough of them. She also recalled, as we talked, that on Tuesday, before the headache came on with full force, she had been seeing the lights and spots in front of her eyes but that they just hadn't really registered in her awareness. She recalled that her boyfriend had asked her at a certain point what she wanted to do for dinner and she had said, "I don't know, I can't think. My mind is a blank."

This was probably the critical point for her. It was an early warning signal from her body that a migraine was coming on. But this time, for some reason, the message just did not get through. She said later that she was probably feeling too busy and rushed and too tired to listen to her body, even though she had had the successful experience of short-circuiting the last one by taking immediate action when she had felt the early warning signs.

After her upset with herself had subsided, she was able to realize that this horrible headache did not mean that she was a failure. If anything, it meant that she might benefit from being even more tuned in to her body's messages. She began to see that perhaps it was unrealistic to expect that after twenty-seven years of problems with migraine headaches, she would learn to control them in four weeks to the point where they would never be a problem for her again, especially given the current upheavals in her life.

By not generalizing from this one headache into making herself a failure, Laurie was able to see that having this *particular* headache at this *particular* time was teaching her something she hadn't yet fully realized and that, in that sense, it could be seen as helpful. It was teaching her that she needed to honor how much of a crisis her life was in at that time, what with court dates coming up and her problems at work and her anger at her ex-husband. It was teaching her that such pressures don't go away just because a holiday is coming up. In fact, they can make the holiday more of a loaded situation emotionally and lead to unconscious but strong expectations and desires that things go a certain way. And most importantly, the headache was teaching her that, at this time in her life especially, she can't afford to override her body's messages. She needs to honor them and be even more prepared than she had been to stop what she is doing when the early warning signs come on, take her medication, and practice the body scan *immediately*. If this is what the full catastrophe of her situation demands of her, then for now nothing less will do if she hopes ultimately to come to greater harmony in her life and to free herself from her headaches, metaphorically and literally.

24

Working with Emotional Pain: Your Suffering Is Not You . . . But There Is Much You Can Do to Heal It

The body has no monopoly on suffering. Emotional pain, the pain in our hearts and minds, is far more widespread and just as likely to be debilitating as physical pain. This pain can take many forms. There is the suffering of self-condemnation, such as when we blame ourselves for something we did or for something we didn't do or when we feel unworthy or stupid and lack confidence in ourselves. If we caused other people hurt, we might also experience the pain of guilt, a combination of self-blame and remorse. There is pain in anxiety, worry, fear, and terror. There is pain in loss and grief, humiliation and embarrassment, despair and hopelessness. We may carry one kind of emotional pain or another deep within our hearts, often for much of our lives, like a heavy and sometimes secret burden, at times unknown even to ourselves.

Just as with physical pain, you can be mindful of emotional pain and can use its energy to grow and heal. The key is to be willing to inquire into your suffering, to observe it, to open up to it consciously, in the present, and work *with* it just as you would with a symptom, with physical pain, or with a thought that surfaces repeatedly.

It is difficult to convey the importance of being able to shift your perspective to an acceptance of the present *as it is* when emotional pain surfaces. Whether, as has happened to people who were in the stress clinic, it is feeling frightened by a medical emergency that takes you to the ICU, or angry and humiliated because the police came to your door and took you away in the middle of the night, or frustrated and depressed because a new doctor yelled at you in front of a waiting room full of people and refused to fill a prescription you had been given routinely in the same clinic for years, it is your willingness to practice mindfulness *in these moments* and in the aftermath of such moments that is most important. Mindfulness *while* you are experiencing pain is critical to working with your emotions.

Of course, the natural tendency is to avoid feelings of pain whenever possible and to wall ourselves off from as much of it as we can, or to be automatically swept away by a tidal wave of feelings. In either case we are too preoccupied, our minds too turbulent, to remember to look directly, with eyes of wholeness, in such moments—that is, unless we have been training the mind to see its own upsets, whatever they may be and however painful, as opportunities to respond in new ways rather than becoming a victim of our own reactions. In the end, the damage that is done when we deny or avoid our feelings or become lost in them only compounds our suffering.

As with physical pain, our emotional pain is also trying to tell us something. It, too, is a messenger. Feelings have to be acknowledged, at least to ourselves. They have to be encountered and felt in all their force. There is no other way through to the other side of them. If we ignore them or repress them or suppress them or sublimate them, they fester and yield no resolution, no peace. And if we exaggerate them and dramatize them and preoccupy ourselves with their turmoil without any awareness of what we are doing, they also linger on and cause us to become stuck.

Even in the tortured throes of grief or anger, in the gnawing remorse of guilt, in the slack tides of sadness and hurt, and in the swells of fear, it is still possible to be mindful, to know that in this moment I am feeling grief, I am feeling anger, I am feeling guilty or sad or hurt or frightened, or confused.

Strange as it may sound, the intentional *knowing* of your feelings in times of emotional suffering contains in itself the seeds of healing. Just as we saw with physical pain, that part of you that can *know* your feelings, that sees clearly what they are, that can accept them in the present, while they are happening, no matter what they are, in their full, undisguised fury if such is the case, or in their many disguises, such as confusion, rigidity or alienation, that awareness itself has an independent perspective that is outside of your suffering. It is not buffeted by the storms of the heart and of the mind. The storms still have to run their course, their pain has to be felt. But they actually unfold differently when cradled in awareness.

For one thing, they are no longer just happening *to* you, like an outside force. You are now taking responsibility for feeling what you are feeling in this moment because this is what is happening now in your life. These moments of pain are as much moments to be lived fully as are any others, and they can actually teach us a great deal, although few of us would seek out these lessons willingly. But relating to your pain consciously, as long as it is here anyway, allows you to be a participant with your feelings rather than a victim of them.

And even though the pain you feel may be as great as if there were no seeing, no conscious awareness of a larger picture at all, this bringing of attention to emotion allows you to see your feelings with a certain degree of wisdom. The pain may be as great, but at least the edge comes off the suffering when we inquire into who is suffering, when we observe our mind flailing about, rejecting, protesting, denying, clamoring, fantasizing, hurting.

Mindfulness allows us to see more clearly into the nature of our pain. Sometimes it helps us to cut through confusion, hurt feelings, and emotional turmoil caused perhaps by misperceptions or exaggerations and our desire that things be a certain way. When you next find yourself in a period of suffering, try listening for a calm inner voice that might be saying, "Isn't this interesting, isn't it amazing what a human being can go through, amazing how much pain and anguish I can feel or create for myself or get bogged down in?" In listening for a calm voice within your own heart, within your own pain, you will be reminding yourself to observe the unfolding of your emotions with wise attention, with a degree of non-attachment. You may find yourself wondering how things will finally be resolved, and knowing that you don't know, that you will just have to wait and see. Yet you can be certain that a resolution will come, that what you are experiencing is like the crest of a wave—it can't keep itself up indefinitely—it has to release. And you will know as well that how you handle what is going on at the crest of this wave can influence what the resolution will be. For instance, if, in a fit of anger, you say or do something that deeply harms another person, you have compounded the suffering of the moment even further and ensured that the resolution will be even further away, and perhaps much less to your liking. So in moments of great emotional pain, perhaps you will come to accept not knowing how things will resolve in the present moment, and in that acceptance, begin the process of healing.

You may discern within your pain, even as you feel it, that some of it is coming from non-acceptance, from rejecting what has *already* happened or what was said or done, from wanting things to be some other way, more to your liking, more under your control. Perhaps you would like another chance. Perhaps you want to turn back the clock and do something differently, or to say something you didn't, or to take back something you did. Perhaps you are jumping to conclusions without knowing the whole story and feeling hurt unnecessarily because of your own premature reactions to things. There are many ways in which we suffer, but usually they are variations on a few basic patterns.

If you are mindful as emotional storms occur, perhaps you will see in yourself an unwillingness to accept things as they already are, whether you like them or not. Perhaps that part of you that does see this has, in one way or another, already come to terms with what has happened or with your situation. Perhaps, at the same time, it recognizes that your feelings still need to play themselves out, that they are not ready to accept or to calm down, and that this is all right.

Just as in the meditation practice, our minds have a strong tendency to reject things as they are when it comes to *my* pain, *my* dilemmas, *my* grief. As Einstein pointed out, this locks us into an identification with our separateness. As we have seen, such a view can cut us off from our ability to see clearly and to heal just when we need it most.

If a momentary insight into the process of your pain unfolding should arise, let it be simply an observation. Do not jump from it to a blanket condemnation of yourself for not "being able" to accept what is or to identify with the greater whole. Your unwillingness to accept may be totally appropriate in this moment. You may feel threatened by an impending calamity or sense of doom. Or perhaps you have suffered a grievous loss, or have been wronged by someone, or you made some error in judgment that you feel remorse for and are unwilling to "just accept."

As we saw in Chapter 2, acceptance does not mean that you *like* what has occurred or that you are merely resigned to it. It does not mean capitulation or surrender. The way we are using the word here, it means only that you admit the bare fact that whatever has happened has *already* happened and is therefore in the past. More often than not, acceptance can only come in time, as the storm plays itself out, as the winds die down. But how much healing takes place after the devastation depends on how much you are able to be awake, face its energies, and observe them with wise attention while they are raging.

Profoundly healing insights may arise if you are willing to look deeply into your own emotional pain as it occurs. One major realization you might come to is the inevitability of change, the direct perception that, whether we like it or not, *impermanence is in the very nature of things and relationships*. We saw this within physical pain when we observed changes in its intensity and the coming and going of different sensations, even the shifting of the pain from one place to another in the body as sometimes happens. We also noted it in our changing thoughts and feelings about pain.

When you look deeply into emotional pain at the time you are feeling it, it is hard to deny that here, too, your thoughts and feelings are coming and going, appearing and disappearing and changing with great rapidity. In times of great stress you may notice certain thoughts and feelings recurring with great frequency. They come back over and over again, causing you to keep reliving what happened or wondering what you might have done differently or how what happened could have come about. You may find yourself blaming yourself or someone else over and over again, or reliving a particular moment again and again, or wondering over and over what will happen next or what will become of you now.

But if you can be mindful at such times, if you are watching carefully, you will also notice that even these recurring images, thoughts, and feelings have a beginning and an end, that they are like waves that rise up in the mind and then subside. You may also notice that they are never quite the same. Each time one comes back, it is slightly different, never exactly the same as any previous wave.

You may also notice that the intensity of your feelings cycles as well. One moment there may be a dull hurt, the next moment intense anguish and fury, the next moment fear, then dullness again or exhaustion. You may even forget you hurt altogether for brief moments. In seeing these changes in your emotional state, you may come to realize that none of what you are experiencing is permanent. You can actually see for yourself that the intensity of the pain is not constant, that it changes, goes up and down, comes and goes, just as your breath comes and goes.

That part of you that is mindful is just seeing what is transpiring from moment to moment, nothing more. It is not rejecting the bad, it is not condemning anything or anybody, it is not wishing that things were different, it is not even upset. Awareness, like a field of compassionate intelligence located within your own heart, takes it all in and serves as a source of peace within the turmoil, much as a mother would be a source of peace, compassion, and perspective for a child who was upset. She knows that whatever is troubling her child will pass, so she can provide comfort, reassurance, and peace in her very being.

When we cultivate mindfulness in our own hearts, we can direct a similar compassion toward ourselves. Sometimes we need to care for ourselves as if that part of us that is suffering is our own child. Why not show compassion, kindness, and sympathy toward our own being, even as we open fully to our pain? To treat ourself with as much kindness as we would another person in pain is a wonderfully healing meditation in its own right. It cultivates lovingkindness and compassion, which know no boundaries.

A "WHAT IS MY OWN WAY?" MEDITATION

One of the major sources of suffering in our lives is that we usually want to have things our own way. Thus when things happen that we like, we feel that everything is going our way and we feel happy. And when things "go against us," when they do not happen the way we want or the way we expected or planned for, then we tend to feel thwarted, frustrated, angry, wounded, unhappy, and we suffer.

The irony is that often we really don't know what our way is, even though we want to have it all the time. If we get what we want, we usually want something else in addition. The mind keeps finding new things that it needs in order to feel happy or fulfilled. In this regard, it is rarely satisfied with things as they are for very long, even if things are relatively peaceful and satisfying.

When little children get upset because they can't have everything they see that they would like to have, we are apt to tell them, "You can't always have your own way." And when they say, "Why not?" we say, "Because" or "You'll understand when you grow up." But this is a fiction we perpetrate on them. In fact, most of the time we grown-ups don't behave as if we understand life any better than our children do. We want to have things our own way too. We just want different things than they do. Don't we get just as upset when things don't turn out as we want them to? We find it easy to smile at their childishness or to get angry at it, depending on our own state of mind. Perhaps we have just learned how to hide our feelings better.

To break out of this trap of always being driven by our own desires, it is not a bad exercise to ask yourself from time to time, "What *is* my own way?" "What *do* I really want?" "Would I know it if I got it?" "Does everything have to be 'perfect' right now, or under my total control right now, for me to be happy?"

Alternatively, you might ask yourself, "Is everything already basically okay right now?" "Am I just *not noticing* the ways in which things are good because my mind keeps coming up with ideas for what it has to have or has to get rid of before I can be happy, just like a child?" Or, if that is not the case, you might go on to ask, "Are there specific steps that I can take, seeing my unhappiness right now, that would help me to move toward greater peace and harmony in my life?" "Are there decisions I could make that would help me to find my own way?" "Do I have any power to chart my own way, or am I fated to live out the rest of my life unable to experience happiness or peace because of fate, because of decisions I made or that were made for me decades ago, perhaps when I was young and silly, or blind, or insecure, or more unaware than I am now?"

If you practice incorporating *asking yourself about your own way* into your meditation practice, you will find that it is very effective in bringing you back to the present moment. You might try sitting with the question "Right now, what is my way?" It is sufficient to ask the question. Trying to answer it is not necessary. It is more fruitful just to ponder the question, keeping it alive from moment to moment, listening for the response from within your own heart. "What is my own way?" "What is my own way?"

◆

Many of the people in the stress clinic rapidly discover that their own way may be the life that they are actually living. What other way could be theirs? They come to see that their pain is a part of their own way, too, and not necessarily an enemy. They also come to see that at least some of their emotional pain, if not most of it, comes from their own actions or inaction and is thus potentially manageable. In seeing with eyes of wholeness, they come to realize that they are not their suffering, just as they are not their symptoms, their physical pain, or their illness.

These realizations are not some abstract philosophy. They have very practical consequences. They lead directly to an ability to do something about your emotional suffering, right in the intensive care unit, right in the police van, right in the doctor's office, or at work or wherever else your life takes an unexpected turn and you find yourself in uncharted territory with very strong feelings surfacing in yourself or in others. Taking responsibility for your own mind at such times provides comforting passageways through what may have seemed like impenetrable barriers, walls of fear or hopelessness or lack of confidence. Such passageways out of suffering appear in those moments when it dawns on you that "this is it," that the life you are actually living right now is your life, the only one you have. When you are willing to see in this way, it becomes possible to accept your life fully in this moment, just as it is, whatever the particulars. For the moment at least, what is happening is what is happening. The future is unknown and the past has already happened.

In coming to your own center of calmness and clear seeing, you become less susceptible to the feelings of fear and hopelessness that might arise in such moments. Right in the pain you are already taking steps toward doing what needs to be done, toward affirming your own integrity, toward healing.

Suggesting that this course is possible and practical is not to belittle either pain or suffering. They are all too real. Rather it is to say that as the emotional upheavals come and go or our bad feelings linger and weigh on us, we also know, because we are tasting it, that our strength and our ability to grow and to make changes, to transcend our hurts and our deepest losses, do not depend on outside forces or on chance. They reside here already, within our own hearts, right now.

PROBLEM-FOCUSED COPING AND EMOTION-FOCUSED COPING

Working mindfully with your emotions begins by acknowledging to yourself what you are actually feeling and thinking in the present. It is helpful to come to a complete stop and, even for short periods, to *sit with the hurt,* breathing with it, feeling it, not trying to explain it or change it or make it go away. This in itself brings calmness.

Once again, it helps to remember to look at your situation with eyes of wholeness. From a systems perspective, there are two major interacting components to emotional pain. One is the domain of your *feelings;* the other is the domain of the situation, or *problem,* which lies at the root of the feelings. In being with your hurt, you might ask yourself whether you can see your emotional state as separate from the details of what has actually happened or is happening. If you can differentiate between these two components of your dilemma, you are more likely to chart your way through to an effective resolution of the entire situation, including your feelings. If, on the other hand, the domain of feelings and the domain of the problem itself get confused, as they often do, it is very difficult to see clearly and to know how to act decisively. This confusion itself generates more pain and more suffering.

Try focusing on the problem. Ask yourself if you are seeing it in its fullness, apart from your strong feelings *about the problem.* Then ask yourself whether there might be actions that you could take that would help solve things in the domain of the problem. If the whole problem seems too big to handle, try breaking it down into manageable parts in your mind. Then act. Do *something.* Listen to and trust your intuition, your heart. You might attempt to correct the problem or to reduce the extent of the damage as best you can. On the other hand, you might see that there are times when absolutely nothing can be done. If this is your perception, then really do *nothing. Do* non-doing! You can use your understanding of non-doing just to be with what is in such moments, intentionally. This is as much of a *response* as anything you might *do.* Sometimes, it is the most appropriate response possible.

By acting mindfully when you can, whether it results in doing or non-doing, you are putting the past behind you. As you act in the present, things change in response to what you choose to do, and this in turn will affect the problem itself. This way of proceeding is sometimes called *problem-focused coping.* It can help you to function effectively in spite of strong emotional reactions; and it can prevent you from doing things that might make matters worse than they already are.

On a parallel track, you can bring awareness to what you are *feeling.* Try to be aware of the source of your suffering. Is it from guilt or fear or loss? What are the thoughts going through your mind? Are they accurate? Can you just watch the play of your thoughts and feelings with full acceptance, seeing them as a storm system or a cresting wave that has a structure and life of its own? Are they affecting your judgment and your ability to see clearly? Are they telling you to do things that you are aware might make things worse rather than better? Bringing wise attention to the domain of feelings is part of what is sometimes called *emotion-focused coping*. As we have seen, just bringing mindfulness to the storm system itself influences how it resolves and so helps you to cope with it. A further step in this process comes when you are able to entertain alternative ways of seeing your feelings, when you are able to hold them in the consciousness of being your own loving parent, when you can bring gentleness and lovingkindness to yourself in the midst of your pain.

Let's look at a concrete example combining problem-focused and emotion-focused coping and see how they might be used together:

I was climbing a mountain with my son, Will, in the spring when he was eleven years old. We had on heavy packs. It was late in the afternoon and it looked like a storm was coming. We were halfway up a difficult series of high ledges and found the going quite rough, especially with the packs. At a certain point we found ourselves holding on to a small tree that was growing out of the rock, looking at the valley beneath us and the storm clouds gathering. All of a sudden we both got scared. It wasn't at all clear how to get up and over the next ledge. It really felt as if one of us could slip and fall very easily. Will was shaking, at that moment frozen by fear. He definitely did not want to go higher.

Our fear was very strong, but it was also an embarrassment. Neither of us wanted to admit to feeling frightened, but there it was. To me, it seemed as if we had only two choices. We could push on and "tough it out" and not pay attention to our feelings, or we could honor them. Especially with the storm coming, it seemed as if our feelings might be telling us something very important. We clung to the little tree and purposefully tuned in to our breathing and to our feelings, suspended somewhere between the top of the mountain and the bottom and not knowing what to do.

As we did this, we calmed down some and were able to think more clearly. We talked about our options, about our strong desire to push on to the top, about not wanting to feel that our fear was "defeating" us, but also weighing our sense of danger and vulnerability at that moment. It didn't take long for us to decide to honor our feelings and to back off from our original intent. We cautiously went back down and found shelter just as the winds and heavy rains let loose. We spent the night snug in a shelter, happy that we had had the sense to honor what we were feeling. But we still wanted to try to climb the mountain. In fact, we wanted to do it more than ever so that, if possible, we would not be left with the feeling that it was our fear that had ultimately prevented us from reaching the summit.

So the next day, as we ate breakfast, we developed a strategy that broke the problem down into pieces. We decided to take each phase of the path up as it came, agreeing that we didn't know how difficult it would be for us to get over the ledges with our packs on. We also agreed that we didn't know what would happen or whether it would be possible for us to make it to the top but that we would try anyway and deal with any problems as we encountered them.

It was very slippery on the rock because of all the rain. This made the going even more difficult than the day before. Almost right away we decided to try going barefoot to see if that would improve our traction. It did. A lot. We climbed as far as we felt comfortable with the packs. When we reached the ledges again, it seemed that Will's pack was just too big and heavy for him and was causing him to be pulled backward as he tried to find fingerholds and footholds up the rock. So we decided to leave the packs and go up as far as we could and just see what things looked like. We got to the little tree again and this time there was no sense of fear in either of us. Barefoot and without the packs, we felt completely secure. What had seemed like an insurmountable obstacle the day before now seemed easy. Now we could see exactly how to go higher from where the tree was. So we climbed on until we reached a place beneath the top where the going got a lot easier.

The view was spectacular. We were above rapidly dissipating storm clouds, watching the mountains as they became bathed in the morning sunlight. After a while, I left Will there, perfectly happy to be alone. He sat perched on a rock in the stillness of the morning, looking out over the valleys and the mountains for well over an hour while I went down to get the packs and bring them up, one at a time. Then we went on our way.

I tell this story because I saw so clearly when we were stopped at the little tree how important it was for us that we got frightened.

It kept us from acting foolishly. I also saw in that moment how important it was going to be *for both of us* to attempt that same route up again the next day, under better conditions and taking a problem-solving approach. When we did so, we dealt with the slipperiness and the weight of the backpacks in imaginative ways. This allowed us to come once more to the point where we had experienced our fear the day before and to see whether we could move through it and beyond it at a different moment in time.

What Will took away from this experience was a sense that fear could be worked with. He learned he could honor feeling frightened, that this feeling could even be helpful and intelligent, and that it was neither a sign of weakness on his part nor an inevitable result of going up the mountain that way. One day things could be frightening, the next day not. Same mountain, same people, but also different. By our willingness to see the problem as separate from our feelings and to honor *both*, we had been able to be patient and to not let the fear mushroom and become dangerous in itself or to defeat our confidence. This strategy enabled us to break down the problem of getting to the top of the mountain into smaller problems that we then took on one at a time, experimenting, seeing how things would go, not knowing whether we would make it but at least trying again and using our imagination, taking things moment by moment.

◆

When you find yourself in times of emotional turmoil and pain, it can be very therapeutic to proceed simultaneously on parallel tracks. One track involves awareness of your thoughts and feelings (the emotion-focused perspective). The other involves working with the situation itself (the problem-focused perspective). Both are essential for responding effectively in stressful and threatening situations.

In the problem-focused approach, as we have just seen, we try to identify the source and scope of the problem with some clarity, independent of our feelings. We try to discern what might need to be accomplished, what actions might need to be taken, what the potential obstacles to progress are, and also what inner and outer resources are available. To proceed in this way, you may need to try things you have never tried before, seek other people's advice and help, even acquire new skills yourself in order to deal with certain problems. But if you break the problem down into manageable pieces and then take them on one at a time, you may find that you can act effectively even in times of emotional pain. In some cases, approaching things in this way can diminish your emotional arousal or suspend it long enough to prevent you from compounding your problems.

There can also be pitfalls to a problem-focused coping approach, especially if you forget that it is only one of two parallel tracks. There are some people who tend to relate to everything in life in an objective, problem-solving mode. In the process, they may cut themselves off from their own feelings about the situations they face and fail to recognize and respond to other people's feelings as well. This habit will hardly lead to a balanced way of life. It can create much unnecessary suffering.

Focusing on our emotions, we observe our feelings and thoughts from the perspective of mindfulness and remind ourselves that we can work *with* our feelings, just as Will and I did at the little tree. You can usually expand your perspective around your feelings and thus cradle them, as we have seen, in awareness. You may sometimes hear this referred to as *reframing*, in other words, putting a larger or different frame around the issue in question. Reframing can be done with either your emotions, the problem itself, or both. Seeing a problem as an opportunity or challenge is an example of reframing. So is seeing your hurt in the frame of the suffering of other people who may be worse off than yourself. Mindfulness itself is the ultimate frame within which to perceive the actuality of things as they are.

◆

Times of great emotional upheaval and turmoil, times of sadness, anger, fear, and grief, moments when we feel hurt, lost, humiliated, thwarted, or defeated, are times when we most need to know that the core of our being is stable and resilient and that we can weather these moments and become more human in the process. It helps to come to stillness in such moments. When we observe our emotional pain as it unfolds, with acceptance, with openness and kindness toward ourselves and at the same time take a problem-focused approach toward the situation itself, we strike a balance between facing, honoring, and learning from our emotional pain moment by moment as it is expressing itself and acting effectively in the world, which itself minimizes the many ways in which we can get stuck in and blinded by emotion. Mindfulness of our thoughts and feelings, particularly those that arise from our relationships with others and in stressful, threatening, and emotionally charged situations, can play a major role in helping us to act effectively in the midst of our deepest emotional pain. At the same time, it sows seeds that heal the heart and the mind.

25

Working with Fear, Panic, and Anxiety

There is a wonderful scene in the movie *Starting Over*, in which Burt Reynolds is in the furniture section of a big department store with a young woman (Jill Clayburgh) when she proceeds to have an anxiety attack right there in the store. As he struggles in a bewildered fashion to help her pull herself together and get her emotions under control, he looks up to find that they are surrounded by a horde of gawking shoppers. He shouts out, "Quick, does anyone have a Valium?" at which point one hundred hands fish frantically into their coat pockets and purses.

This is certainly an age of anxiety. Many of the people in the stress clinic have problems related to anxiety, caused by the rampant stress in their lives and compounded by their medical problems. Anxiety is one of the most pervasive mind states we encounter in the clinic. This is hardly surprising, since most of our patients are sent precisely because either they or their doctors think they need to learn how to relax and how to handle stress better.

If we are honest with ourselves, most of us will have to admit that we live out our lives on an ocean of fear. From time to time, in even the hardiest of us, feelings of fear surface. They may be about death or being abandoned by someone. They may be about being abused or violated or tortured, or about feeling pain or being alone or being sick or disabled, or about someone you love being hurt or killed. We may have fears of failure or fears of success, fears of letting other people down or about the fate of the earth. Most of us carry such fears within us. They are always present but they only surface under certain circumstances.

Some people handle feelings of fear much better than others do. Commonly, we cope with our fears by ignoring such feelings

334 TAKING ON THE FULL CATASTROPHE

when they surface or denying them altogether, or concealing them from other people. But to cope in this way increases the likelihood that damage will be done in some other way, either by developing habitual maladaptive behavior patterns such as passivity or aggressiveness to compensate for our insecurities, by becoming overwhelmed and incapacitated by the very feelings themselves when they do surface, or by focusing on physical symptoms or other less threatening aspects of our lives that we feel more able to control. And many people are unable to cope even in these questionable ways. They find it difficult, if not impossible, to deny or ignore or conceal their anxiety. Without effective means for dealing with it, their anxiety can have significant detrimental effects on their ability to function. And of course, it causes people to pursue many of the maladaptive coping avenues we reviewed in Chapter 19.

Mindfulness practice can have a positive impact on anxiety reactions via the stress-response pathway discussed in Chapter 20. As you might imagine, the application of mindfulness to chronic anxiety involves allowing the anxiety itself to become the object of our non-judgmental attention. We intentionally observe fear and anxiety when they come up, just as we do with pain. When you move in close to your fears and observe them as they surface in the form of thoughts, feelings, and bodily sensations, you will be in a much better position to recognize them for what they are and know how to respond to them appropriately. Then you will be less prone to become overwhelmed or swept away by them or to have to compensate in self-destructive or self-inhibiting ways.

The word *fear* implies that there is something specific that is causing this emotional state to arise. Under certain threatening circumstances, all of us might experience fear, even terror. It is a major characteristic of the fight-or-flight reaction. Suddenly being unable to breathe would trigger it, for example. People with lung disease have to face this kind of fear and learn to work with the panic it induces. Being the object of an attack or learning that you have a fatal disease would be other examples.

Under such circumstances, frightening thoughts or experiences can easily lead to a state of panic, driven by desperation and feelings of complete loss of control. But to panic in a threatening situation is a very dangerous and unfortunate reaction, because it is disabling just at the time that you most need to keep your wits about you and problem-solve with extreme rapidity and clarity.

When we speak of "anxiety," we are talking about a similar

strongly reactive emotional state but without a clearly identifiable impending cause or threat. Anxiety is a generalized state of insecurity and agitation that can be triggered by almost anything. Sometimes it seems as if there is nothing triggering it at all. You can feel anxious and not really know why. As we saw in Chapter 23 when we discussed headaches, it is possible to wake up feeling shaky, tense, and frightened. If you are plagued by anxious feelings, your anxiety may frequently seem out of proportion to the actual pressures you are under. You may have a hard time putting your finger on the root cause of your feelings. You may find yourself worrying all the time, even when there is nothing the matter or there is no major threat. You may be tense all the time and feeling that "If it's not one thing, then it's another," that there is always *something* to be worried about. If this state of mind becomes a chronic condition, it is referred to as generalized anxiety. Its symptoms may include trembling, shakiness, muscle tension, restlessness, easy fatigability, shortness of breath, rapid heartbeat, sweating, dry mouth, dizziness or light-headedness, nausea, the feeling of a "lump in the throat," feeling keyed up, being easily startled, difficulty concentrating, trouble falling asleep or staying asleep, and irritability.

In addition to generalized anxiety, some people suffer from what are called anxiety attacks, or panic attacks. These are episodes in which a person experiences a discrete period of intense fear and discomfort for no apparent reason. Often people who suffer from panic attacks have no idea why they get them or when one will happen. The first time it happens, you can think you are having a heart attack since it is frequently accompanied by acute physical symptoms including chest pains, dizziness, shortness of breath, and profuse sweating. There may be feelings of unreality and you may also think that you are dying or that you are going crazy or that you may lose control of yourself. It may be very disconcerting rather than reassuring if your doctor tells you that you are not having a heart attack and you are not going crazy, because it is apparent that *something* is very wrong. If you are cared for by a doctor who can recognize these symptoms as a panic attack, you may be on the road to getting the right kind of help in bringing them under control. Unfortunately, many people with panic attacks continue to visit emergency rooms and wind up being told that "there is nothing wrong" and being sent home with no assistance or with a prescription for tranquilizers.

While it can be reassuring to know what a panic attack is and that you are not going to die from it or go crazy, what is most important is that you know that you can work with these mind-body storms by changing the way you see and pay attention to the very processes of thought and reactivity within your own mind. It is to undertake such work that physicians send their patients with chronic panic attacks to the stress clinic.

MINDFULNESS CAN REDUCE ANXIETY AND PANIC

In collaboration with Drs. Linda Peterson and Ann Massion in the department of psychiatry, and Drs. Jean Kristeller and Lori Pbert in behavioral medicine at the University of Massachusetts Medical School, we studied the effects of mindfulness training in the stress clinic on people referred for anxiety and panic attacks. This study came about because we were seeing dramatic improvements in people with anxiety conditions, improvements that we thought merited a more systematic investigation. In addition to people's reports that they were feeling more in control of their panicky feelings, they were showing major reductions in measures of anxiety, phobic anxiety, and medical symptoms following the program. We wanted to put these results to a more stringent test, using even more sophisticated measures to monitor psychological status. We also felt the need to confirm independently that the people who were being referred to the stress clinic primarily for anxiety and panic attacks were being correctly diagnosed. We began the study by inviting people referred to the stress clinic by their doctors for problems associated with anxiety or panic to participate. Each person who agreed was interviewed at length by either a psychiatrist or a clinical psychologist to establish a precise psychological diagnosis. Their levels of anxiety, depression, and panic were then assessed weekly while they were undergoing training in the stress clinic and for three months after the program ended. Twenty-three people were followed in this way.

We found that both anxiety and depression dropped markedly in virtually every person in the study. So did the frequency and severity of their panic attacks. The three-month follow-up showed that they maintained their improvements after completion of the program. Most individuals were virtually free of panic attacks by the end of the follow-up period.

This study clearly showed that people who have panic attacks and anxiety disorders are able to put mindfulness training to practical use in regulating their feelings of anxiety and panic. It also showed that what they learned in the program had a lasting positive effect, just as we saw with the people with chronic pain conditions over a much longer period in Chapter 22.

During this study, the instructors in the stress reduction classes did nothing special with these patients. The program was not altered in any way to try to get good results with anxiety patients. They were mixed in with everybody else—people with chronic pain, heart disease, and all the other problems that people come with. And although the results of the study showed major improvements among the twenty-three people who were followed in this way on the various symptom measures we used, the most interesting part is that, ultimately, as with each person who goes through the clinic, they all had their own unique experiences and stories to tell. Although the results suggest that practicing mindfulness can dramatically reduce anxiety and the frequency and severity of panic attacks, it is in their individual stories that we can best see how meditation practice can help someone who is suffering from anxiety. The following is an account of how one person successfully resolved her problems after eleven years of chronic anxiety and panic.

CLAIRE'S STORY

Claire, a thirty-three-year-old happily married woman with a seven-year-old son, came to the stress clinic when she was six months pregnant with her second child. She had been having feelings of panic and actual panic attacks on and off for the past eleven years, since her father died. In the last four years the attacks had gotten much worse and were preventing her from living a normal life. Claire described herself as having been raised in an overprotective ethnic family. She was twenty-two and engaged to be married when her father died. She had promised him that she would get married right away, even if he were to die before the wedding, which is what happened. Her father died on a Thursday, he was buried on Saturday, and on Sunday she was married. She said she knew nothing about the world at that time, having always been protected from problems by living at home.

Until that time, Claire had thought of herself as happy and well adjusted. Her problems with anxiety started shortly after her father's death and getting married. She would find herself feeling nervous and worked up about little things that she knew weren't important or even real, and she felt unable to either explain or control these feelings. She began to think she was "going crazy." This pattern of anxious thoughts and feelings got worse over the years. She felt less and less in control. Four years prior to her coming to the stress clinic, she began having attacks in which she actually passed out. At that point she went to see a neurologist, who gave her tranquilizers and told her that her problems were due to anxiety.

From then on, her biggest fear was that she would make a fool of herself by passing out in a crowd of people. She was afraid to drive or to go places alone. She began seeing a psychiatrist, who continued her on the tranquilizers. He also urged her to take antidepressants as well, but she refused.

After some time in treatment, Claire and her husband came to feel that the therapeutic approach being taken with her amounted to trying to "brainwash" her into taking medication rather than taking her seriously as a person.

Her psychiatrist saw her only to change her medication and worked in conjunction with a counselor who saw Claire regularly. She recalled that both the psychiatrist and the counselor repeatedly told her that the medication was the solution to her problems, that she was "just that kind of person," the kind that needs to take tranquilizers every day to get through the day. They used the argument that her situation was no different than people with high blood pressure or with a thyroid condition. These people need to take medication every day to keep their conditions regulated, and she did too. The message was that she should stop resisting their efforts to help her and just be cooperative. They kept insisting that her panic attacks could only be controlled if she would take the drugs. And for the most part she did, at least at first.

But in her heart Claire was feeling that her doctor and counselor had no interest in her unless she was willing to accept their position on her need for medication. When she would go in and tell them that the medication wasn't working, that she was still having panic attacks, the psychiatrist would simply increase the dose. She just didn't feel heard as a person.

She also felt blamed. She was accused of being stubborn and unreasonable for refusing to go on antidepressants and for questioning the need to be on the tranquilizers for an indefinite period. It bothered her that they would never tell her how long she would have to be on them. She felt they were implying that she would probably be on them for decades and that she would always have to be in counseling. When she asked about alternative approaches that might replace the drugs, such as stress reduction, yoga, relaxation, and biofeedback, she was told that she could do that if she wanted, that "It won't hurt, but it won't help your problem."

The last straw for her came when she learned she was pregnant. Looking back, she feels that this pregnancy was a blessing because it resulted in a dramatic change in her relationship to the medical world. She insisted on getting off all her medication as soon as she found out she was pregnant, against the advice of her psychiatrist and counselor. She saw another counselor for a while who supported her position and she finally decided to stop seeing the psychiatrist altogether because it was always such a battle of viewpoints about the medication. So she started looking for alternatives. She found someone who did hypnosis with her to control the anxiety, and that helped some. At least she felt supported in the therapy itself. But she was still very nervous and panicky. Finally her neurologist suggested that she go to the stress clinic.

She was at a point where her anxiety made it difficult for her to get in her car and go anywhere. She couldn't stand to be in crowds. Her heart was always pounding. She was totally unused to dealing with any kind of stress on her own. So, six months pregnant, she enrolled in the stress reduction program.

In the first class she found that she was able to relax into the body scan. She had no anxiety while she was doing it, even though she was lying on the floor with thirty total strangers packed in like sardines on foam mats. Her usual anxious thoughts and feelings had somehow disappeared for those two hours in the first class.

Claire was thrilled to have such an experience. It confirmed her belief that there was something she could do herself to free herself from her chronic nervousness. She practiced every day with the tapes and each week had some progress to report. She was ebullient and enthusiastic and appeared quite confident when she spoke in class. She told us one day that she had stopped playing the radio in her car and was following her breathing instead. She said she felt more calm that way.

No one had told her to do that. She came to it on her own as she experimented with integrating her meditation practice into her everyday life. When she feels herself getting tense, she now lets herself go *into* the tension and observe it. During the eight weeks of the program she had only one very mild panic attack, a dramatic change from the period when she was on the tranquilizers and having several every day.

She says she feels a lot better now. She is much more confident and is no longer preoccupied with the fear that she might lose control in public. She no longer fears parking in parking lots or walking on a crowded street. In fact, now she deliberately tries to park her car several blocks from where she is going so that she can walk the rest of the way and slow things down by walking mindfully. She is also sleeping soundly, which she was unable to do before.

In summary, Claire says she feels better about herself now than she has ever felt in her life, although she points out that her problems haven't changed at all. Somehow, even though she has fears about the baby she is expecting because of the drugs she took in the early weeks of her pregnancy, her fearful thoughts have not been leading to nervousness and panic. Things do not seem so overwhelming anymore. She has confidence in her ability to cope with things if she has to, "when the time comes." This was something she was never able to feel or say before. In the past, the slightest negative thought would have sent her right into a state of nervous agitation and panic.

Currently, although she is nine months pregnant, she is practicing her meditation every day. She gets up an hour early to do it. She sets her alarm for 5:30 A.M., lies in bed for fifteen minutes, and then goes into another room and does the tape. She alternates the yoga one day and the meditation the other day. She likes the sitting meditation more than the body scan and practices that the most.

Postscript: I spoke with Claire a year later and got an update on her life. At that point, she had been off all medications for a year and had not had a panic attack. She did have about six miniepisodes of anxiety, all of which she was able to control on her own. It turned out that her baby had to have surgery eighteen days after birth for repair of pyloric stenosis (a condition in which there is a narrowing of the valve between the stomach and the intestines that causes the baby to vomit up feedings and may prevent adequate nourishment and weight gain). During that time, Claire virtually lived at the hospital to be with her baby and found herself concentrating almost constantly on her breathing to remain calm and clearsighted and to remind herself not to let her mind wander to "what ifs." Her baby is fine now and growing well. Claire feels she could never have handled a situation like this effectively had she not learned what she did in the stress clinic.

◆

Claire's story illustrates that chronic anxiety and panic are potentially controllable through the practice of meditation, at least for a highly motivated person. Her experience and that of many other people in the stress clinic suggest that meditation might be a good first line of treatment for such conditions rather than going to drug treatment right away, especially for people who do not want to take medications.

This is not to suggest that there are not appropriate uses of medications in the treatment of anxiety and panic. Certain tranquilizers and antidepressants have proved extremely useful in managing acute anxiety disorders and panic attacks and helping to bring people out of them and back to self-regulation. Medications are also often used effectively *in combination* with good psychotherapy and behavioral counseling, using a range of different techniques such as cognitive therapy, hypnosis, and stress-reduction methods. However, Claire's experience is far from atypical, unfortunately. Many patients with anxiety disorders do feel that the drugs they are on do not help them that much, and that medication is often used *instead* of listening to people and guiding them to find the domain of self-regulation and inner balance. Claire was determined to face her anxiety and try to manage it herself because she saw so clearly how it was ruining her life. She felt that her dependency on tranquilizers was just reinforcing the view of herself as a nervous wreck, a basket case. And she proved to herself that her instincts were right all along, that she didn't have to live her whole life as an invalid, taking medication forever to manage her own mental states as if they were a thyroid deficiency.

◆

Let us now explore in detail how the meditation practice might be used to work with feelings of panic and anxiety so that they no longer control your life. These suggestions go hand in hand with the approaches we explored in the last chapter on handling emotional pain.

HOW TO USE THE PRACTICE TO WORK WITH ANXIETY AND PANIC

Your meditation practice is a perfect laboratory for working with anxiety and panic. In the body scan, the sitting meditation, and the yoga, we work at recognizing and accepting any feelings of tension we find in our body and any agitated thoughts and feelings that occur as we dwell in the domain of being. The meditation instructions emphasize that we don't have to *do* anything about bodily sensations or anxious feelings except to become aware of them and desist from judging them and condemning ourselves.

In this way, practicing moment-to-moment awareness amounts to a systematic way of teaching your body and mind to develop calmness within or beneath anxious feelings. This is exactly what Claire did in her practice. The more you practice, the more comfortable you become in your own skin. The more comfortable you feel, the closer you come to perceiving that your anxiety and fears are not you and that they do not have to rule your life.

As you come to taste even brief moments of comfort and relaxation, you may notice, both during meditation and at other times, that you are not *always* feeling anxious. In observing this, you see that anxiety varies in intensity and comes and goes just like everything else. It is a temporary mental state, just like boredom or happiness.

Recall from Chapter 3 the story of Gregg, the firefighter, who was incapacitated by anxiety and unable to breathe when he tried to put on his mask. When he started the stress clinic, just watching his breathing during the body scan would induce feelings of agitation and panic. Yet by working with his aversive reaction to his own breathing, he quickly taught himself to relax. He learned how to go "underneath" his agitation into a state of deeper calmness.

With regular practice, you learn to get in touch with and draw upon your own deep capacity for physiological relaxation and calmness, even at times when there are problems that have to be faced and resolved. In doing so, you also learn that it is possible to trust a stable inner core within yourself that is reliable, dependable, unwavering. Gradually the tension in your body and the worry and anxiety in your mind become less intrusive and lose some of their force. While the surface of your mind can still be choppy and agitated at times, like the surface of the ocean, you can learn to accept the mind's being that way and experience at the same time an underlying inner peace in a domain that is always right here, a domain in which the waves are damped to gentle swells at most.

An important part of this learning process is coming to see, as we have now emphasized many times, that you are not your thoughts and feelings and that you do not have to believe them or react to them or be driven or tyrannized by them. As you practice, focusing on whatever you are paying primary attention to in your meditation practice, you are likely to come to see your thoughts and feelings as discrete, short-lived events, as individual waves on the ocean. These waves rise up in the ocean of your awareness for a moment and then fall back. You can watch them and perceive them as "events in the field of your consciousness."

When you observe the unfolding of your own thinking, moment by moment, you may come to notice that thoughts carry different levels of emotional charge. Some are highly negative and pessimistic, loaded with anxiety, insecurity, fear, gloom, doom, and condemnation. Others are positive and optimistic, joyful and open, accepting and caring. Still others are neutral, neither positive nor negative in emotional content, just matter-of-fact thoughts. Our thinking proceeds in rather chaotic patterns of reactivity and association, elaborating on its own content, building imaginary worlds, and filling the silence with busyness. Thoughts with a high emotional charge have a way of recurring again and again. When they come up, they grab hold of your attention like a powerful magnet, carrying your mind away from your breathing or from awareness of your body.

When you look at thoughts as just thoughts, purposefully not reacting to their content and to their emotional charge, you become at least a little freer from their attraction or repulsion. You are less likely to get sucked into them quite as much or as often. The more powerful the charge, the more the content of the thought is likely to capture your attention and draw you away from just being in the moment. Your work is simply seeing and letting go, seeing and letting go, sometimes ruthlessly and relentlessly if need be, always intentionally and courageously. Just seeing and letting go.

When you practice this way with *all* of the thoughts that come up during meditation, whether they are "good," "bad," or "neutral" in content, with the highly charged ones and with the weakly charged ones, you will find that the ones that are anxious and fearful in content will seem less powerful and less threatening. They will have less of a hold over your attention because now you are seeing them as "just thoughts" and no longer as "reality" or "the truth." It becomes easier to remind yourself that you don't have to get caught up in their content. It becomes easier to see how you contribute to the ongoing strength of certain thoughts by fearing them and, ironically, by holding on to them.

Seeing them in this light breaks the insidious chain by which one anxious thought leads to another and to another until you become lost in a self-created world of fear and insecurity. Instead, it will be just one thought with anxiety content, seeing it, letting it go, returning to calmness; another thought with anxiety content, seeing it, letting it go, calmness; over and over and over, thought by thought by thought, holding on to the breath (for dear life if you must) to get you through the choppier times.

◆

Working mindfully with highly charged thoughts and feelings does not mean that we do not value the expression of strong feelings or that strong feelings are bad, problematic, or dangerous and that every effort should be made to "control" them or get rid of them or suppress them. Observing your feelings mindfully and accepting them and then letting go of them does not mean that you are trying to invalidate or get rid of them. It means that you know what you are experiencing. It also does not mean that you won't act on your thoughts and feelings or express them in their full power! It simply means that when you do act, you are more likely to do so with clarity and inner balance because you have some perspective on your own experience and are not just being driven by mindless reactivity. Then the force of your feelings can be applied creatively to solve or dissolve problems rather than compounding difficulties and causing harm to yourself or others, as so often happens when you lose your center. This is another example of the way in which the emotion-focused perspective and the problem-focused perspective can complement each other in mindfulness.

As we change our relationship to our thoughts by paying attention to the process of thinking, we will also come to see that perhaps we should change the way we think and speak about our thoughts and feelings altogether. Rather than saying "I am afraid" or "I am anxious," both of which make "you" *into* the anxiety or fear, it would actually be more accurate to say "I am having a lot of fear-filled (or fearful) thoughts." In this way you are emphasizing that you are not the content of your thoughts and that you do not have to identify with their content. Instead you can just be aware of it, accept it, and listen to it caringly. Then your thoughts will not drive you toward even more fear, panic, and anxiety but can be used instead to help you see more clearly what is actually on your mind.

◆

As you look deeply into the process of your own thinking from the perspective of calmness and mindfulness, you may come to see, as we noted in Chapters 15 and 24, that much of your thinking and emotions occur in recognizable patterns that are driven by discomfort of one kind or another. There is the discomfort of being dissatisfied with the present and wanting something more to happen, to possess something more that would make you feel better, more complete, more whole. This pattern could be described as the impulse to get what you want and to hold on to it, much like the monkey we saw in Chapter 2, who holds on to the banana and is trapped.

If you look deeply into it, you will probably find that, at a deep level, such impulses are driven, much as we might hate to admit it, by a kind of greediness, the desire for "more for me" in order to be happy. Perhaps it is money or control or recognition or love that you want. Whatever it is you are craving at the moment, to be driven by such impulses means that, on a deep level, you don't believe that you are whole as you are.

Then there is the opposite pattern, dominated by thoughts and feelings of wanting certain things *not* to happen or to stop happening, the desire to get rid of certain things or elements in your life that you think are preventing you from feeling better, happier, more satisfied. These patterns of thought can be described as driven by hatred, dislike, rejection, or a need to get rid of what you don't want or don't like so that you can be happy.

Mindfulness brought to our actual behavior may drive home the realization that we can be caught, in our mind and actions, between these two driving motives of liking/wanting (greed) and disliking/not wanting (aversion)—however subtle and unconscious they may be—to the point that our lives become one incessant vacillation between pursuit of what we like and flight from what we don't like. Such a course will lead to few moments of peace or happiness. How could it? There will always be cause for anxiety. At any moment you might lose what you already have. Or you might never get what you want. Or you might get it and find out it wasn't what you wanted after all. You might still not feel complete.

Unless you can be mindful of the activity of your own mind, you won't even notice that this is going on. A blanket of unawareness, our old acquaintance the automatic-pilot mode, will ensure that you will continue to bounce from pillar to post, feeling out of control much of the time. This is basically because you think happiness is solely dependent on whether you are getting what you want. (See the section in Chapter 24, "A 'What Is My Own Way?' Meditation.")

This process winds up consuming a great deal of energy. It can blanket so much of our life with unawareness that we hardly ever perceive that we may actually be basically okay right now, that it may be possible to find a core of harmony within ourselves in the midst of the full catastrophe of our fear and anxiety. In fact, when you think about it, where else could it possibly be found?

The only way to free yourself from a lifetime of being tyrannized by your own thought processes, whether you suffer from excessive anxiety or not, is to come to see your thoughts for what they are and to discern the sometimes subtle—but most often not-so-subtle—seeds of craving and aversion at work within them. When you can successfully step back and see that you are not your thoughts and feelings and that you do not have to believe them and you certainly do not have to act on them, when you see, vividly, that many of them are inaccurate, judgmental, and fundamentally greedy, you will have found the key to understanding why you feel so much fear and anxiety. At the same time you will have found the key to maintaining your own equilibrium. Fear, panic, and anxiety will no longer be uncontrollable demons. Instead you will see them as natural mental states that can be worked with and accepted just like any others. Then, lo and behold, the demons may not come around and bother you so much. You may find that you don't see them at all for long stretches. You may wonder where they went or even whether they ever existed. Occasionally you may see some smoke, just enough to remind you that the lair of the dragon is still occupied, that fear is a natural part of living, but not something you have to be afraid of.

◆

Believing in your capacity to take on whatever comes up is fundamental to the healing power you are cultivating. A woman named Beverly who recently took the stress reduction program was living with the uncertainty of a very frightening situation. She had had a cerebral aneurysm (broken blood vessel in the brain) the year before, which was surgically repaired but left a weakened place in an artery that might lead to a second aneurysm. She came to the stress clinic because she was experiencing a lot of anxiety. She felt that she was no longer her old self and that her body and her nervous system were sometimes out of control. She was having unpredictable, frightening seizures, dizzy spells, and problems with her eyes. She felt unsure of herself now with other people. She also thought that she was much more emotional than she had been before, but she wasn't sure of this. She was confused and frightened.

Numerous CAT scans were required to monitor her condition. They made her anxious and uncomfortable. She did not like having her head inside a big machine and having to lie perfectly still for long periods. Of course she also feared the results of these tests.

Two weeks into the stress reduction program, another CAT scan was scheduled. She was not looking forward to it at all. Yet as her head was being slowly glided into the cavity of the machine, somehow the thought came to her to try to put her mind in her toes as she had been practicing in the body scan for two weeks. She wound up keeping it there for the entire test and breathing in and out from her toes, which were farthest from the machine. Focusing on her toes, she felt more in control and could stay relaxed. She came through totally calm and panic-free. Her calmness amazed both her and her husband. She came to the next class thrilled with the discovery of her newfound ability to control what had seemed uncontrollable.

Beverly's body still continues to do strange things that worry her a great deal but she now feels that she has some tools that she can use daily to keep her in balance. In particular, she finds helpful the image of the mountain, stable and unmoving amidst all the changes in the weather that engulf it, and she often invokes this "inner mountain" during her meditation and at other times. She says that she is now accepting the uncertainty of her condition. This alone gives her more peace of mind. The full catastrophe hasn't gone away. But she is handling it in a way that enables her to feel better about herself now and more optimistic about the future.

Having the confidence and the imagination to take on and work with whatever comes up requires that you have powerful "tools" to work with and enough experience with them to know how to use them, as well as the flexibility and presence of mind to remember them under trying circumstances. Beverly displayed these qualities when she decided to focus her mind on her toes and use her meditation while she was in the CAT scanner.

A few weeks following her CAT scan, she had to have another type of brain-imaging test called an MRI scan. She thought she would use the same method that had helped during the CAT scan, but when she tried to concentrate on her toes, she found she couldn't do it this time because the sound of the machine bothered her too much. Instead of panicking, she switched her attention to the sounds themselves and again found that she was able to dwell in a state of calm during the procedure. So, in addition to developing a set of tools to handle her anxiety, she was also imaginative and flexible in the use of them. She responded to the MRI scan as a challenge instead of merely reacting automatically in this stressful situation. Flexibility of this kind is essential if you hope to be able to maintain your balance in the face of the unexpected.

Another example of successfully working with anxiety comes from a man who told the following story to his class in the stress clinic. He had always had a tendency to panic and to feel frightened in crowds but had not had a panic attack in about six months. He was taking the program for a medical problem unrelated to anxiety. At one point during the program he went with friends to a Celtics basketball game in the Boston Garden. As he sat down in his seat, high above the parquet floor, he felt the old familiar feelings of claustrophobia and fear of being trapped in a closed space with a throng of people. In the past, that feeling would have presaged a full-blown panic attack. It would have caused him to bolt for an exit. In fact, fear of it would have kept him from going to the game in the first place.

Instead of bolting, he reminded himself that he was breathing. He sat back and rode the waves of his breathing for a few minutes, focusing on them and letting go of his panicky thoughts. After a few minutes the feeling passed and he enjoyed the rest of the evening thoroughly.

These are just a few examples of how people have used the meditation practice to work with and calm anxiety and panic. Together with some of the other stories in this book, they may give you a handle on how to come to your own center of stability and calmness of mind within the storms of fear, panic, and anxiety that sometimes blow in our lives, and on how to emerge from their hold wiser and freer.

26
Time and Time Stress

"Practice not-doing and everything will fall into place."
—Lao-tzu, *Tao Te Ching*

In our society, time has become one of our biggest stressors. At some stages of life it may feel as if there is never enough time to do what we need to do. Often we don't know where time has gone, the years pass by so fast. At other stages, time may weigh heavily upon us. The days and the hours can seem interminable. We don't know what to do with all our time. Crazy as it may sound, we are going to suggest that the antidote to time stress is intentional non-doing, and that non-doing is applicable whether you are suffering from not having "enough time" or suffering from having "too much time." The challenge here is for you to put this proposition to the test in your own life, to see for yourself whether your relationship to time can be transformed through the practice of non-doing.

If you feel completely overwhelmed by the pressures of time, you might wonder how it could possibly help to take time away from what you "have to do" in order to practice non-doing? And on the other hand, if you are feeling isolated and bored and have nothing but time on your hands, you might wonder how it could possibly help to fill this burden of time unfilled with "nothing"?

The answer is simple and not at all farfetched. *Inner peace exists outside of time*. If you commit yourself to spending some time each day in inner stillness, even if it is for two minutes, or five, or ten, for those moments you are stepping out of the flow of time altogether. The calmness, relaxation, and centering that come from letting go of time transform your experience of time when you go back into it. Then it becomes possible to flow along with time during your day rather than constantly fighting against it or feeling driven by it, simply by bringing awareness to present-moment experience.

The more you practice making some time in your day for non-doing, the more your whole day becomes non-doing; in other words, is suffused with an awareness grounded in the present moment and therefore outside of time. Perhaps you have already experienced this if you have been practicing the sitting meditation or the body scan or the yoga. Perhaps you have observed that being aware takes no extra time, that awareness simply rounds out each moment, makes it more full, breathes life into it. So if you are pressed for time, being in the present gives you more time by giving you back the fullness of each moment that you have. No matter what is happening, you can be centered in perceiving and accepting things as they are. Then you can be aware of what still needs to be done in the future without it causing you undue anxiety or loss of perspective. Then you can move to do it, with your doing coming out of your being, out of peace.

On the other hand, let's suppose you are in a life situation in which you don't know what to do with all the time you have. Time weighs on your hands. Perhaps you feel empty, disconnected from the world and from all the meaningful things being done in it. Perhaps you can't go out, or hold down a job, or get out of bed for long, or even read much to "pass the time." Perhaps you are alone, without friends and relatives or far from them. How could non-doing possibly help you? You are already not doing anything and it is driving you nuts!

Actually you are probably doing a lot even though you are unaware of it. For one thing, you may be "doing" unhappiness, boredom, and anxiety. You are probably spending at least some time, and perhaps a great deal of time, dwelling in your thoughts and memories, reliving pleasant moments from the past or unhappy events. You may be "doing" anger at other people for things that happened long ago. You may be "doing" loneliness or resentment or self-pity or hopelessness. These inner activities of mind can drain your energy. They can be exhausting and make the passage of time seem interminable.

Our subjective experience of time passing seems linked to the activity of thought in some way. We *think* about the past, we *think* about the future. Time is measured as the space between our thoughts and in the never-ending stream of them. As we practice watching our thoughts come and go, we are cultivating an ability to dwell in the silence and stillness behind the stream of thought itself, in a timeless present. Since the present is always here, now, it is already outside of time passing.

Non-doing means letting go of *everything*. Above all, it means seeing and letting go of your thoughts as they come and go. It means letting yourself be. If you feel trapped in time, non-doing is a way that you can step out of all the time on your hands by stepping into timelessness. In doing so you also step out, at least momentarily, from your isolation and your unhappiness and from your desire to be engaged, busy, a part of things, doing something meaningful. By connecting with yourself outside of the flow of time, you are already doing the most meaningful thing you could possibly do, namely coming to peace within your own mind, coming into contact with your own wholeness, reconnecting with yourself.

> Time past and time future
> Allow but a little consciousness.
> To be conscious is not to be in time.
> T. S. Eliot, "Burnt Norton," *Four Quartets*

You could look at all the time you have as an opportunity to engage in the inner work of being and growing. Then, even if your body doesn't work "right" and you are confined to the house or to a bed, the possibility is still there to turn your life into an adventure and to find meaning in each moment. If you commit yourself to the work of mindfulness, your physical isolation might take on a different meaning for you. Your inability to be active in outer ways and the pain and regret that you may feel from it may become balanced by the joy of other possibilities, by a new perspective on yourself, one in which you are seeing optimistically, reframing the time that weighed on your hands as time to do the work of being, the work of non-doing, the work of self-awareness and understanding.

There is no end to this work, of course, and no telling where it might lead. But wherever that is, it will be away from suffering, away from boredom and anxiety and self-pity and toward healing. Negative mental states cannot survive for long when timelessness is being cultivated. How could they when you are embodying peace? Your concentrated awareness serves as a crucible in which negative mental states can be contained and then transmuted.

And if you are able-bodied enough to do at least some things in the outside world, dwelling in non-doing will likely lead to insights as to how you might connect up with people and activities and events that might be meaningful to you as well as helpful and useful to others. Everybody has something to offer to the world—in fact, something that no other person can offer, something unique and priceless, *one's own being*. If you practice non-doing, you may find that, rather than having all this time on your hands, the days may not be long enough to do what needs doing. In this work, you will never be unemployed.

◆

If you take a more cosmic perspective on time, none of us is here for very long anyway. The total duration of human life on the planet has itself been the briefest of eye blinks, our own individual lives infinitesimal in the vastness of geological time. Stephen Jay Gould, the paleontologist, points out that "the human species has inhabited this planet for only 250,000 years or so—roughly 0.0015 percent of the history of life, the last inch of the cosmic mile." Yet the way minds represent time, it feels as if we have a long time to live. In fact we often delude ourselves, especially early in life, with feelings of immortality and of our own permanence. At other times we are only too keenly aware of the inevitability of death and the rapidity of the passage of our lives.

Perhaps it is the knowledge of death, conscious or unconscious, that ultimately drives us to feel pressed for time. The word *deadline* certainly carries the message. We have many deadlines, those imposed by our work and by other people and those we impose on ourselves. We rush here and there, doing this and that, trying to get it all done "in time." Often we are so stressed by the squeeze of time that we do what we are doing just to get through with it, to be able to say to ourselves, "At least *that* is out of the way." And then it's on to the next thing that needs doing, pressing on, pressing through our moments.

Some doctors believe that time stress is a fundamental cause of disease in the present era. Time urgency was originally featured as one of the salient characteristics of coronary-disease-prone, or Type A, behavior. The Type-A syndrome is sometimes described as "hurry sickness." People who fit into this category are driven by a sense of time pressure to speed up the doing of all their daily activities and to do and think more than one thing at a time. They tend to be very poor listeners. They are constantly interrupting and finishing other people's sentences for them. They tend to be very impatient. They have great difficulty sitting and doing nothing or standing in lines, and they tend to speak rapidly and to dominate in social and professional situations. Type A's also tend to be highly competitive, easily irritated, cynical and hostile. As we have seen, the evidence to date seems to be pointing toward hostility and cynicism as the most toxic elements of coronary-prone behavior. But, even if further research shows that time urgency by itself is not a major factor in heart disease, it nevertheless has a toxicity of its own. Time stress can easily erode the *quality* of a person's life and threaten health and well-being.

Dr. Robert Eliot, a cardiologist and well-known stress researcher, described his own mental state and his relationship to time prior to his heart attack as follows:

> My body cried out for rest, but my brain wasn't listening. I was behind schedule. My timetable read that by the age of forty I should be the chief of cardiology at a major university. I was forty-three when I left the University of Florida at Gainesville and accepted the position of chief of cardiology at the University of Nebraska in 1972. All I had to do was run a little faster and I'd be back on track.

Yet he found himself running into roadblocks of various kinds in his efforts to establish an innovative cardiovascular research center.

> I came to feel that the walls were closing in on me and that I would never break free to make my dream a reality.
>
> Desperately I did what I had been doing all my life. I picked up the pace. I tried to force things through. I crisscrossed the state to provide on-the-spot cardiology education to rural Nebraska physicians and build support among them for the university's cardiovascular program. I scheduled academic lectures across the country, continually flying in and out at a moment's notice. I remember that on one trip on which my wife, Phyllis, helped with the business arrangements, a seminar went superbly, and on the plane ride home Phyllis wanted to savor the memory. Not me. I was rushing through the evaluation forms, worrying about how to make the next seminar better.
>
> I had no time for family and friends, relaxation and diversion. When Phyllis bought me an exercise bike for Christmas, I was offended. How could I possibly find time to sit down and pedal a bicycle?

I was often overtired, but I put that out of my mind. I wasn't concerned about my health. What did I have to worry about ? I was an expert in diseases of the heart, and I knew I didn't have any of the risk factors. My father had lived to be seventy-eight and my mother, at eighty-five, showed no sign of heart disease. I didn't smoke. I wasn't overweight. I didn't have high blood pressure. I didn't have high cholesterol. I didn't have diabetes. I thought I was immune to heart disease.

But I was running a big risk for other reasons. I had been pushing too hard for too long. Now all my efforts seemed futile. . . . A feeling of disillusionment descended on me, a sense of *invisible entrapment*.

I didn't know it then, but my body was continuously reacting to this inner turmoil. For nine months I was softened for the blow. It came two weeks after my forty-fourth birthday.

As he described it, after a disappointing confrontation one day, he got very angry and was unable to calm down. After a sleepless night and a long drive to a speaking engagement, he gave a medical lecture. Following a heavy lunch, he tried to diagnose cases, but his mind was foggy, his eyes were blurry. He felt dizzy. These were the conditions immediately preceding his heart attack.

Dr. Eliot's heart attack led him to write a book called *Is It Worth Dying For?* in which he describes how he came to answer that question with a resounding *no* and went on to change his relationship to time and to stress. He described his life leading up to his heart attack as "a joyless treadmill."

Norman Cousins described the conditions leading up to his heart attack in much the same way in his book *The Healing Heart:*

The main source of stress in my life for some years had been airports and airplanes, necessitated by a heavy speaking and conference schedule. Battling traffic congestion en route to airports, having to run through air terminals . . . , having to queue up for boarding passes at the gate and then being turned away because the plane had been overbooked, waiting at baggage carousels for bags that never turned up, time-zone changes, irregular meals, insufficient sleep—these features of airline transportation had been my melancholy burdens for many years and were especially profuse in the latter part of 1980. . . . I returned from a hectic trip to the East Coast just before Christmas only to discover that I was due to leave again in a few days for the Southeast. I asked my secretary about the possibility of a postponement or a cancellation. She carefully reviewed with me the special facts in each case that made it essential to go through with the engagements. It was obvious . . . that only the most drastic event would get me out of it. My body was listening. The next day I had my heart attack.

Notice the sense of time pressure and urgency in the words themselves in both these passages: "behind schedule," career "timetable," "I picked up the pace," "I tried to force things through," "no time for family or friends," "joyless treadmill," "battling traffic," "having to run" to make the plane, "having to queue up," "waiting" for baggage, dealing with "time-zone changes."

Time pressures are not the limited province of successful executives, physicians, and academicians who travel a lot. In our postindustrial society, all of us are exposed to the stress of time. We strap on our watches in the morning and we get *going*. We conduct our lives by the clock. The clock dictates when we have to be where, and woe to us if we forget too often. Time and the clock drive us from one thing to the next. It has become a "way of life" for many of us to feel driven every day by all our obligations and responsibilities and then to fall into bed exhausted at the end of it all. If we keep up this pattern for long stretches without adequate rest and without replenishing our own energy reserves, breakdown will inevitably occur in one way or another. No matter how stable your homeostatic mechanisms are, they can eventually be pushed over the edge if they are not reset from time to time.

Nowadays we even transmit time urgency to our children. How many times have you found yourself saying to little children, "Hurry up, there's no time" or "I don't have time"? We hurry them to get dressed, to eat, to get ready for school. By what we say, by our body language, by the way we rush around ourselves, we are giving them the clear message that there is simply never enough time.

This message has been getting through to them all too clearly. It is not uncommon now for children to feel stressed and hurried at an early age. Instead of being able to follow their own inner rhythms, they are scooped up onto the conveyor belt of their parents' lives and taught to hurry and to be time-conscious. This may ultimately have deleterious effects on their biological rhythms and cause various kinds of physiological disregulation as well as psychological distress, just as it does in adults. For instance, high blood pressure begins in childhood in our society, with small but significant elevations detectable even in five-year-olds. This is not true in nonindustrial societies, where high blood pressure is virtually unknown. Something in the stress of our way of life beyond just dietary factors is probably responsible for this. Perhaps it is the stress of time.

◆

In earlier times our activities were much more in step with the cycles of the natural world. People stayed put more. They didn't travel very far. Most died in the same place they were born and knew everybody in their town or village. Daylight and night dictated very different life rhythms. Many tasks just could not be done at night for lack of light. Sitting around fires at night, their only sources of heat and light, had a way of slowing people down—it was calming as well as warming. Staring into the flames and the embers, the mind could focus on the fire, always different, yet always the same. People could watch it moment by moment and night after night, month after month, year after year, through the seasons— and see time stand still in the fire. Perhaps the ritual of sitting around fires was mankind's first experience of meditation.

In earlier times, the rhythms of people were the rhythms of nature. A farmer could only plow so much by hand or with an ox in one day. You could only travel so far on foot or even with a horse. People were in touch with their animals and their needs. The animals' rhythm dictated the limits of time. If you valued your horse, you knew not to push him too fast or too far.

Now we can live largely independent of those natural rhythms. Electricity has given us light in the darkness, so that there is much less of a distinction between day and night—we can work after the sun goes down if we have to, or want to. We never have to slow down because the light has failed. We also have cars and tractors, telephones and jet travel, radios and televisions, photocopying machines, and now personal computers and fax machines. These have shrunk the world and reduced by a staggering amount the time that it takes to do things or find things out or communicate or go someplace or finish a piece of work. Computers have amplified to such an extent the ability to get paperwork and computations done that, although they are tremendously liberating in some ways, people can find themselves under more pressure than ever to get more done in less time. The expectations of oneself and of others just increase as the technology provides us with the power to do more faster. Instead of sitting around fires at night for light and warmth and something to look into, we can throw switches and keep going with whatever we have to *do*. Then, too, we can watch television and think we are relaxing and slowing down. Actually it is just more sensory bombardment.

And in the future, what with cellular phones in our cars and even on our bodies, with portable computers, electronic mail, computer shopping, smart television, narrowcasting, and personal robots, we will have more and more ways to stay busier and busier and to do more and more things simultaneously, with expectations rising accordingly. We can drive *and* do business, we can exercise *and* process information, we can read *and* watch television, or have split screens so that we can watch two or three or four things at once on television. We will never be out of touch with the world. But will we ever be in touch with ourselves?

FOUR WAYS TO FREE YOURSELF FROM THE TYRANNY OF TIME

Just because the world has been speeded up through technology is no reason for us to be ruled by it to the point where we are stressed beyond all limits and perhaps even driven to an early grave by the treadmill of modern life. There are many ways you might free yourself from the tyranny of time. The first is to remind yourself that time is a product of thought. Minutes and hours are conventions, agreed upon so that we can conveniently meet and communicate and work in harmony. But they have no absolute meaning, as Einstein was fond of pointing out to lay audiences. To paraphrase what he was supposed to have said in explaining the concept of relativity, "If you are sitting on a hot stove, a minute can seem like an hour, but if you are doing something pleasurable, an hour can seem like a minute."

Of course we all know this from our own experience. Nature is in fact very equitable. We all get twenty-four hours per day to live. How we see that time and what we do with it can make all the difference in whether we feel we have "enough time" or "too much time" or "not enough." So we need to look at our expectations of ourselves. We need to be aware of just what we are trying to accomplish and whether we are paying too great a price for it or, in Dr. Eliot's words, whether it is "worth dying for."

A second way of freeing yourself from the tyranny of time is to live in the present more of the time. We waste enormous amounts of time and energy musing about the past and worrying about the future. These moments are hardly ever satisfying. Usually they produce anxiety and time urgency, thoughts such as "time is running out" or "those were the good old days." As we have seen now many times, to practice being mindful from one moment to the next puts you in touch with life in the only time you have to live it, namely right now. Whatever you are engaged in takes on a greater richness when you drop out of the automatic-pilot mode and into awareness and acceptance. If you are eating, then really eat in this time. It might mean *choosing* not to read a magazine or watch TV while half-consciously "shoveling" food into your body. If you are baby-sitting for your grandchildren, then really *be* with them, become engaged. Time will disappear. If you are helping your children with their homework or just talking with them don't do it on the run. Make the effort to be fully present. Make eye contact. Own those moments. Then you will not see other people as "taking time" away from you. All your moments will be your own. And if you want to reminisce about the past or plan for the future, then do *that* with awareness as well. Remember *in the present*. Plan *in the present*.

The essence of mindfulness in daily life is to make every moment you have your own. Even if you are hurrying, which is sometimes necessary, then at least hurry mindfully. Be aware of your breathing, of the need to move fast, and do it with awareness until you don't have to hurry anymore and then let go and relax intentionally. If you find your mind making lists and compelling you to get every last thing on them done, then bring awareness to your body and the mental and physical tension that may be mounting and remind yourself that some of it can probably wait. If you get really close to the edge, stop completely and ask yourself, "Is it worth dying for?" or "Who is running where?"

A third way of freeing yourself from the tyranny of time is take some of it intentionally each day to just be, in other words to meditate. We need to protect our time for formal meditation practice because it is so easy to write it off as unnecessary or a luxury; after all, it is empty of doing. When you do write it off and give this time over to doing, you wind up losing what may be the most valuable part of your life, namely time for yourself to just be.

As we have seen, in practicing meditation you are basically stepping out of the flow of time and residing in stillness, in an eternal present. That doesn't mean that every moment you practice will be a moment of timelessness. That depends on the degree of concentration and calmness that you bring to each moment. But just making the commitment to practice non-doing, to let go of striving, to be non-judgmental, slows down that time for you and nourishes the timeless in you. By devoting some time each day to slowing down time itself, for giving yourself time for just being, you are strengthening your ability to operate *out of* your being, in the present, during the rest of your day, when the pace of the outer and inner worlds may be much more relentless. That is why it is so important to organize your life around preserving some time each day for just being.

A fourth way of freeing yourself from time is to simplify your life in certain ways. As already noted, we once held an eight-week stress reduction program just for judges. Judges tend to be sorely stressed by overwhelming caseloads. One judge complained that he never had enough time to review cases and to do extra background reading to prepare for them and that he didn't feel he had enough time to be with his family. When he explored how he used his time when he was not at work, it turned out that he religiously read three newspapers every day and also watched the news on television for an hour each day. The newspapers alone took up an hour and a half. It amounted to a kind of addiction.

Of course he knew how he was spending his time. But for some reason, he hadn't made the connection that he was choosing to use up two and a half hours a day with news, almost all of which was the same in each newspaper and on TV. When we discussed it, he saw in an instant that he could gain time for other things he wanted to do by letting go of two newspapers and the TV news. He intentionally broke his addictive news habit and now reads one paper a day, doesn't watch the news on TV, and has about two more hours a day to do other things.

Simplifying our lives in even little ways can make a big difference. If you fill up all your time, you won't have any. And you probably won't even be aware of why you don't. Simplifying may mean prioritizing the things that you have to and want to do and, at the same time, *consciously choosing to give certain things up.* It may mean learning to say no sometimes, even to things you want to do or to people you care about and want to help so that you are protecting and preserving some space for silence, for non-doing.

After an all-day session, a woman who had been in pain for a number of years discovered that the next day she had no pain at all. She also woke up feeling differently about time that morning. It felt precious to her in a new way. When she got a routine call from her son, saying that he was bringing over the children so that she and her husband could baby-sit for them, she found herself telling him not to bring them, that she couldn't do it, that she needed to be alone. She felt she needed to protect this amazing moment of freedom from pain. She felt she had to preserve the preciousness of the stillness she was experiencing that morning rather than to fill it, even with her grandchildren, whom she of course loved enormously. She wanted to help her son out, but this time she needed to say no and to do something for herself. And her husband, sensing something different in her, perhaps her inner peacefulness, uncharacteristically supported her.

Her son couldn't believe it. She had never said no before. She didn't even have anything she was doing that day. To him it seemed nuts. But she knew, perhaps for the first time in quite a while, that some moments are worth protecting, just so that nothing can happen. Because that "nothing" is a very rich nothing.

◆

There is a saying: "Time is money." But some people may have enough money and not enough time. It wouldn't hurt them to think about giving up some of their money for some time. For many years I worked three or four days a week and got paid accordingly. I needed the full-time money, but I felt the time was more important, especially when my children were very little. I wanted to be there for them as much as I could. Now I work full-time. This means I'm away from home more and I feel the pressure of time more in many ways. But I try to practice non-doing within the domain of doing and to remember not to overcommit myself.

I was lucky enough to have some outer control over how much I worked. Most people don't. But there are still many ways in which it is possible to simplify your life. Maybe you don't need to run around so much or have so many obligations or commitments. Maybe you don't have to have the TV on all the time in your house. Maybe you don't need to use your car so much. And maybe you don't really need so much money. Giving some thought and attention to the ways in which you might simplify things will probably start you on the road toward making your time your own. It is yours anyway, you know. You might as well enjoy it.

Mahatma Gandhi was once asked by a journalist, "You have been working at least fifteen hours a day, every day for almost fifty years. Don't you think it's about time you took a vacation?" To which Gandhi replied, "I am always on vacation."

Of course, the word *vacation* means "empty, vacant." When we practice being completely in the present, life in its fullness is totally accessible to us at all times, precisely because we are out of time. Time becomes empty and so do we. Then we, too, can always be on vacation. We might even learn how to have better vacations if we practiced all year long.

> But only in time can the moment in the rose-garden
> The moment in the arbour where the rain beat,
> The moment in the draughty church at smokefall
> Be remembered; involved with past and future.
> Only through time is time conquered.
>   —T. S. Eliot, "Burnt Norton," *Four Quartets*

27

Sleep and Sleep Stress

Of all the things we do on a regular basis, sleeping is one of the most extraordinary and least appreciated. Imagine, once a day, on the average, we lie down on a comfortable surface and leave our bodies for hours at a time. It is sacred time too. We are very attached to sleeping and we almost never consider giving up some sleep on purpose to accomplish personal goals. How many times have you heard people say, "I need my eight hours or I'll be a basket case"? And if you suggest to people that they might get up an hour earlier or even fifteen minutes earlier to make time to do other things that they value but have no time for, you will find lots of resistance. People feel threatened when you tamper with their sleep time.

Yet ironically, one of the most common and earliest symptoms of stress is trouble with sleep. Either you can't get to sleep in the first place because your thinking mind won't shut down, or you wake up in the middle of the night and can't get back to sleep. Or both. Usually you toss and turn, trying to clear your mind, telling yourself what a big day you have tomorrow, how important it is to be rested, all to no avail. The more you try to get back to sleep, the more awake you are.

As it turns out, you can't *force* yourself to go to sleep. It is one of those states, like relaxation, that you have to let go into. The more you try to get to sleep, the more you create tension and anxiety, which wake you up.

When we talk about "going to sleep," the language itself suggests "getting somewhere." Perhaps it would be more accurate to say that sleep "comes over us" when the conditions are right. Being able to sleep is a sign of harmony in your life. Getting enough sleep is a basic ingredient of good health. When we are sleep-deprived, our thinking, our moods, and our behavior can become erratic and unreliable, our body becomes exhausted and we become more susceptible to "getting" sick.

Our sleep patterns are intimately related to the natural world. The planet turns on its axis once every twenty-four hours, giving us cycles of light and darkness, and living organisms seem to cycle with it, as seen in diurnal changes known as *circadian rhythms*. These rhythms show up in daily fluctuations in the release of neurotransmitters in the brain and nervous system and in the biochemistry of all our cells. We have these basic planetary rhythms built into our systems. In fact, biologists speak of a "biological clock," controlled by the hypothalamus, which regulates our sleep-wake cycle and which can be disrupted by jet travel, by working the night shift, and by other behavior patterns. We cycle with the planet, and our sleep pattern reflects this connection. When it is disrupted, it takes us some time to readjust, to get back to our normal pattern.

A seventy-five-year-old woman was sent to the stress clinic with a sleep problem that had started a year and a half previously. She had also had a recent onset of hypertension that was under control with medication. She had been employed in the public schools and had retired ten years before. She reported that most nights she just wasn't able to sleep and would spend the whole night "perfectly comfortable, not restless" but awake. Her doctor had prescribed a very low dose of Xanax to help her relax, but she still thought of the medication with "fear and trembling." She tried it a few times, taking half a pill. It did help her to sleep, but she hated taking it and stopped. She came to the stress clinic hoping she could learn to sleep better without depending on medication.

She did. She kept up the meditation practice faithfully throughout the course. She didn't like the sitting meditation because she said her mind wandered too much, but she loved the yoga and did it every day, much more than we required. By the end of the eight weeks, she was sleeping, as she put it, "marvelously" every night and was very pleased with her ability to do it without medication.

◆

If you are having a lot of trouble sleeping, your body may be trying to tell you something about the way you are conducting your life. As with all other mind-body symptoms, this message is worth listening to. Usually it is just a signal that you are going through a stressful time in your life and you can expect that if and when it is resolved, your sleeping pattern will improve by itself. Sometimes it helps to look at how much exercise you are getting. Regular exercise, such as walking or yoga or swimming, can make a major difference in your ability to sleep soundly, as you can discover by experimenting for yourself.

Sometimes people get caught up in thinking they need more sleep than they really do. Our need for sleep changes as we grow and is known to diminish as we get older. Some people can function well on four hours of sleep per night, but they may feel that they "should" be able to sleep longer.

We recommend that when you can't sleep, you get out of bed and do something else for a while, something you like doing or that you might feel good about getting done. I like to assume that if I can't sleep, it may be because I don't need to be sleeping just then, even if I really want to be. When I have trouble sleeping, the second thing I do is meditate. (The first is toss and turn and feel upset until I realize what I'm doing.) I get out of bed, wrap myself up in a warm blanket, sit on my cushion, and just watch my mind. This gives me a chance to look carefully at what is so pressing and agitating that it is keeping me from peaceful sleep.

Sometimes meditating for a half hour or so will calm the mind to the point where you can go back to sleep. Other times it may lead you to do something else, such as work on a favorite project, make lists, read a good book, listen to music, or just accept the fact that you are upset, angry, fearful, whatever it may be, and be mindful of that. The middle of the night is also a good time to do yoga if you happen to be up.

To handle sleeplessness in this way requires that you recognize and accept that you are already awake. Catastrophizing about how bad your day is going to be because you'll be so exhausted if you don't get back to sleep doesn't help. And forcing sleep doesn't help. So why not let the future take care of itself, especially since the fact is that right now you are already awake! Why not be fully awake?

◆

As was mentioned briefly in the introduction, mindfulness practice comes primarily out of the Buddhist meditative tradition, although it is found in one form or another in all spiritual traditions and practices. Interestingly enough, there is no God in Buddhism, which makes it an unusual religion. Buddhism is really based on reverence for a principle, embodied in a historical person known as the Buddha. As the story goes, someone approached the Buddha, who was considered a great sage and teacher, and asked him, "Are you a god?", or something to that effect, to which he replied, "No, I am awake." The essence of mindfulness practice is to work at waking up from the self-imposed half sleep of unawareness in which we are so often immersed.

♦

We function on automatic pilot so much of the time that it might well be said that we are more asleep than awake, even when we are awake. If we make a commitment to ourselves to be *fully* awake when we are awake, then our view of not being able to sleep at certain times will change along with our view of everything else. Whenever we happen to be awake in the twenty-four-hour cycle of the planet's turning can be seen as an opportunity to practice being fully awake and accepting things as they are, including the fact that your mind is agitated and you are unable to sleep. When you do this, more often than not, your sleeping will take care of itself. It just may not come when you think it should and it may not last as long as you think it should. So much for "shoulds."

If this approach sounds radical to you, it might be valuable to think of the alternatives for a moment. There is a multimillion-dollar industry built around drugs to regulate sleep. This industry is a testament to our collective loss of homeostasis, to how widespread this single example of disregulation is. Many people regularly rely on pills to help them to get to sleep or to stay asleep. Control and regulation of their internal rhythms and cycles are given over to a chemical agent to restore homeostasis. Shouldn't this be the recourse of last resort, after all else has failed?

In the stress clinic, we put a lot of people to sleep, not that we mean to. It's just that the body scan can be very relaxing. If you do it when you are tired, it is easy to fall into sleep rather than finding a deep state of relaxed awareness. This is why some people have to really work at staying awake through the entire body scan. Some don't hear the end of the tape for weeks. Some are even "out" by the time they reach the left knee!

When people come to the stress clinic primarily for help with sleep problems, we give them permission to use the body-scan tape to help them to fall asleep at night as long as they promise that they will also use it once a day at some other time to "fall awake." And it works! Most people with sleep disturbances report a marked improvement after a few weeks practicing the body scan (for one example, see Mary's sleep graphs in Figure 3, Chapter 5) and many give up their sleeping pills before the eight weeks are up.

Some find it equally effective and easier when they want to go to sleep or to get back to sleep to just focus on their breathing as they lie in bed, letting the mind follow the breath as it moves into the body and then following it back out all the way and letting the body just sink into the mattress each time. You can think of it as breathing out to the ends of the universe, and breathing in from there, all the way back to your body.

Let's think for a moment about how we "go to sleep." At a certain time we lie down on a padded surface, close our eyes, and relax. Things start to feel hazy and off we "go." When we practice the body scan, particularly because it is done lying down with the eyes closed, we have to learn to travel along the road of deepening relaxation and recognize when we are coming to a fork. In one direction lies haziness, loss of awareness, and sleep. This is an extremely good road to take on a regular basis. It helps us to stay healthy and to restore our physical and psychological resources. In the other direction lies meditation, a condition of relaxation and *heightened* awareness. This is also an extremely restorative state, worth cultivating on a regular basis. Physiologically and psychologically it differs greatly from sleep. The ideal is to cultivate both and to know when one is more important than the other.

Our great attachment to sleep usually causes us to worry a lot about the consequences of losing sleep. But if you subscribe to the belief that your body and mind can self-regulate and correct for some of these disturbances we experience, then you can use your sleep imbalance as a vehicle for further growth, just as we have seen that you can use other symptoms, even pain or anxiety, to come to deeper levels of wholeness.

In my own case, I recently came out of a period of eleven years of disrupted sleep. During those years, there were very few nights of totally uninterrupted sleep. First, the children were nursing, and then they seemed to have a gene that caused each of them to wake up frequently from the time they were born until the age of four or five. My wife and I decided at the very beginning to try to accept this in them rather than to force our *idea* of what their sleep pattern should be on to them. This meant learning to live with getting up, sometimes three or four different times in one night, night after night, year after year. Every once in a while I would go to bed really early and catch up that way. But mostly, my system seemed to adjust to getting less sleep and less dreaming, and I managed quite well in those years.

I think one reason it didn't exhaust me completely and that I didn't get sick as a result was that I didn't fight it. I accepted it and used it as part of my meditation practice. I mentioned in Chapter 7 that I frequently found myself walking the floors at night with one of them, comforting, chanting, rocking, and using the walking, the singing, the rocking and the patting as opportunities to re-mind myself to be aware of them as my children, of their feelings, of their bodies, of my own body, of my being their father. True, I would just as soon have been back in bed, but since I wasn't and couldn't be, I used being awake as an opportunity to practice being really awake. Seeing it this way, being up at night became just another form of training and growth as a person and as a father.

And now that the children sleep very well, I find that every so often I still wake up in the middle of the night. Sometimes it's because I have a lot of things on my mind that won't leave just because I want them to. So I get out of bed and I sit or do some yoga or both. Then, depending on how I feel, I either go back to bed or I might work on projects that I want to complete and that don't make noise. I find it very peaceful and quiet in the middle of the night. No phone calls, no disturbances. The stars and the moon and the dawn can be spectacular and give a feeling of connectedness that you don't get if you are unaware of the heavens at night. The mind usually relaxes once I stop trying to get back to sleep and focus on using this time to be mindful.

Of course, people are different and we have different rhythms. Some people function best late at night, others early in the morning. It's very useful to find out how you might use the twenty-four hours you have each day in the way that works best for you. And you can only find this out by listening carefully to your mind and your body and letting them teach you what you need to know. As usual, this means letting go of some of your resistance to change and experimentation and giving yourself permission to get enthusiastic about exploring the boundaries of your life. Your relationship to sleep is a very fruitful object of mindfulness. It will teach you a lot about yourself if you worry less about losing sleep and instead pay more attention to being fully awake.

28

People Stress

Other people can be a big source of stress in our lives. We all have times when we feel that others are controlling our lives, making demands on our time, are being unusually difficult or hostile, don't do what we expect them to, or don't care about us and our feelings. We can probably all think of particular people who cause us stress, people we prefer to avoid if we can but often can't because we live with them or work with them or have obligations that have to be met. In fact, many of the people who cause us the most stress may be people we love very deeply. We all know that love relationships can occasion deep emotional pain as well as joy and pleasure.

Our relationships with other people provide us with unending opportunities for practicing mindfulness and thereby reducing "people stress." As we saw in Part III, our stress cannot be said to be due solely to external stressors, because psychological stress arises from the *interaction* between us and the world. So in the case of people who "cause us stress," we need to take responsibility for our part in those relationships, for our own perceptions, thoughts, feelings, and behavior. Just as in any other unpleasant or threatening situation, we can react unconsciously with some version of the fight-or-flight reaction when we are having a problem with another person, and this usually makes matters worse in the long run.

Many of us have developed deeply ingrained habits for dealing with interpersonal unpleasantness and conflict. These habits are often our inheritance, molded by the ways our parents related to each other and to other people. Some people are so threatened by conflict or angry feelings in others that they will do anything to avoid a blowup. If you have this habit, you will tend not to show or tell people how you are really feeling but will try to avoid conflict at all costs by being passive, placating the other person, giving in to them, blaming yourself, dissimulating—whatever it takes.

Others may deal with their insecure feelings by creating conflict wherever they go. They see all their interactions in terms of power and control. Every interaction is made into an occasion for exerting control in one way or another, for getting their own way, without thinking or caring about others. People who have this habit of relating tend to be aggressive and hostile, often without any awareness of how it is perceived from the outside. They can be abrasive, abusive, insensitive out of sheer habit. Their speech tends to be harsh, both in their choice of words and in their tone of voice. They may act as if all relationships are struggles to assert dominance. As a result they usually leave a wake of bad feelings behind them in other people.

As we saw in Chapter 19, the deeply automatic impulse for fight-or-flight influences our behavior even when our lives are not in danger. When we feel that our interests or our social status is threatened, we are capable of reacting unconsciously to protect or defend our position before we know what we are doing. Usually this behavior compounds our problems by increasing the level of conflict. Or alternatively, we might act submissively. When we do, it is often at the expense of our own views, feelings, and self-respect. But since we also have the ability to reflect, think, and be aware, we have a range of other options available to us that go well beyond our most unconscious and deeply ingrained instincts. But we need purposefully to cultivate these options. They don't just magically surface, especially if our mode of interpersonal relating has been dominated by automatically defensive or aggressive behavior that we have not really bothered to look at. Again, it is a matter of choosing a response rather than being carried away by a reaction.

Relationships are based on connectedness. When people communicate, an exchange of perspectives takes place that can lead to new ways of seeing and being together for the people involved. We are capable of communicating far more than fear and insecurity to each other when our feelings become part of the legitimate scope of our awareness. Even when we are feeling threatened, angry, or frightened, we have the potential to improve our relationships dramatically if we bring mindfulness into the domain of communication itself. As we saw in Chapter 15, the motive of affiliative trust, for instance, which got stronger in people who took the stress reduction program, might be a healthy alternative to the relentlessly one-pointed pursuit of power in relationships.

◆

The word *communication* suggests a flow of energy through a common bond. As with *communion*, it implies a union, a joining or sharing. So to communicate is to unite, to have a meeting or union of minds. This does not necessarily mean agreement. It does mean seeing the situation as a whole and understanding the other person's view as well as one's own.

When we are totally absorbed in our own feelings and our own view and agenda, it is virtually impossible to have a genuine communication. We will easily feel threatened by anyone who doesn't see things our way and we will tend to be able to relate to only those people whose view of the world coincides with our own. We will find our encounters with people who hold strongly opposing views to be stressful. When we react by feeling personally threatened, it is easy to draw battle lines and have the relationship degenerate into "us" against "them." This makes the possibility of communication very difficult. When we lock in to certain restricted mind-sets, we cannot go beyond the nine dots and perceive the whole system of which we and our views are only a part. But when both sides in a relationship expand the domain of their thinking and are willing to consider the other side's point of view and keep in mind the system as a whole, then extraordinary new possibilities emerge as imaginary but all-too-limiting boundaries in the mind dissolve.

The possibility of attaining harmony in communication applies to large collections of people, such as nations, governments and political parties, as well as to individuals. How else to explain that countries that were only a short time ago enemies, such as the United States and Germany and Japan, are now closely allied, and that the United States and the USSR are beginning to see and communicate about common interests and problems in ways that acknowledge the paradigm of wholeness and interdependence rather than just self-interest and mutually assured destruction?

Even when one party takes responsibility for thinking of the whole system and the other does not, the whole system is altered and new possibilities for conflict resolution and understanding may emerge. Of course these possibilities can also be damaged by unilateral reversions to an older way of thinking and acting, the massacre of Chinese demonstrators in Beijing by the Chinese army in June 1989 and the subsequent crackdown on the new democracy movement being one poignant example.

◆

When we come to the topics of people stress and difficulties in communication in the stress clinic, sometimes we have the whole class break up into pairs to do a number of awareness exercises originally adapted from the martial art of aikido by the author and aikido practitioner, George Leonard. These exercises help us to act out with our bodies, in partnership with another person, the experience of responding instead of reacting in threatening and stressful situations. We get to simulate different possible energy relationships between the two people and to look at these relationships and feel how they feel "from the inside."

In aikido, the goal is to practice maintaining your own center and calmness under physical attack, and to make use of the attacker's own irrational and imbalanced energy to dissipate his or her energy without getting hurt yourself and also without harming the attacker. This involves being willing to move in close to the attacker and actually make contact with him or her while at the same time not placing yourself directly in the path of greatest danger, that is, right in front of the oncoming person.

The way we do these exercises in class, the partner who is "attacking" always represents a situation or person who is "running you over," in other words, causing you stress. The attacker comes at the other person with arms outstretched in front and going straight for the other person's shoulders, to give that person a significant "hit."

In the first scenario, as the attacker comes at you, you just lie down on the floor and say something like, "It's okay, do whatever you want, you're right, *I'm* to blame," or "Don't do it, it wasn't my fault, someone else did it." We observe what that feels like with a partner, with each of us taking each role in turn. People invariably find this scenario distasteful in both roles but admit that it is frequently acted out in the "real" world. Many people share their stories of feeling like the doormat in the family or feeling trapped in their own passive behavior, intimidated by powerful others. The attackers usually admit feeling pretty frustrated by this scenario.

Then we proceed to a scenario in which, when the attacker comes at you, you move out of the way *at the last minute* as fast as you can so that he or she goes right by you. There is no physical contact. This usually causes the attackers to feel even more frustrated. They were expecting contact and they didn't get it. The people who got out of the way feel pretty good this time. At least they didn't get run over. But they also realize that you can't relate like this all the time or you will be constantly running away and avoiding people. Couples often get into this kind of behavior with each other, one pursuing contact, the other rejecting or avoiding it at all costs. These aggressive and passive (and sometimes, as when you are always avoiding contact as a way of getting back at another person, passive-aggressive) roles, when they become deep habits, can be very painful for both parties because there is no contact, no communication. It is lonely and frustrating. Yet people can and do live out their lives relating to other people through these basic passive and aggressive stances, even toward those they are closest to.

In another exercise, you push back when you are attacked instead of getting out of the way. You dig in your heels and resist. Both parties wind up pushing against each other. To intensify the situation and make it more emotionally charged, we might have people yell "I'm right, you're wrong" at each other as they are doing this. When we stop action, close our eyes, and bring our attention to our bodies and feelings, people invariably say, after they have caught their breath, that this scenario feels better than the one in which one person was being passive. At least in this one there is contact. They discover that, while struggling is exhausting, it can also be exhilarating in its own way. We are making contact, standing up for ourselves, letting our feelings out, and that feels good. When we do this exercise, it always seems a little clearer *why* so many of us are virtually addicted to—and stuck in—this way of relating. It can actually feel good, in a limited way.

But this exercise leaves us feeling empty too. Usually both people in a struggle think they are right. Each is trying to force the other to see it "my way." Both know deep down that the other person is not likely to come to see it differently, not out of forcing and intimidation and struggle. What does happen is that either we adjust to a life of perpetual struggle or one person submits every time, usually claiming that he or she is doing it to "save the relationship." We can even get caught in thinking that these patterns in our relationships are the way things have to be. Even if they are painful and exhausting, in some ways we might tend to feel comfortable and secure with what we already know, with the familiar. At least we don't have to face the unknown risks of choosing to see or do things differently and thereby threaten the status quo.

Too often we forget the physical and psychological costs of living like this, not only for the two parties in the relationship but for others who are connected to it as well, such as children and grandparents, who may be observing this kind of relating day in, day out, and even taking the brunt of it. In the end, our lives can become bogged down in a very limited view of ourselves, our relationships, and our options. Perpetual struggle hardly seems a very good model for communication or for growth or change.

The last exercise in this series is called *blending* in aikido. This option represents the *stress response* as opposed to the various stress reactions we have just reviewed in the other scenarios. It is based on being centered, on being awake and mindful. It requires that we be aware of the other person as a stressor without losing our own balance of mind. We are grounded in our breathing and in our seeing the situation as a whole without reacting totally out of fear, even if fear is present, which it very likely is in our real-life stressful encounters with people. Blending, or responding, involves stepping into the attacker, positioning your feet so that you step toward but also slightly to the side of the attacker at the same time that you take hold of one of his or her outstretched wrists. This movement is called *entering* in aikido. By entering the attack, you manage to sidestep the brunt of it at the same time that you move in close and make contact. The very positioning of your body is making a statement that you are willing to encounter and work with what is happening, that you will not be run over. You don't try to control the attacker with brute force. Instead you take hold of his or her wrist and "blend" with the attacker's energy by turning with his or her momentum so that you are both facing in the same direction, still holding on to the wrist. At this moment you are both seeing the same thing because you are looking in the same direction. In blending, you avoid a head-on impact, in which you might be badly hurt or overwhelmed by the sheer momentum of the other person, yet you do make firm contact and also show, by moving *with* his or her momentum and turning, that you are willing to see things from his or her perspective, that you are receptive and willing to look and listen. This allows the attacker to maintain his or her own integrity, but at the same time it communicates that you are not afraid of making contact nor are you willing to let his or her energy over-whelm or harm you. At this moment you become partners rather than adversaries, whether the other person wants to or not.

You don't know what will happen in the next moment, but you have a lot of options. One possibility is to turn the attacker as his or her energy winds down and show that person how *you* see things now by both of you facing another direction. What happens next becomes a dance. You are not totally in control and neither is the other person. But by maintaining your center, you are at least in control of yourself and much less vulnerable to harm. You can't have much of a plan for what to do next because so much depends on the situation itself. You have to trust in your own imagination and your ability to come up with new ways of seeing right in that moment.

I once had an immediate supervisor whose way of relating was to say things like "you son of a bitch" with a big smile on his face. He caused me a lot of stress because his hostility prevented us from having an effective working relationship. But I came to realize that he had no idea that he was being hostile. He would drive many of the people he supervised to distraction and often they would have terrible arguments with him and go away feeling angry, hurt, and, above all, frustrated at not being supported. One day, when he smiled as he said something hostile to me, I decided to call him on it. Very gently but matter-of-factly, I asked him if he was aware that every time he related to me he put me down. I also told him how it looked from my perspective, that I felt he really didn't like me and disapproved of the work I was doing. His response to this was utter amazement. He genuinely had no idea that he had been calling me names and had been giving me the feeling that he didn't like me and disapproved of the work. As a result of this conversation, our working relationship improved a good deal and became much less stressful for me. We had come to understand each other better, in part because I chose to blend with his attacks rather than resist them and mount an all-out assault of my own in return because I felt angry, hurt, and frustrated.

The path of blending obviously involves taking certain risks, since you don't know what the attacker will do next nor how you will respond. But if you are committed to meeting each moment mindfully, with as much calmness and acceptance as you can muster and with a sense of your own integrity and balance, new and more harmonious solutions often come to mind as you need them. Partly this requires being in touch with your feelings and accepting them, even acknowledging them and sharing them as appropriate. When one person in an adversarial relationship takes responsibility for doing this, the entire relationship changes, even if the other person is completely unwilling to engage in this way. The very fact that you are seeing differently and holding your own center means that you are much more in control than if you were merely reacting and forcing. Why let the momentum of another person's agenda cata-pult you into your own imbalance of body and mind just at the moment when you need all your inner resources for being clear and strong?

The patience, wisdom, and firmness that can come out of a moment of mindfulness in the heat of a stressful interpersonal situation yield fruit almost immediately because the other person usually senses that you cannot be intimidated or overwhelmed. He or she will feel your calmness and self-confidence and will in all likelihood be drawn toward it because it embodies inner peace.

When you are willing to be secure enough in yourself to listen to what other people want and how they see things without constantly reacting, objecting, arguing, fighting, resisting, making yourself right and them wrong, they will feel heard, welcomed, accepted. This feels good to anybody. They will then be much more likely to hear what you have to say as well, maybe not right away, but as soon as the emotions recede a little. There will be more of a chance for communication and for an actual communion of sorts, a meeting of minds, and an acknowledging and coming to terms with differences. In this way, your mindfulness practice can have a healing effect on your relationships.

◆

Relationships can heal just like bodies and minds can heal. Fundamentally, this is done through love, kindness and acceptance. But in order to promote healing in relationships or to develop the effective communication such healing depends on, you will have to cultivate an awareness of the *energy* of relationships, including the domains of minds and bodies, thoughts, feelings, speech, likes and dislikes, motives and goals—not only other people's but also your own—as they unfold from moment to moment in the present. If you hope to heal or resolve the stress associated with your interactions with other people, whoever they may be, whether they are your children or your parents, your spouse, your ex-spouse, your boss, your colleagues, your friends, or your neighbors, mindfulness of communication becomes of paramount importance.

◆

One good way to increase mindfulness of communication is to keep a log of stressful communications for a week. We have people do this in the week preceding the class on communication (fifth week). The assignment is to be aware of one stressful communication per day at the time that it is happening. This involves an awareness of the person with whom you are having the difficulty, how it came about, what you really wanted from the person or situation, what the other person wanted from you, an awareness of what was actually happening and what came out of it, as well as how you were feeling at the time it was happening. These items are recorded each day in a workbook and we then share and discuss them in class. (See the sample calendar in the Appendix.)

People come in with many rich observations about their patterns of communication that they had not been very conscious of before. Just keeping track of stressful communications and your own thoughts, feelings, and behavior while they are happening provides major clues about how you might behave differently to achieve your ends more effectively. Some people come to realize that much of their stress comes from not knowing how to be assertive about their own priorities when interacting with others. They may not even know how to communicate what they are really feeling, or they feel that they don't have a right to feel what they are feeling. Or they may feel afraid about expressing their feelings. Some feel absolutely incapable of ever saying no to other people, even though they know that to say yes means that their own resources will be taxed to the limit or beyond. They feel guilty doing something for themselves or having plans of their own. They are always ready to serve others at the expense of themselves, not because they have transcended their own physical and psychological needs and have become saints, but because they believe that that is what they "should" do to be a "good person." Sadly, this often means that they are always helping other people but feel incapable of nourishing or helping themselves. That would be too "selfish," too self-centered. Thus they put other people's feelings first, but for the wrong reasons. Deep down they may be running away from themselves by serving other people, or they may be doing it to gain approval from others or because they were taught and now think that that is the way to be a "good person."

This behavior can create enormous stress because you are not replenishing your own inner resources nor are you aware of your own attachments to the role you have adopted. You can exhaust yourself running around "doing good" and helping others and in the end be so depleted that you are incapable of doing any good at all and unable to help even yourself. It's not the doing things for others that is the source of the stress here. It is the lack of peace and harmony in your own mind as you engage in all the doing.

If you decide that you have to say no more often and define certain limits in your relationships so that you might bring your life into balance, you will discover that there are a lot of ways you might do it. Many ways of saying no cause more problems than they solve. If you react to demands upon you from others by saying no in an angry way, you create bad feelings all around and more stress. Often when we feel put upon, we automatically attack the other person in return, making them feel blamed or threatened or inadequate. The use of abrasive language and tone of voice contribute to this attack. Usually the first thing we do is to *react* by saying no. Adamantly. In some circumstances you might even find yourself calling the other person names. Here is where authentic assertiveness training can be very useful. What assertiveness training amounts to is mindfulness of feelings, speech, and actions.

Assertiveness is predicated on the assumption that you can be in touch with what you are actually feeling. It goes far beyond whether you can say no when you want to. It concerns your deepest ability to know yourself and to read situations appropriately and face them consciously. If you have an awareness of your feelings *as feelings*, then it becomes possible to break out of the passive or hostile modes that so automatically rear up when you feel put upon or threatened. So the first step in becoming more assertive is to practice knowing how you are actually feeling. In other words, practice mindfulness of your own feeling states. This is not so easy, especially if you have been conditioned your whole life to believe that it is wrong to have certain kinds of thoughts or feelings in the first place. Every time they come up, the reflex is to go unconscious and lose your awareness completely. Alternatively, you may condemn yourself inwardly, feel guilty about what you are feeling, and try to hide what you are really feeling from others. You may get stuck in your own beliefs about good and bad and end up denying or suppressing your feelings.

The first lesson in assertiveness is that your feelings are simply *your feelings*! They are neither good nor bad. "Good" and "bad" are just judgments that you or others impose *on* your feelings. To act assertively really requires a non-judging awareness of your feelings as they are.

Many men grew up in a world in which there was an overriding message that "real men" don't have—and therefore should not show—certain kinds of feelings. This social conditioning makes it very difficult for boys and men to be aware of their true feelings a lot of the time because their feelings are "unacceptable" and therefore very quickly edited out, denied, or repressed. This makes it particularly difficult to communicate effectively at highly emotionally charged times, such as when we are feeling threatened or vulnerable and when we experience grief or sorrow or hurt.

Our best chance of breaking out of this dilemma is for us to suspend the judging and editing of our feelings as we become aware of doing this and instead, to risk listening to our feelings and accepting them because they are already here. But, of course, this means we have to want to be more open, at least with ourself, and perhaps, also, to communicate differently.

Even in situations that are not threatening, men can have a hard time communicating their feelings. We have been so conditioned to devalue communicating our true feelings that we often forget that it is even possible. We just plunge ahead with what we are doing and expect people to *know* what we want or what we are feeling without our having to say it. Or we don't care; we do what we do and let the consequences fall where they may. It can threaten our autonomy to tell other people our plans or our intentions or our feelings. This behavior can be a source of endless exasperation to women.

When you know what you are feeling and have practiced reminding yourself that your feelings are just feelings and that they are okay to have and to feel, then you can begin to explore ways of being true to your feelings without letting them create more problems for you. They create problems both when you become passive and discount them and when you become aggressive and inflate and overreact to them. To be assertive means to know your feelings *and* to be able to communicate them in a way that allows you to maintain your integrity without threatening the integrity of others. For example, if you know that you want to or need to say no in a particular situation, you can practice saying it in such a way that you are not using it as a weapon. You might try first telling the other person that you would be glad to fulfill the request if the circumstances were different (if this is in fact the case), but . . . , or you might in some other way acknowledge that you respect the other person and his or her needs. You do not have to tell the other person why you are saying no, but you can choose to if you want to.

When being assertive, it is very helpful to remember to say how you are feeling or seeing the situation by making *"I" statements* rather than *"you" statements*. "I" statements convey information about your feelings and views. Such statements are not wrong; they are simply statements of *your* feelings. But if you are uncomfortable with your feelings, you might wind up blaming how you are feeling on the other person without even knowing it. Then you may find yourself saying things like "*You* make me so angry" or "*You* are always making demands on me."

Can you see that this is saying that the other person is in control of *your* feelings? You are literally handing power over your feelings to another person and not taking responsibility for your end of the system, which includes you both.

The alternative is to say something like "I feel so angry when you say this or do that." This is more accurate. It says how *you* feel in response to something. This leaves the other person room to hear what you are saying about how you see and feel without feeling blamed or attacked and without being told that he has more power than he actually has.

Maybe the other person won't understand. But at least you have made the attempt to communicate without doing battle. This is where the dance begins. What you do or say next will depend on the particular circumstances. But if you maintain mindfulness of the entire situation and of your own thoughts and feelings, you will be much more likely to steer your way through to some kind of understanding, or accommodation, or agreement to disagree, without losing or surrendering your own dignity and integrity, either through being passive or being aggressive.

The most important part of effective communication is to be mindful of your own thoughts, feelings, and speech as well as of the situation. It is also crucial to remember that you and your "position" are part of a social system. If you expand the field of your own awareness to include the whole system, this will allow you to see and honor the other person's point of view as well. Then you will be able to listen and really hear, to see and comprehend, to speak and know what you are saying, and to act effectively and assertively, with dignity. Most of the time cultivating this approach—which we might call *the way of awareness*—will resolve potential conflicts and create greater harmony and mutual respect. In the process, you are much more likely to get what you want and what you need from your encounters with other people. And so are they!

29

Role Stress

One of our biggest obstacles to effective communication, one that prevents us from even *knowing* our true feelings, is that we easily get stuck in our various personal and professional roles. Either we have no awareness of this or we feel helpless to break out of the rigid constraints they can impose on our attitudes and behaviors. Roles have a momentum of their own, the momentum of the past, the way other people have done things, the expectations we hold for ourselves and how we should do things or that we think other people hold for how we should act. Men can unconsciously take on habitual roles with women, and women with men, parents with their children, and children with their parents. Work roles, group roles, professional roles, social roles, roles we might adopt in illness—all can be confining if we have no awareness of them and how they mold our behavior in so many different situations.

Role stress is a side effect of our ingrained habits of doing when the domain of being gets lost. It can be a major obstacle to our continued psychological growth and the source of much frustration and suffering. We all have strong views about our situations, about what we do and how things should be done, what the parameters are within which we can work, what the rules of the game are. Usually these are colored by very strong beliefs about what can and cannot be done, what constitutes appropriate behavior in a particular situation, what we would feel comfortable with, and what it means to be a ————, where you fill in the blank: mother, father, child, sibling, spouse, boss, worker, lover, athlete, teacher, lawyer, judge, priest, patient, man, woman, manager, executive, doctor, surgeon, politician, artist, banker, conservative, radical, liberal, capitalist, socialist, success.

All these domains of doing, of acting in the world, have a stylized component to them, often a set of unwritten expectations that one has of oneself about what it means to be "good" at what one is doing. They convey a kind of a mantle of importance or authority or power to the role of being a good this or a good that. While some of this is basic to knowing the role or "job," much of it is merely posturing, a creation of our own mind more than anything else, an attaching of a particular view and expectation to ourself that we then act out and get caught up in. If we fail to perceive that we may be treading this path, such entanglements can wind up causing us much distress and prevent us from being who we really are while doing what we do. The momentum and demands of our roles, coupled with these self-imposed unconscious expectations, can drive us to the point where our roles become prisons rather than vehicles for expressing our being and our wisdom.

Mindfulness can help us to extricate ourselves from the negative effects of excessive role stress because, once again, much of the stress comes from unawareness, partial seeing, or misperception. When we are able to observe our own involvement in the stress that we blame on our roles, then we will be able to act in imaginative ways to restore balance and harmony and get unstuck.

This happened dramatically in class one day during the pushing exercises. Abe, a sixty-four-year-old rabbi who came to the clinic with heart disease and who was recently having a lot of trouble in his relationships with people, had a difficult time with the blending exercise described in the last chapter. After attempting it with a partner, he just stood still, looking bewildered. His body reflected his state of confusion. Then all of a sudden he exclaimed, "That's what it is! I never turn! I'm afraid I will get hurt if I turn!"

He had realized that he wasn't *turning* when he was being attacked, that his body was rigid when he attempted to take hold of the other person's wrist. This was why there was no harmonious blending of his energy with the attacker's.

In a metaphorical flash of insight, he connected this to his relationships in general. He saw that he never "turns" in his relationships, that he is *always* rigid, that he only holds *his* point of view, even as he plays at seeing the other person's. And all because he has a fear of being hurt himself.

Then Abe took it one step further. He said, pointing to his partner in the exercise, "I could *trust* him. He's trying to help me."

Abe shook his head, dumbfounded, as the whole experience took hold and he saw its ramifications. He called it a new type of learning for him. His body had taught him something in a matter of minutes that words could never have accomplished. For one moment, it had released him from a role he is so emeshed in that he can almost never see it. Now he has to keep this newfound awareness alive and find alternative ways of relating to people and to potential conflict.

◆

Sometimes it is easy to feel that the role you feel confined in is the worst possible role. We readily project that other people in other roles never have the kinds of problems that we do, but it's not true. Just talking with other people who are in your situation or to people who are feeling stress in entirely different situations can be healing, because it puts things in a larger perspective. We feel less isolated and less alone in our suffering. We learn that other people feel as we do, that they are in or have been in similar roles.

If you are willing to discuss your roles, other people can mirror your situation back to you and help you to see new options, ones your mind may have edited out for you as being "unthinkable." They are unthinkable only because your mind is so attached to one way of seeing or because you are so unconscious of your roles that you can't see them at all.

One day in class, a woman in her mid-forties who was referred with heart disease and panic attacks recounted her trials with one of her grown-up sons, who was being extremely abusive of her but who refused to move out of the house, although she and her husband wanted him to. They were in an ongoing stalemate, with the son refusing to leave, and the mother alternatively telling him to leave and feeling guilty about not wanting him around and fearful about what might happen to him if he did leave. Her disclosure occasioned a spontaneous outpouring of sympathy and advice from other people in the class who had been through similar situations. They tried to help her to see that her love for her child was preventing her from seeing clearly that he needs to leave and is even asking her, by his behavior, to kick him out into the world. But the love of a parent is so strong that it can often lead to being stuck in a role that is no longer working, no longer helpful to either the child or the parent.

We suffer in all sorts of roles. Usually it is not the role per se but rather our relationship to it that makes it stressful. Ideally we want to make use of our roles as opportunities to do good work, to learn and to grow and to help others. But we need to be wary of identifying so strongly with one view or one feeling that it blinds us to seeing the full extent of what is actually happening and narrows our options, confining us to self-created ruts that ultimately frustrate us and prevent us from growing.

Every role has a particular set of potential stressors that goes with the territory. For instance, let's say you are in a role at work that identifies you as a leader and innovator, as a hard-driving problem solver. If you succeed in bringing your enterprise to the point where things are more or less under control, it may leave you feeling uncomfortable and out of sorts. You may be one of those people who function best under pressure, with constant threats, crises, and impending "disasters" to which they can devote their full energies. You may not know how to accommodate yourself to situations in which you have already succeeded at bringing some stability to the scene. You may continue to be hard-driving and seek out new windmills to joust at just to feel comfortable and engaged. Such a pattern may be a sign that you are becoming stuck in a particular role. Perhaps you are now only feeding a chronic addiction for work while devaluing your other roles and obligations.

If this work addiction results in an erosion of the quality of family life, for instance, it may be sowing the seeds of much unhappiness. You may find that you are very successful in some arenas while at the same time you are not relating well to your children or to your spouse anymore. You may find a gulf broadening between you. Your mind may be full of details about work, absorbed in your own problems that they don't even know about or wouldn't find interesting. You may not be around very much, either physically or psychically. You may not even know that much about their lives anymore, about what they are feeling and what they are going through each day. Without even knowing it, you may gradually have lost your ability to tune in to the people you love and who love you the most, perhaps even your ability to express your feelings for them. You may have become stuck in your work role and unable to operate in your many other life roles comfortably. And you may even have forgotten what is most important to you. You may even have forgotten who you are.

All people who are in positions of power and authority in their work lives run the risk of this kind of alienation. We call this "the stress of success." The power and the control, the attention and respect that you get in your professional role can become intoxicating and addicting. It's hard to make the transition from the authority who commands, dictates, and makes consequential decisions that influence people and institutional policies to one's position as father or mother, husband or wife, a position in which you are just a regular person, not some major authority. Your family won't be too impressed that you make million-dollar decisions or are an important and influential person. You still have to take out the garbage, do the dishes, spend time with the kids, be a regular person, just like everybody else. Your family knows who you really are. They know the good, the bad, and the ugly, the kind of things you can conceal in your work life to make yourself look a certain way, more perfect, more authoritative. They see you when you are confused and unsure of yourself, stressed, sick, upset, angry, depressed. They love you for who you are, not for what you do. But they may miss you deeply and become alienated from you if you undervalue your role in the family and forget how to let go of your professional persona. In fact, if you get *too* lost in your work role, you may wind up jeopardizing your relationships to the point where the gulfs you create may become impossible to bridge. By that time, of course, no one may want to even make the effort anymore.

The clash of your multiple roles and their tug in different directions is one ongoing manifestation of the full catastrophe. It has to be faced and worked with. Some kind of balance has to be struck. Without awareness of the potential dangers of role stress, the damage may be done long before you come to realize what is happening. This is one reason why there is so much alienation between men and women in families and between parents and young children and adult children and elderly parents. It is certainly possible to grow and change within our roles without abandoning them. But roles can become confining and can limit further growth if we lock ourselves or each other into them.

If we bring awareness to our various roles, we will be more likely to function effectively without getting stuck in them. We might even risk being ourselves in *all* our various roles. We might at some point feel secure enough to be true to ourselves and be more authentic in everything we choose to do. Of course this means being willing to see and let go of old baggage that no longer works for us. Perhaps you have gotten stuck in a bad-guy role, a victim role, a doormat role, a weak-person role, the role of the incompetent, the dominant one, the big authority, the hero, the sick person, or the sufferer. Whenever you have had enough of this, you can decide to bring an element of wise attention to these roles. You can practice letting go of them and allowing yourself to expand to the full extent of your being by changing the way you actually *do* things and respond to things. There is really only one way to do this. It takes a ruthless commitment to seeing your own impulses to go for the familiar, to fall into habitual patterns and confining mind-sets, and a willingness to let go of them in the very moments when they arise. As Abe saw so clearly, you have to turn, turn, turn to stay fresh and avoid the ruts.

30
Work Stress
—

All the potential stressors that we have examined so far, including time pressures, other people, and confining roles, converge in the work arena. They can be sorely compounded by our need to make money. Most of us have to do something to earn money to live and most jobs are at least potentially stressful in a variety of ways. But work is also a way of connecting with the larger world, a way of doing something useful, of making some kind of contribution of labor and effort to something meaningful, which hopefully has its own rewards beyond those of a paycheck. The sense of contributing something, of creating, of helping others, of putting our knowledge and skills to work can help us to feel a part of something bigger, something worth working for. If we could see our own work in this way, it might make it more tolerable, even under difficult circumstances.

People who can't work at all because of illness or injury often feel they would give anything to be working, to not have to stay in bed or go stir-crazy around the house. When you are limited in your ability to get out and connect in this way, almost any job can seem worth having, even tolerable. We often forget or take for granted that work can lend meaning and coherence to our lives. The meaning and coherence it provides is in proportion to how much we care about and believe in it.

As we know, some jobs are particularly demeaning and exploitative. Some working conditions are highly toxic to either physical or psychological health or both. Work can be dangerous to your health. Some studies show that men (these particular studies were done on men) in jobs that have little decision-making latitude but have high standards of performance—such as a waiter, an office computer operator, or a cook—show a higher prevalence of heart attacks than men in jobs with more control. This is true independent of age and other factors, such as cigarette smoking.

But even if you have a job with a lot of autonomy and a good salary and you are doing things that you care about, even love to do, you are never completely in control. The law of impermanence still applies. Things still change. You can't control that. There are always people or forces that can disrupt your work and threaten your job and your role, or make what you said one day "inoperable" the next, no matter how much power you may think you have accumulated. Moreover, there are usually intrinsic limits to how much you can do to change things or resist certain changes within organizations, even if you have a lot of power and influence.

A person can experience job stress, insecurity, frustration, and failure at any level, from janitor to chief executive, from waiter, factory worker, or bus driver to lawyer, doctor, scientist, or politician. Many jobs are intrinsically stressful because of the combination of low decision-making latitude and high responsibility. To correct this requires reorganizing the job itself or compensating the employees better to make it more tolerable. Yet, given that many job descriptions will not be rewritten in the short run to lower employee stress, people are forced to cope as best they can using their own resources. The degree to which you are affected by stressful circumstances can be influenced positively by your own coping skills. As we saw in Part III, the level of psychological stress you experience depends on how you interpret things, in other words on your attitude, and on whether you are able to flow with change or, on the other hand, make every ripple in the way things are unfolding into an occasion for fighting or worrying.

♦

To cope effectively with work stress as an individual practically *requires* that you look at your situation with eyes of wholeness, no matter what the particulars of your job may be. It helps to keep things in perspective if you ask yourself from time to time, "What is the job I am really doing and how can I best do it under the circumstances I find myself in?" As we have seen, we can easily fall into ruts in our roles, especially if we have held the same job for a long time. If we do not guard against it, we may stop seeing each moment as new, each day as an adventure. Instead, we may become susceptible to feeling drowned in the repetitiveness and predictability of each day. We may find ourselves resisting innovation and change and becoming overly protective of what we have built because we feel threatened by new ideas or requirements or by new people.

It is not uncommon for us to operate at work the same way we do at other times in our lives, namely on automatic pilot. Why should we expect to be fully awake and living in the moment at work if mindfulness is not something we value in our lives as a whole? As we have seen, the automatic-pilot mode may get us through our days but it won't help with feeling worn down by the pressure, the routine, the sameness of what we are doing. We can feel just as stuck at work as in other domains in our lives. Or more so. We may feel that we don't have many alternatives, that we are limited by economic realities, by our own earlier life choices, by all sorts of things that prevent us from changing jobs or advancing or doing what we really want to be doing. But we may not be as stuck as we think. Work stress can be greatly reduced in many cases simply by an intentional commitment to cultivate calmness and awareness in the domain of work and by letting mindfulness guide our actions and responses.

As we have seen over and over again, our own mind can produce more limitations for us than are really there. While we all live within certain "economic realities" and the need to make a living doing what we are able to do, we often don't know what those limits really are, just as we don't know what the limits of our body's ability to heal really are. What we do know is that clarity of vision usually doesn't hurt, and it may provide fresh insights as to what might be possible.

Bringing the meditation practice to bear on your work life can make for major improvements in the quality of your life at work no matter what your job. You do not always have to get out of a stressful job for your work life to start to change in positive ways. Sometimes simply deciding, as an experiment, to make your work part of your meditation practice, part of your work on yourself, can shift the balance from a sense of being done in by the job to a sense of knowing what you are doing and choosing to do it. This change in perspective can lead directly to a change in what your job means to you. Work can become a vehicle that you are purposefully using to learn and to grow. Obstacles then become challenges and opportunities, frustrations occasions to practice patience, what other people are doing or not doing occasions to be assertive and communicate effectively, and power struggles occasions to watch the play of greed, aversion, and unawareness in other people and in yourself.

Of course, sometimes you may have to leave a job because it is not worth the effort to pursue such a path, given the circumstances.

When you introduce mindfulness as the thread guiding your seeing and your actions from moment to moment and from day to day, at work, as you get up in the morning and prepare to go to work, and as you leave to come home, work really becomes something you are *choosing* to do every day in a way that goes beyond the necessity of having a job to make money or to "get somewhere" in life. You are bringing the same attitudes that we have been cultivating as the foundation of mindfulness in other aspects of life into your work life in a seamless merging of moments. Rather than having work run your life completely, you are now in a position to be in greater balance with it.

True, there are obligations and responsibilities and pressures that you have to face and deal with and that may be beyond your control and may cause you stress, but is that not the same in every other aspect of your life as well? If it were not one set of pressures, would it not be another after a short time? You need to eat. You need connection to the larger world one way or another. There will always be some aspect of the full catastrophe to be faced somewhere, sometime. It is *how* you will face it that matters.

When you begin to look at work mindfully, whether you work for yourself, for a big institution, or for a little one, whether you work inside a building or outside, whether you love your job or hate it, you are bringing all your inner resources to bear on your working day. This will allow you to take more of a problem-solving approach as you go along, and thus to cope better with the stressors at work. Then, even if you come to a point where you have to face a big life transition, perhaps because you were fired from your job or were laid off or you decided to quit or to go out on strike, you will be better prepared to meet these changes, hard as they are, with balance, strength, and awareness. You will be better prepared to handle the emotional turmoil and reactivity that invariably accompany major life crises and transitions. Since you have to go through difficult times anyway if such things happen to you, you might as well have all your resources and strength at your disposal to deal with them as best you can.

◆

Many people in the stress clinic are sent by their doctors because of stress-related problems stemming from pressures at work. Not uncommonly, they go to the doctor with one or more physical complaints, such as palpitations, nervous stomach, headache, and insomnia, and expect the doctor to diagnose them and treat what is wrong with them. When the physician suggests that it is "just stress," these people can feel incensed and indignant.

One man, the plant manager of the largest high-tech manufacturing firm of its kind in the country, came to the stress clinic with complaints of dizzy spells at work and a feeling that his life was "spinning out of control." When his doctor suggested that his symptoms were due to job stress, he wouldn't believe it at first. Even though he had responsibility for the production efficiency of the entire plant, he denied feeling stressed. While there were certainly things that bothered him at work, they were "no big deal." He suspected he might have a brain tumor or something "physical" causing his problems. He said, "I thought there had to be something wrong with me internally. . . . When you feel like you're about to fall down on the job and you're looking to grab something, you say, 'Stress is one thing, but there has got to be something *really wrong* for this to happen.'" He felt so bad physically at work and was wound up so tight mentally by the time he left to go home at night that he would frequently have to pull his truck over to the side of the road to regain control of himself. He thought he was losing his mind. He also thought he was going to die from lack of sleep. He described himself as being up for days at a time. He would watch the news until 11:30 and then go to bed. He might sleep for one hour, perhaps from 2:00 to 3:00 A.M. Then he would be awake thinking about what the next day was going to bring. His wife recognized that he was under a lot of stress, but somehow he was unwilling to see it that way, perhaps because he just couldn't believe that stress could make him feel so bad. It was also inconsistent with his role, his image of himself as a strong leader. When he was referred to the stress clinic, he had been having problems at work for about three years and things were reaching a breaking point.

By the time the course ended, he was no longer having dizzy spells and he was sleeping soundly through the night. Things changed about the fourth week, when he heard other people in his class describing the same things he was feeling and their success at controlling them. He began to believe that perhaps he, too, could do something to control his own body and its problems. He realized that his symptoms really *were* directly related to stress at work. He began to see that he felt worse toward the end of the month when the shipments had to go out, the profits had to be made, and the pressure was on. At those times, he would find himself running around like crazy getting his employees "cooking." But because he was practicing the meditation daily, he was now aware of what he was doing and feeling and he could use awareness of his breathing to relax and break the stress-reaction cycle before it built up too much.

Looking back on it when the course was over, he felt that it was his attitude toward his work, more than anything else, that had changed. He attributed this to the fact that he was paying more attention to his body and to what was bothering him. He began to see himself and his own mind and behavior in a new light and realized that he didn't have to take things so seriously. He would tell himself, "The most they can do is fire me. Let's not worry about it. I'm doing the best I can. Let's take it day by day." He would use his breathing to keep himself calm and centered, to keep himself from reaching what he called "that point of no return." When he recog-
· nizes that he is in a stressful situation, he can now immediately feel himself tensing up in the shoulders and he says to himself, "Slow down, let's gear it back a little." He said, "I can back right off it now. I don't even have to go sit down. I can just do it. I can be talking to someone and go right into a state of relaxation."

His change in perspective is reflected in how he goes to work in the morning. He started taking back roads, driving more slowly, doing his breathing on the way in to work. By the time he gets there, he is ready for the day. He used to take the main roads through the city, as he put it, "fighting with people at the lights." Now he can see and admit to himself that in the past he was actually a nervous wreck even before he reached work. He feels like a different person now, ten years younger, he says. His wife can't believe it and neither can he.

He was shocked to think that things could have gotten as bad as they did, that he could have gotten into such an "unbelievable state of mind." "I used to be the calmest person when I was a kid. Then gradually things at work crept up on me, especially as the money got bigger and bigger. I wish I had taken this program ten years ago."

But it wasn't just his attitude toward work and his awareness of his own reactivity that changed. He took steps to communicate more effectively with his employees and made real changes in the way things were getting done. "After I was practicing the meditation for a few weeks, I came to the decision that it was time to start putting more trust into the people who work for me, that I just had to. I called a big meeting and said, 'Look, you guys, you are getting paid a lot of money to do these jobs and I'm not carrying you anymore. This is what I expect, bang bang bang bang, and if it's too much, we'll get more people, but this is what has to be done and we're all going to get it together and we are going to work as a team.' And it's working out all right. They don't do it one hundred percent the way you'd like, but it gets done anyway and you have to be willing to bend and live with that. That's life, I guess. I am able to be much more efficient, and we are making big money." So now he feels that he is more productive on the job even though he is experiencing far less stress. He had seen that he was wasting a lot of time doing things that other people should have been doing. "To be a manager of a plant, you have to be doing the right things to keep the ship floating and going in the right direction all the time. I find that although now I'm not working as hard, I get more done. Now I have time to sit at my desk and plan, whereas before I used to have fifty people always on my back, constantly coming to me with this or that."

This is an example of how one person was able to bring the meditation practice into his work life. He came to see what was actually happening at work with greater clarity and, as a result, was able to reduce his stress and get rid of his symptoms without having to run away from his job. If we had told him at the beginning that this would have happened as a result of lying down and scanning his body for forty-five minutes a day for eight weeks or from following his breathing, he would have thought we were crazy, and with good reason. But because he was at his wit's end, he made the commitment to do what his doctor and we were recommending in spite of its apparent "craziness." As it was, it took four weeks for him to begin to see how the meditation practice was relevant to his situation. Once that connection was made, he was able to tap his own inner resources. He was able to slow down and appreciate the richness of the present, listen to his body, and put his own intelligence to work.

◆

Few of us on the planet, regardless of the work we do, would not benefit from greater awareness. It is not just that we would be calmer and more relaxed. In all likelihood, if we saw work as an arena in which we could hone inner strength and wisdom moment by moment, we would make better decisions, communicate more effectively, be more efficient, and perhaps even leave work happier at the end of the day.

HINTS AND SUGGESTIONS FOR REDUCING WORK STRESS

1. When you wake up, take a few quiet moments to affirm that you are choosing to go to work today. If you can, briefly review what you think you will be doing and remind yourself that it may or may not happen that way.
2. Bring awareness to the whole process of preparing to go to work. This might include showering, dressing, eating, and relating to the people you live with. Tune in to your breathing and your body from time to time.
3. Don't say good-bye mechanically to people. Make eye contact with them, touch them, really be "in" those moments, slow them down just a bit. If you leave before other people wake up, you might try writing them a brief note to say good morning and express your feelings toward them.
4. If you walk to public transportation, be aware of your body walking, standing and waiting, riding, and getting off. Walk into work mindfully. Breathe. Try smiling inwardly.

   If driving, take a moment or two to come to your breathing before you start the car. Remind yourself that you are about to drive off to work now. Some days at least try driving without the radio on. Just drive and be with yourself, moment by moment. When you park, take a moment or two to just sit and breathe before you leave the car. Walk into work mindfully. Breathe. If your face is already tense and grim, try smiling, or try a half smile if that is too much.
5. At work, take a moment from time to time to monitor your bodily sensations. Is there tension in your shoulders, face, hands, or back? How are you sitting or standing in this moment? What is your body language saying? Consciously let go of any tension as best you can as you exhale and shift your posture to one that expresses balance, dignity, and alertness.

6. When you find yourself walking at work, take the edge off it. Walk mindfully. Don't rush unless you have to. If you have to, know that you are rushing. Rush mindfully.

7. Use any breaks you get to truly relax. Instead of drinking coffee or smoking a cigarette, try going outside the building for three minutes and walking or standing and breathing. Or do neck and shoulder rolls at your desk (see Figure 7). Or shut your office door if you can and sit quietly for five minutes or so, following your breathing.

8. Spend your breaks and lunchtime with people you feel comfortable with. Otherwise, maybe it would be better for you to be alone. Changing your environment at lunch can be helpful. Choose to eat one or two lunches per week in silence, mindfully.

9. Alternatively don't eat lunch. Go out and exercise, every day if you can, or a few days per week. Exercise is a great way of reducing stress. Your ability to do this will depend on how much flexibility you have in your job. If you can do it, it is a wonderful way of clearing the mind, reducing your tension, and starting the afternoon refreshed and with a lot of energy. I try to get out of the hospital and run in the middle of the day for from half an hour to an hour, depending on my schedule. Many work places have organized employee exercise programs, such as aerobics, weight lifting, yoga, and dance, both at lunchtime and before and after work. If you have the opportunity to exercise at work, take it! But remember, an exercise program takes the same kind of commitment that the formal meditation takes. And when you do it, do it mindfully.

10. Try to stop for one minute every hour and become aware of your breathing. We waste far more time than this daydreaming at work. Use these mini-meditations to tune in to the present and just be. Use them as moments in which to regroup and recoup. All it takes is remembering to do it. This one is not easy, since we so easily get carried away by the momentum of all the doing.

11. Use everyday cues in your environment as reminders to center yourself and relax—the telephone ringing, down time at the computer terminal, waiting for someone else to finish something before you can start. Instead of relaxing by "spacing out," relax by tuning in.

12. Be mindful of your communications with people during the

work day. Are they satisfactory? Are some problematic? Think about how you might improve them. Be aware of people who tend to operate in a passive mode or a hostile mode with you. Think about how you might approach them more effectively. Think about how you might be more sensitive to other people's feelings and needs. How might you help others at work by being more mindful? How might awareness of tone of voice and body language help you when communicating?

13. At the end of the day, review what you have accomplished and make a list of what needs to be done tomorrow. Prioritize the items on your list so that you know what is most important.

14. As you are leaving, bring your awareness to walking and breathing again. Be aware of the transition we call "leaving work." Monitor your body. Are you exhausted? Are you standing erect or bent over? What expression is on your face?

15. If you are taking public transportation, bring your attention to your walking, standing, and sitting. Notice if you are rushing. Can you "back it down a bit" and own those moments between work and home as much as any of your other moments to live?

   Or, if you are driving, take a moment or two once again to sit in your car before you start it up. Drive home mindfully.

16. Before you walk in the door, realize that you are about to do so. Be aware of this transition we call "coming home." Try greeting people mindfully and making eye contact rather than shouting to announce your arrival.

17. As soon as you can, take your shoes off and get out of your work clothes. Changing to other clothes can complete the transition from work to home and allow you to integrate more quickly and consciously into your non-work roles. If you can make the time, take five minutes or so to meditate before you do anything else, even cooking or eating dinner.

The foregoing are offered as hints and suggestions, not as a daily program. Ultimately the challenge is yours to decide what might best help you to reduce your work stress.

31
Food Stress

You cannot live a healthy life in our complex society without paying at least some attention to what you put into your body. Our relationship to food has changed so much in the past few generations that the exercise of a new form of intelligence, still developing, may be necessary to sort out what is of value from the incredible choices that are presented to us.

For example, gone are the days when we ate directly off the land, consuming a small number of foods that had been the exclusive and unchanging staples of the culture over millennia. Until this century our diet had changed little from generation to generation. It was intimately dependent on an individual's ability to acquire food through hunting and gathering and to cultivate it through farming. Over the years, we came to know what was edible in nature and what was not, and our bodies adapted to the diet of particular isolated regions, climates, groups, and cultures. Getting or growing food took most of the energy of all of the members of the social group. We ate what we could obtain from the local environment to live as best we could. For better or for worse, subject to all its unpredictability and fickleness, we lived in an intrinsically homeostatic balance with the natural environment. We lived within nature, not apart from it.

We are still very much a part of nature, but we may be less aware of our intimate connections with it now because we are able to manipulate it so much of the time to our own ends.

Our relationship to food in the so-called developed countries has recently undergone an enormous transformation toward greater complexity. The majority of the members of our society live physically and psychologically far from food production. Although biologically we still eat in order to live, psychologically many people could be said to live in order to eat instead, so great are our psychic preoccupations with food that have little to do with actual hunger.

Moreover, we are now continually exposed to foods that didn't exist even five or ten years ago, foods that are synthesized or processed in factories, that are only distantly related to anything we might recognize as grown or cultivated. In the developed countries, it is now possible to obtain any food we want in any season, thanks to a distribution system that transports it over huge distances in a matter of days. Very few people in these societies any longer depend completely on growing food for themselves or hunting or foraging it off the land. We no longer have to expend all our time and energy acquiring food to have enough to eat.

As a population, we have become a nation of food consumers. Only a small percentage of the population is involved in food production, a great change from earlier days. Now we buy food in large stores, veritable cornucopias, temples of abundance and consumerism. Our experience is that there is always food on the supermarket shelves, thousands of different kinds of foods to choose from. This arrangement liberates us from having to acquire it every day. All we need is enough money to purchase it. Refrigeration and freezing, canning and packaging, have made it possible for us to store food in our homes so that we can actually eat whatever we want whenever we want.

Our food production and distribution system is a perfect example of our collective interdependence and interconnectedness. The conduits of food distribution are the arterial circulation of the social body, and the refrigerator trucks, railroad cars, and planes are the specialized transport vehicles for supplying the tissues and cells of the society with vital nourishment. A massive trucker strike would result in cities empty of food within a matter of days. There would simply be no food left in the stores for people to acquire. We tend not to think about such things.

◆

The fact is, as a population, we are probably healthier than ever before. While many people would ascribe much of this to our diets, it turns out that this may be only partially true. In fact much evidence suggests that the health of Americans is now being impaired by diseases associated with an overconsumption of food in general and of certain foods in particular, diseases occasioned by our affluence and abundance.

Our health may also be threatened by exposure to at least some of the hundreds of chemicals that human bodies never ingested over the course of evolution because they were only recently invented. Many of these chemicals, residues from fertilizers and pesticides, additives and preservatives put there by the food industry, and pollutants that make their way into the food chain from an increasingly contaminated environment, put our homeostatic biochemical networks at unknown risk for cellular and tissue disruption and damage. We simply do not know, no matter what the experts say, what exposure to some of these chemicals in food will lead to in coming generations or over a lifetime of ingestion. What we do know is that we are playing a kind of chemical Russian roulette with our own bodies, in almost all instances without the consumer knowing that he or she is an involuntary participant in this game.

Since the food we eat over a lifetime has a major influence on our health, we need to pay attention in a sensible, non-alarmist, non-fanatical way to the whole domain of what we put into our bodies, if we haven't already begun to do so. The adage "you are what you eat" has more than a modicum of truth to it.

For example, it is not an exaggeration to say that the average American diet is a major factor in, and in some cases, even a prescription for, heart disease. This is due in large part to the high levels of cholesterol and fat, in particular animal fat, in our diets. Dietary cholesterol is a fatty substance only found in foods of animal origin. It appears to play a major role in heart disease. When scientists want to create coronary artery disease in animals, they just put them on a diet that is the equivalent of bacon, eggs, and butter for six months or so. This diet is very effective in clogging the arteries of the heart.

There are very high levels of cholesterol and animal fat in butter, red meat, hamburgers, hot dogs, and ice cream—all popular staples of the American diet. In countries such as China and Japan, which have diets with less meat and animal fat and more fish and rice, the incidence of heart disease is much lower. However, these countries have high rates of certain cancers, such as esophageal and stomach cancer, which are thought to be related to a high consumption of salt-cured, salt-pickled, and smoked foods.

While the relationship of diet to cancer is less clear than in the case of heart disease, there is considerable evidence that points to a role of diet in cancers of the breast, colon, and prostate. Here, too, the total amount of fat in the diet seems to play a significant role. There is some evidence that people who have a high-fat diet have lower levels of some immune functions (for instance, natural killer cell activity which, as we have seen, is thought to play a role in protecting the body against cancer) and that when they change to a diet with a lower total fat content (including fats of both animal *and* vegetable origins), they show increases in natural killer cell activity. Many studies in animals also show a link between diet and cancer and here, too, dietary fat plays the largest role. Excessive consumption of alcohol, particularly in conjunction with cigarette smoking, also appears to increase the probability of some cancers in people.

In 1977, the Senate Select Committee on Nutrition declared that Americans were killing themselves by overeating. It recommended that we reduce the calories we obtain from fat from about 40 percent to about 30 percent, of which only 10 percent should come from saturated fat and the other 20 percent from mono- and poly-unsaturated fats. They recommended that the loss of calories from fat should be compensated for by increasing the calories we obtain from complex carbohydrates. They made this recommendation because they thought it was achievable, not because they thought that 30 percent was the optimal level of fat in the diet. The Chinese consume only 15 percent of their total calories as fat. Societies such as the Tarahumara Indians of Mexico only obtain 10 percent of their total calories from fat, and almost none of it is from animal fat. Scientists who have studied the Tarahumara have shown that they have virtually no heart disease or high blood pressure in their population. In this country, the Seventh Day Adventists have been studied by scientists interested in nutrition because most of them are vegetarians. They, too, have a very low incidence of heart disease and cancer.

Recently, Dr. Dean Ornish of the Preventive Medicine Research Institute in Sausalito and his collaborators, in a revolutionary study, demonstrated conclusively and for the first time, using highly sophisticated methods for measuring changes in the heart, including quantitative angiography (to precisely measure the size of the blockages in the coronary arteries) and PET scans (to measure blood flow to the heart past the blockages), that heart disease can be *reversed* in people without using drugs when they change the way they live and eat. They showed that by eating an almost exclusively vegetarian diet with about 10 percent of calories from fat, plus walking regularly and practicing yoga and meditation regularly over a period of one year, people who had severe coronary artery disease showed significantly increased blood flow to their hearts. In other words, the blockages in their coronary arteries, which restricted the flow of blood to the heart muscle, were reduced. They also had enormous drops in their levels of blood cholesterol, far bigger reductions than had ever been shown without using cholesterol-lowering drugs.

Dr. Ornish's work is a dramatic demonstration of the resiliency and flexibility of the human body and its ability to heal itself (in this case, reverse the disease process of atherosclerosis) if given a chance. Since atherosclerosis (narrowing of the arteries of the heart) is a disease that progresses over decades in our bodies before we suffer the ill effects of it, this discovery is very promising. It suggests that even after years of a chronic and pathological process, something can be done to stop it and reverse its damage. And this something can be accomplished, not with drugs, but by people changing the way they live their lives and what they choose to eat and not eat.

In Dr. Ornish's study, those people who were in the control group received excellent traditional medical care for their heart disease over the same period. They followed the latest conventional recommendations espoused by most cardiologists, namely to lower their intake of fat in their diet to about 30 percent and to exercise regularly. However, they did not make the radical life-style changes that the other group did. The people in the control group, in spite of following these recommendations, showed progression of their disease. Their coronary arteries were, on the average, more clogged a year later, as might be expected of a progressive disease such as coronary heart disease.

This study marks the first time that it has been demonstrated that changing the way you live can improve the functioning of your heart and actually reverse atherosclerosis. You might say that these men and women were able actually to induce their own hearts to heal by changing the way they lived through the regular practice of meditation and yoga (one hour per day) and walking (three times per week), by getting together regularly to practice and to support each other, and of course by changing what they ate. At the time of writing, this study has only been going on for one year. It seems more than likely that if these people keep up their new diet and life-style changes, their heart disease will continue to diminish year by year, but this remains to be investigated in follow-up studies.

In an earlier experiment, mentioned in Chapter 20, Dr. Ornish and his collaborators showed that it was possible to obtain significant changes in heart functioning, reductions in blood pressure reactivity under stressful situations, and dramatic reductions in chest pain in people with severe coronary blockages by putting them on this low-fat diet for twenty-four days while they stayed in a resort setting in which they practiced yoga and meditation daily. This earlier study had shown that in even a short time, given the right conditions, life-style changes can have a profound effect on the physiology of the heart and on overall mental and physical health.

◆

But changing your relationship to food is not so easy, even if you decide that you want to or that you need to in order to be healthier. This is evident from all the failed efforts that people make to lose weight. If, for whatever reason, you decide that you need to change your diet in order to promote increased health and to prevent or slow down the disease process, you will have to go about it with a profound commitment and inner discipline that is born of intelligence rather than fear or paranoia. This will involve becoming mindful of your relationship to food at all levels. You will need to become more aware of your automatic behaviors around eating, of your thoughts and feelings, and of the social customs associated with food and eating. These are areas in which we are unlikely to observe our behavior systematically and non-judgmentally unless we make a strong commitment to liberate ourselves from our mal-adaptive patterns and to develop a healthier, more coherent and integrated way of living.

As we have seen, the systematic training of the mind can be profoundly beneficial when we seek to encounter and free ourselves from our automatic and unconscious behaviors and from the under-lying motivations and impulses that drive them and cause us in-creased suffering. Our relationship to food is no exception. For this reason, the practice of mindfulness can be particularly useful for making and then maintaining healthy changes in your diet. In fact, awareness, and to a certain extent change as well, come naturally to the domain of food and eating as your meditation practice grows stronger and as you practice bringing mindfulness to all the ac-tivities of daily living. Perhaps you have already noticed this for yourself. We can hardly avoid looking at the domain of eating when we start paying attention in daily life.

Food certainly occupies a central role in most of our lives. Effort and energy go into buying food, preparing it, serving it, eating it, attending to the physical and social environments in which we eat, and cleaning up afterward. All of these activities involve behaviors and choices that we might pay attention to. In addition, we might be more conscious of domains such as the quality of the food we eat, how it was grown or made, where it comes from, and what is in it. We might also pay attention to how much we eat, how frequently we eat, when, and how we feel as a consequence of eating. For instance, we could be mindful of how we feel *after* we eat certain foods or certain amounts of food, and whether we feel differently when we eat quickly or slowly or at particular times. We can bring mindfulness to the attachments and cravings we may have for particular foods, to what we, as well as our children, will and won't eat, and to the habits the family has toward food. All of these areas come into vivid focus when you bring mindfulness to the domain of food.

Most of us find it quite difficult to change our habits, and dietary habits are no exception. Eating is a highly emotionally charged social and cultural activity. Our relationship to food has been conditioned and reinforced over our entire lifetime. Eating holds many different meanings for us. We have emotional associations with particular types of food, with eating a certain amount of food, with eating in particular places and at particular times and with particular people. These associations with food can be part of our sense of identity and well-being. They can make changing our diet even more difficult than making other kinds of life-style changes.

◆

Perhaps the best place to begin is not by trying to make any changes at all but simply by paying close attention to exactly what you are eating and how it affects you. Try observing exactly what your food looks like and how it tastes *as you are eating it*. The next time you sit down to a meal, really *look* at what is on your plate. What is its texture? Look at the colors, the shapes of the food. How does it smell? How do you feel as you look at it? How does it taste? Is it pleasurable or unpleasant? How do you feel right after eating it? Is it what you wanted? Does it agree with you?

Notice how you feel an hour or two after eating. How is your energy level? Did eating what you ate give you energy or did it make you feel sluggish? How does your belly feel? What do you think now about what you ate then?

When people in the stress clinic start paying attention to their eating in this way, they report some interesting observations. Some discover that they eat particular foods more out of habit than from liking them or wanting to eat them. Others notice that eating certain foods upsets their bellies or results in fatigue later on, connections they never noticed before. Many report that they enjoy eating much more because they are aware of it in a new way.

Many of the patients in the stress clinic make major changes in their diets long before we go into the question of diet in detail, which doesn't happen until the end of the program. These changes come about simply by bringing mindfulness to their eating as part of their daily informal meditation practice. Almost none of our patients come to the clinic seeking to lose weight or change their diets. Nevertheless, many start eating more slowly. They find they are satisfied eating less and are more aware of their impulses to use food to satisfy psychological needs. Some people actually lose weight over the eight weeks simply by paying attention in this way and without consciously *trying* to lose weight.

For example, Phil, the truck driver with back pain whom we met in Chapters 13 and 23, also changed his relationship to food while he was in the stress reduction program. In fact, he lost fourteen and a half pounds. In his own words, "Actually I'm not on any special diet. I'm paying attention when I eat. I catch myself sometimes after I start to eat, get the breathing down pat, slow down a bit. Life is such a rat race even if you're not going anywhere, always running, running, running. You do everything fast, you just slop the food in your mouth and two hours later you're hungry again because you didn't taste nothing, you just went right by it. You're full but, like I say, the taste bud has a lot to do with everything. If you didn't taste it, you'll be hungry again because you didn't taste anything you had. That's the way I look at it now. I eat less if I slow myself down because I chew my food better, I taste it. I've never been able to do that before, ya know. I'd like to lose another fifteen pounds. If I keep slowing down, ya know, losing just a little like I am now every week, then I'll probably be able to keep it down after, ya know. It's like, if you lose in a hurry, when dieting is over, you put it right back on. With the meditation I learned that you gotta set goals for yourself, ya know, and once you set your goal, go for it, don't get away from it. When you go somewhere, you see it all the time, it's in your mind. You reflect on it."

We spend at most part of one class focusing on our relationship to food and merely touching on what is known of the relationship between diet and health. We do this so that our patients can begin to make more informed decisions about diet and nutrition out of awareness. We do not advocate a particular diet. We *do* advocate that people pay attention in this domain of their lives as well as in all others instead of leaving it in the control of the automatic-pilot mode. We encourage people to inform themselves and to make whatever changes they think are important, intelligently and over a relatively long period of time, in order to shift the odds more in their favor in terms of health. The mindful eating of the raisins and the early homework assignment to eat at least one meal mindfully and in silence sow seeds that blossom when we discuss diet and nutrition. By that time, most people are convinced that there is a lot of room for making healthy changes in their diet, and quite a few have already changed their eating patterns to some extent.

But even if you have decided that you want to make changes in your diet to improve your health and to reduce the risks of heart disease and cancer, or even simply to enjoy your food more, it is not always easy to know how to initiate healthy changes. Nor is it easy to stick with them over time. Our habits and customs of a lifetime have a momentum of their own that needs to be respected and worked with intelligently. In Dr. Ornish's study, the participants received a great deal of support in changing their diets and in sticking with their new regimen. They were taught vegetarian cooking, had to give up many foods entirely, and were supplied with a range of frozen dinners and snacks to keep in the freezer to use when they ran out of ideas.

It's hardly the same if you, as an individual, want to make changes on your own to lower your cholesterol and fat intake or to cut down on the amount of certain foods you eat or the amount of food you eat, period. Habits and customs of a lifetime are hard to change without outside support. To change your eating patterns, you need to really know *why* you are trying to make those changes in the first place. Then you will have to *remember* why from day to day and even from moment to moment, as you encounter a myriad of impulses, opportunities, and frustrations that can throw you off the track. In other words, you will need to believe really deeply in yourself and in *your* vision of what is healthy and important for you. You will certainly need reliable information about food and nutrition and an awareness of your own relationship to food and to eating so that you can make intelligent choices about where to shop, what to buy, and how best to prepare it.

This is where simply applying moment-to-moment awareness to food and to eating can be crucial for bringing about positive changes. In the same way that mindfulness can have a positive influence on our relationships with pain, fear, time, and people, it can also be used to transform our relationship to food.

For instance, many people use eating as a major form of stress reduction. When we are anxious, we eat. When we are lonely, we eat. When we are bored, we eat. When we feel empty, we eat. When all else fails, we tend to eat. That is a lot of automatic eating. We don't do it to nourish the body. We mostly do it to make ourselves feel better emotionally, and also to fill up time.

What we eat at those times can add up to an unhealthy diet. The rewards and treats we give ourselves to feel better tend to be rich and sweet, such as cookies, candy, cake, pastries, and ice cream. These are all high in hidden fat and loaded with sugar. Or they tend to be salty, such as chips and dips of various kinds. These are also loaded with hidden fat.

We also have to deal with what is available and convenient. Fast-food chains specialize in foods that are high in animal fat, cholesterol, salt, and sugar, although even they are now changing to provide more healthy alternatives, such as salad bars and baked instead of fried foods. Although many restaurants are now highlighting heart-healthy foods, such as baked fish and chicken, most still do not pay attention to such matters and prepare food in ways that can make it higher in fat than it need be. It is still not easy to find healthy food if you are away from home and trying to find something to eat. Sometimes it may be healthier *not to eat* until you find what you really want to put into your body. At such times we can fall back to practicing patience and work at letting go of feeling incomplete or deprived.

If you want to improve your health, looking at your diet becomes extremely important. It's not just a question of animal fat and cholesterol, heart disease and cancer. There is considerable evidence that Americans overeat, period. We ordinarily eat about 3,000 calories per day. Yet as a society we are relatively sedentary. We don't burn up calories working to the same extent as people did in previous generations. We do a lot of driving in cars to go places and a lot of sitting at work. Driving and sitting do not burn calories the way walking and manual labor do.

It is very likely that just by eating a little less, you will be healthier, even if you don't change your diet in any other way. Some animal studies have shown that lifetimes can be extended considerably on a diet that supplies needed nutrients but is restricted in calories. Some researchers believe that this is also true for people and have presented evidence that immune function can be improved by restricting caloric intake while providing all required nutrients. However, in our society it has become dangerous even to suggest that we might be overeating. The prevalence of eating disorders, especially among young girls and women, has sensitized us to how neurotic people can become about their body image. Sometimes people's relationship to eating becomes disregulated to the point of either starving themselves and thinking that their emaciated bodies are still overweight (*anorexia nervosa*) or bingeing on food they cannot resist eating and then purposefully purging (vomiting) so that they won't gain weight (*bulimia*). Usually there is a strong underlying emotional component to these disorders as well.

These eating disorders may be, in part, an unhappy consequence of the gross preoccupation of our postindustrial society with outward appearance as well as its tendency to objectify bodies and notions of beauty, especially in women. Rather than paying attention to inner experience and being kind and accepting of oneself, we tend to condemn ourselves if we do not fit the established norms of weight, height, and outward appearance. So we have become a society alienated from our bodies as they are and in search of some eternal, unaging ideal, a society of crash dieters and failed dieters, of consumers of chemical cocktails known as diet sodas—all in the quest for the "perfect" body.

Yet there is little wisdom in all the fads associated with food and dieting. Why don't we drink water instead of diet soda? Why do we go on elaborate diets and then binge on what we have deprived ourselves of? Perhaps it is time to realize that our energy is being misdirected. Perhaps we are overly preoccupied with our weight and our appearance rather than with healing ourselves and optimizing our well-being. If we start paying attention to the basics, such as *what the mind is up to* and what we are putting into our bodies and why, we might make more substantial progress toward realizing greater health with a lot less neuroticism and wasted energy. This can be accomplished by a combination of paying attention to how much you eat and making sensible choices of what to eat. It has more to do with striking an informal balance than with being artificially rigid. If you eat eggs every day, cutting back to eating them once a week would be a big improvement. You might take a similar approach toward red meat and other foods that have been associated with increased risk of certain diseases.

We review with our patients the guidelines from the national scientific and professional societies that concern themselves with the American diet. For example, the National Academy of Medicine recommends that people reduce their consumption of pickled foods, smoked foods, and prepared meats or avoid them altogether because of their likely relationship to certain cancers. In practical terms this means giving up or drastically reducing consumption of salami, bologna, corned beef, sausage, ham, bacon, and hot dogs. The American Heart Association recommends reducing red-meat consumption, drinking low-fat or skim milk, and eliminating whole milk and cream, cutting down on fatty cheeses, and restricting the intake of eggs, which contain about 300 milligrams of cholesterol per egg! (The Ornish diet contains about 2 milligrams of cholesterol per day.)

What do these organizations recommend that you eat to replace the foods they are telling you to avoid or cut down on? They recommend increasing your consumption of fresh fruits and vegetables, preferably raw or carefully cooked so that their nutrients are not destroyed or dissolved away. Some vegetables, such as broccoli and cauliflower, seem to have a protective effect against certain kinds of cancer, perhaps from the naturally occurring antioxidants they contain. These organizations also recommend introducing more whole grains, such as wheat, corn, rice, and oats into your diet. These can be eaten in breads, as cereals for breakfast or snacks, and as an important part of dinners. They are the best sources of complex carbohydrate, which should constitute approximately 75 percent of the calories in our daily intake of food.

In addition to providing complex carbohydrate and nutrients, whole grains, fruits, and vegetables also lend bulk to the diet because they contain the outside husks of the grain and plant tissues, known as roughage or *fiber*. Fiber gives the intestinal tract, which after all, is a long coiled tube whose walls are living muscle, something to squeeze on in order to move the food along from one end to the other. When the food we eat has bulk to it from fiber, its transit time through the digestive tract is altered. Under the right conditions, the time that the tissues of the digestive tract are exposed to the waste products of digestion, which can be toxic and which the body needs to eliminate efficiently, can be reduced.

♦

In summary, paying attention to your relationship to food is important for your health. Listening to your body and observing the activity of your mind in relationship to food can help you to make and maintain healthy changes in your diet. If your meditation practice is strong, you will naturally be more in touch with your food and how it affects you. You will naturally be more mindful of your desires and cravings for food and you will be able to see them more readily *as thoughts and feelings* and to let them go *before* you act on them.

When we are on automatic pilot, we tend to act (in this case, eat) first and only then become aware of what we have done and remember why we actually didn't really want to do it. Mindfulness of when we eat, what we eat, how it tastes, where it comes from, what is in it, and how we feel after we eat it, if practiced consistently, can go a long way toward bringing change naturally to this highly charged and extremely important domain of our lives.

HINTS AND SUGGESTIONS FOR MINDFULNESS OF FOOD AND EATING

1. Start paying attention to this whole domain of your life, just as you have been doing with your body and your mind.
2. Try eating a meal mindfully, in silence. Slow down your movements enough so that you can watch the entire process carefully. See the description of eating the raisins mindfully in Chapter 1. Try shutting off your phone while you are eating.
3. Observe the colors and textures of your food. Contemplate where this food comes from and how it was grown or made. Is it synthetic? Does it come from a factory? Was anything put into it? Can you see the efforts of all the other people who were involved in bringing it to you? Can you see how it was once connected to nature? Can you see the natural elements, the sunlight and the rain, in your vegetables and fruits and grains?
4. Ask yourself if you want this food in your body before you eat it. How much of it do you want in your belly? Listen to your body while you are eating. Can you detect when it says "enough"? What do you do at this point? What impulses come up in your mind?
5. Be aware of how your body feels in the hours after you have eaten. Does it feel heavy or light? Do you feel tired or energetic?

Do you have unusual amounts of gas or other symptoms of disregulation? Can you relate these symptoms to particular foods or combinations of foods to which you might be sensitive?

6. When shopping, try reading labels on food items such as cereal boxes, breads, frozen foods. What is in them? Are they high in fat, in animal fat? Do they have salt and sugar added? What are the first ingredients listed? (By law they have to be listed in decreasing order of amounts, with the first ingredient the most plentiful, etc.).

7. Be aware of your cravings. Ask yourself where they come from. What do you *really* want? Are you going to get it from eating this particular food? Can you eat just a little of it? Are you addicted to it? Can you try letting go of it this once and just watch the craving as a thought or a feeling? Can you think of something else to do at this moment that will be healthier and more personally satisfying than eating?

8. When preparing food, are you doing it mindfully? Try a peeling-potatoes meditation or a chopping-carrots meditation. Can you be totally present with the peeling, with the chopping? Try being aware of your breathing and your whole body as you peel or chop vegetables. What are the effects of doing things this way?

9. Look at your favorite recipes. What ingredients do they call for? How much cream, butter, eggs, lard, sugar, and salt is in them? Look around for alternatives if you decide that they are no longer what you want to be cooking. Many delicious recipes are now available that are low in fat, cholesterol, salt, and sugar. Some use low-fat yogurt instead of cream, olive oil instead of lard or butter, and fruit juices for sweetening.

32

World Stress

It will never be possible to control our diet completely in a polluted world. There are too many factors we don't know about yet that nevertheless could have long-term toxic effects. For instance, you could be eating a healthy, low-cholesterol, low-fat, low-salt, low-sugar diet high in complex carbohydrates, fruits, vegetables, and fiber and still be at risk for illness if your water supply is contaminated with chemicals from illegal dumping, if the fish you eat is polluted with mercury or PCBs, or if there are pesticide residues on the fruits and vegetables you are eating.

So when you think about the relationship of health to diet, it is important to think about diet in a broader sense than the way we usually do. The *quality* of the food, where it was grown or caught, how it was raised, and what was added to it are important variables. Awareness of these interconnected aspects of diet and health will at least allow us to make intelligent decisions about what to eat a lot of and what to eat only once in a while, to hedge our bets so to speak in the absence of absolute knowledge about the state of particular foods.

Perhaps we need to expand our definition of food and what we include within it. I like to think of anything that we take in and absorb and that gives us energy or allows us to make use of the energy in other foods as food. If you think in this way, you certainly need to consider water in this category. It is an absolutely vital food. So is the air we breathe. The quality of the water we drink and the air we breathe directly affects our health. In Massachusetts, some town water supplies have been contaminated to the point where towns have had to import water from other towns. Many local wells in the state are now highly polluted too. There are many days in Los Angeles when there are air pollution alerts due to high concentrations of chemicals in the air. Children, elderly people, and pregnant women are advised to stay indoors on those days. And driving into Boston from the west, there are many days when you can *see* the air overhanging the city. It has a yellowish-brown tinge to it. It is hard to believe that it is healthy to be breathing that air day in and day out, as a steady diet over a lifetime. Many of our cities are like this now, some even most of the time.

Clearly we as individuals have to start thinking about our air and water as food and pay attention to their quality. You can filter the tap water you use for drinking and cooking just to be on the safe side, or buy bottled water. While it seems a shame to have to pay even more for water than you might be paying now, in the long run it may be intelligent to do so, especially if you are pregnant or if you are trying to encourage your children to drink water rather than soda. Of course, this will depend on knowing how good your water is and whether bottled water is any better. In some cases, it may not be.

Protecting yourself from air pollution is another matter. If you live downwind from power plants or other industry or even just live in a city, there is little you can do as an individual, except to stay away from people who are smoking and maybe hold your breath when a city bus goes by. Only legal and political action over an extended period will have an effect on air and water quality. These are dramatic reasons why people who care about their health might want to put some of their energy into action for social change. It is in everybody's self-interest to care for the natural world. The environment is easily polluted, but it is not so easy to clean it up. We as individuals cannot detect pollution in our food. We have to depend on our institutions to keep the food supply uncontaminated. If they do not, or if they fail to establish appropriate standards or testing procedures, our health and the health of future generations may be at significantly greater risk in countless ways that we are only now coming to realize.

For instance, the pesticide DDT and PCBs from the electronics industry are now found everywhere in nature, including our own body fat and, sadly, in mother's milk. Pesticides that have been banned in the United States, such as DDT, continue to be sold by American manufacturers to Third World countries. Ironically, these pesticides are used on crops that are grown for export to the United States, such as coffee and pineapples, so that we get back, in our own food, residues of the poisons we exported for use elsewhere. (This has been described in a compelling account in *Circle of Poison*, by David Weir and Mark Schapiro).

The trouble is that while the manufacturers of the pesticides know about this, consumers in general do not. We think we are being protected by our laws about what can be used on crops and what cannot, but our laws do not govern pesticide levels used on food grown in other countries, such as Costa Rica, Colombia, Mexico, Chile, Brazil, and the Philippines, where our coffee, bananas, pineapples, peppers, and tomatoes often come from. What is more, pesticides used in the Third World are usually applied in the field by farm workers who are not given any instruction in the safe use of these products to minimize the contamination of the food, nor are they even told how to protect themselves while using these chemicals. According to the World Health Organization, there are 500,000 cases of people being poisoned by pesticides in the Third World, and thousands die from pesticide poisoning each year. Meanwhile, the global environment is rapidly becoming overloaded with pesticides: four billion pounds were produced worldwide in 1981 alone. The continued effect of this kind of saturation of the environment and of our food chain with pesticides is unknown, but is not likely to be beneficial.

We have only recently come to realize that we live on and share a small planet that can be stressed and ultimately overwhelmed by our activities. We now know that our interconnectedness extends to the planet itself. Our ecosystem, just like the human body, is a dynamic system, robust but also fragile, with its own homeostatic mechanisms that can be stressed. It has its own limits beyond which it can rapidly break down. If we fail to realize that our collective human activity is capable of throwing its cycles out of balance, then we may very well be creating the seeds of our own destruction, not just as individuals but even as a species.

Many scientists think we have already gone dangerously far along that road. The world is slowly coming to recognize that human activity can pollute the oceans to an unthinkable extent, denude the forests of Europe from acid rain, and raze the remaining tropical rain forests that provide a significant fraction of the oxygen we breathe and that cannot be replaced. Human activity also degrades croplands to the point where they cannot produce food. It pollutes the atmosphere with carbon dioxide, thereby raising the average temperature of the earth's surface. It destroys the ozone layer of the earth's atmosphere by producing and releasing fluorocarbons, thereby increasing our exposure to dangerous ultraviolet radiation from the sun. It pollutes our water and the air we breathe and contaminates the soil and the rivers and wildlife with toxic chemicals.

While such issues, when we read about them or hear them on TV, may seem remote to us or appear to be the quaint saber-rattling of romantic and hysterical wildlife and nature lovers, their effects on us may not be remote at all in the next decade or two if the destruction of the environment is not slowed. These problems could be major stressors in our lives and in the lives of future generations and a source of significant increases of disease. In this category would be the increased incidence of skin cancer that might be expected if the atmosphere becomes less and less able to filter out the harmful ultraviolet rays in the sun's light, and increased rates of cancer, miscarriages, and birth defects from greater lifetime exposures to chemicals in the environment and perhaps in food as well.

Although you can find these issues discussed and reported on in the newspapers daily, much of the time we pay them little heed, as if they don't really concern us or as if it is hopeless. Sometimes it does feel as if there is nothing that we as individuals can do.

But just becoming more aware and informed about these problems and their relationship to our health as individuals and to the health of the planet as a whole may be a significant positive first step toward bringing about change in the world. At least you have changed yourself when you become more informed and aware. You are already a small but significant part of the world, perhaps more significant than you think. By changing yourself and your own behavior in even modest ways, such as recycling reusable materials, you do change the world.

These issues affect our lives and our health even now, whether we know it or not. And they are a source of psychological as well as physical stress. Our psychological well-being may depend on being able to find someplace in nature where we can go and just hear the sounds of the world itself, without the sounds of human activity, of airplanes, cars, and machines. And, more ominously, knowing that a nuclear war between the superpowers could destroy life as we know it within twenty minutes is a psychological stress we all live with but don't like to think about. But our children know it, and some studies show that they are deeply disturbed by the possibility that their parents' generation could blow up the planet.

Unless we radically change the course of history with a new kind of thinking based on understanding wholeness, the examples of the past give us little cause for optimism. After all, there has never been a weapons system that has been invented that has not been used, except for the intermediate-range ballistic missiles. The recent destruction of these weapons by the United States and USSR is certainly a step toward eliminating the possibility of nuclear war, but it is only a first step. We ourselves found it possible to incinerate two entire cities of people, so it is not just "the other side" that is capable of unleashing violence on civilian populations, given the right combination of circumstances. We are "the other side." Perhaps what is required is to stop thinking in terms of "us" and "them" and to start thinking more in terms of "we." Recent events in the USSR and in Eastern Europe, catalyzed in part by Mikhail Gorbachev's new ways of thinking and acting, are a hopeful sign that major changes toward greater harmony on the planet are possible.

We also need to be more conscious as a society of the threat to the environment and to our health posed by the radioactive wastes produced in nuclear-weapons manufacturing and in nuclear power plants. We have no realistic ways at present of preventing contamination of the environment from these highly radioactive wastes, which remain toxic for hundreds of thousands of years. The nuclear industries and the government have always downplayed the danger to civilian populations from radioactivity and they continue to do so to this day. But the danger is undeniable. Plutonium is the most toxic substance known to man. It is manmade. One atom of it inside your body can kill you. Hundreds of pounds of it, enough to make many homemade nuclear bombs, have disappeared from weapons plants.

Such concerns are definitely deserving of our conscious attention. We encounter information about these issues every day, whether we are aware of it or not. Perhaps we should expand our concept of our diet to recognize that it also includes the information, images, and sounds that we take in and absorb in one way or another, usually without the least awareness. We live immersed in a sea of information. The new technology has made this an information age. Are we not exposed to a steady "diet" of information, which we take in daily through newspapers, the radio, and television? Does it not influence our thoughts and feelings and shape our view of the world and even of ourselves much more than we are apt to admit? Does not information constitute, in and of itself, a major stressor in many ways?

Take, for example, the fact that we are constantly taking in the details of mostly bad news from all around the world. We are usually immersed in a sea of information about death, destruction, and violence. It is a steady diet, so much so that we hardly notice it. During the Vietnam war, it was not uncommon for families to think nothing of eating dinner while watching the battle footage of the day and hearing about the body counts. Keep your radio on for a while on any day and it is likely that you will hear graphic details of rape and murder.

We consume this diet daily. You can't help but wonder what kind of effects it has on us, individually and collectively, to have such graphic and up-to-the-minute knowledge of all these disturbing problems but with virtually no power to influence them. One likely effect is that we might gradually become insensitive to what happens to other people. The fate of others may become just another part of the sea of background violence within which we live. Unless it is particularly gruesome, we may not even notice it at all.

But it does go inside us, just as all the advertisements we are exposed to are taken in. You notice this when you meditate. You begin to see that your mind is full of all sorts of things that have crept into it from the news or from advertisements. In fact, advertising people are paid very high salaries to figure out effective ways of getting their message inside your head so that you will be more likely to want and choose what they are selling.

Television and movies also figure as a large part of our standard diet nowadays, even more so with the advent of cable TV and VCRs. In the average American household, the television is on for seven hours per day according to some studies, and many children watch four to seven hours per day, more time than they spend doing anything else in their lives except sleeping. They are exposed to staggering amounts of information, images, and sounds, much of it frenetic, violent, cruel, and anxiety-producing, and all of it artificial, two-dimensional, not related to actual experiences in their lives other than TV watching itself.

Children are also exposed to images of extreme violence and sadism in popular horror movies. Grotesque and graphic simulations of reality involving killing, raping, maiming and dismemberment have become extremely popular among the young. These vivid simulations have now become part of the diet of young minds, minds that have few defenses against this kind of reality distortion.

These images have enormous power to disturb and distort the development of a balanced mind, particularly if there is nothing of equal strength in the child's life to counterbalance them. For many children, real life pales in comparison to the excitement of the movies, and it becomes harder and harder, even for the moviemakers, to maintain their viewers' interest unless they make the images more graphic and more violent with each new release.

We have no idea what this new diet for American children in the 1980s will yield in the coming decades, but there are already far too many reports of adolescents and young adults killing other people after seeing movies that they used as inspiration, as if real life were just an extension of the movies in their own minds, and as if other people's lives and fear and pain were of no value or consequence. This diet seems to be catalyzing a profound disconnection from human feelings of empathy and compassion, to the point where many children no longer identify with the pain of someone who is being victimized. One recent news article on teenage violence reported that by the time they are sixteen years old, American children have passively witnessed on the average approximately 200,000 acts of violence, including 33,000 murders on television and in the movies.

The bombardment of our nervous system with images, sounds, and information is particularly stressful if it never lets up. If you switch on the television the moment you wake up, and you have the radio on in the car on the way to work, and you watch the news when you get home, and then watch television or movies in the evening, you are filling your mind with images that have no direct relationship to your life. No matter how wonderful the show or how interesting the information, it will probably remain two-dimensional for you. Little of it has enduring value. But in consuming a steady diet of this "stuff," which feeds the mind's hunger for information and diversion, you are squeezing out of your life some very important alternatives: time for silence, for peace, for just being without anything happening; time for thinking, for playing, for doing real things. The constant agitation of our thinking minds, which we encounter so vividly in the meditation practice, is actually fed and compounded by our diet of television, radio, newspapers, and movies. We are constantly shoveling into our minds more things to react to; to think, worry, and obsess about; and to remember, as if our own daily lives did not produce enough. The irony is that we do it to get some respite from our own concerns and preoccupations, to take our mind off our troubles, to entertain ourselves, to carry us away, to help us relax.

But it doesn't work that way. Watching television hardly ever promotes physiological relaxation. Its purview is more along the lines of sensory bombardment. It is also addicting. Many children are addicted to TV and don't know what to do with themselves when it is off. It is such an easy escape from boredom that they are not challenged to find other ways of dealing with time, such as through imaginative play, drawing, painting, and reading. Television is so mesmerizing that parents use it as a baby-sitter. When it is on, at least they might get a few moments of peace. Many adults are themselves addicted to soap operas and sitcoms or news programs in a similar way. One can't help wondering about the effects of this diet on family relationships and communication.

◆

. All these observations are food for thought. Every issue we have raised here can be seen in many different lights. There are no "right" answers, and our knowledge of the intricacies of these issues is always incomplete. They are presented here as examples of our interface with what we might call world stress. They are meant to provoke and challenge you to take a closer look at your own views and behaviors and at your own local environment, so that you might cultivate mindfulness and conscious living in these areas.

Each one of us needs to come to our own way of seeing world stress. It affects us whether we like it or not and whether we ignore it or not. We touch on these issues in the stress clinic precisely because we do not live in a vacuum. The outer world and the inner world are no more separate than the mind and the body. We believe that it is important for our patients to develop conscious approaches for recognizing and working with these problems as well as with their more personal problems if they are to bring mindfulness to the totality of their lives and cope effectively with the full range of forces at work within them.

World stress will only become more intense in the future. According to Stewart Brand of *Whole Earth Catalog* fame, the not-too-distant future will bring narrowcasting and smart televisions, which will deliver to you all the information you want to know when you get home at the end of the day. The computers of the future and cellular phones and smart televisions and personal robots, all interconnected of course, will make sure that your access to information never sleeps and that it is always right at your fingertips. While this may turn out to be liberating in some ways and give us more freedom and flexibility, we will also have to be on our guard against being sucked into a mode of living in which each of us is reduced to being a walking information processor and entertainment consumer.

The more complicated the world gets and the more intrusive it becomes on our own personal psychological space and privacy, the more important it will be to practice non-doing. We will need it just to protect our sanity and to develop a greater understanding of who we are, beyond our roles, beyond our computer-access code numbers and our Social Security numbers and our credit card numbers and our secret passwords. It may be that meditation will become an absolute necessity in order for us to encounter the stressors of the twenty-first century and to remind ourselves of what it means to be human once we have one more level of smart solid-state adult toys to play with.

None of the problems we have touched on here is insurmountable. They have all been created by the human mind and by its expressions in the outer world. These problems can also be resolved by the human mind if it learns to value and develop wisdom and harmony and to see its own interests in terms of wholeness and connectedness. To do so requires us to leap beyond the impulses of mind we call fear, greed, and hatred. We can all play significant roles in making this happen by working on ourselves and on the world, too. If we can come to understand that we cannot be healthy in a world that is stressed beyond its capacity to respond and to heal, perhaps we will learn to treat our world and ourselves differently. Perhaps here, too, we will learn not to treat the symptoms, trying to make them go away, but to come to grips with their underlying causes. As with our own inner healing, the outcome will depend on how effectively we tune the instrument. To have a positive effect on the problems of the larger environment, we will need continually to tune and retune to our own center, cultivating awareness and harmony in our individual lives. Information itself is not the problem. What we must learn is to bring wise attention to the information that is at our disposal and to contemplate it and discern order and connectedness within it so that we can put it to use in the service of our own health and healing, both individual and collective.

And so we come full circle, from the outer world back to the inner world, from the larger whole back to the individual person, facing his or her own life, with his or her own breathing and body and mind. The world we live in is changing very rapidly, and we are inexorably enmeshed in those changes, whether we like it or not, whether we know it or not. Many of the changes in the world today are definitely in the direction of greater peace and harmony and health. Others clearly undermine it. All are part of the full catastrophe.

The challenge, of course, is how we are to live as people. Given world stress and food stress, work stress and role stress, people stress and sleep stress and time stress and our own fears and pain, what are we going to do this morning when we wake up? How will we conduct ourselves today? Can we be a center of peace right now? Can we live in harmony with our own being right now? Can we put our intelligence to work for us, in our inner lives and in the outer world?

The thousands of extraordinary "ordinary" people who have been through the stress clinic in the past ten years have come to face these challenges of living with greater confidence and success by cultivating awareness within themselves, by discovering for themselves that there is a healing power in mindfulness.

We cannot predict the future of the world, even for a few days, yet our own futures are intimately connected to it. But what we can do, and so often fail to do, is to own our own present, fully, as best we can, moment by moment. As we have seen, it is *here* that the future gets created, our own and the world's. What we choose to do is important. It makes a difference.

So, having looked at a number of concrete applications of mindfulness, it is time for us to come back to the practice itself and to close with a final section in which you will find further suggestions for how to make mindfulness a part of your life and how to connect up with others who share this way of being.

◆

HINTS AND SUGGESTIONS FOR DEALING WITH "WORLD STRESS"

1. Pay attention to the quality and source of your water and your food. How is the air quality where you live?

2. Be aware of your relationship to information. How much do you read the newspapers and magazines? How do you feel afterward? When do you choose to read them? Is this the best use of these moments for you? Do you act on the information you receive? In what ways? Are you aware of cravings for news and information, to the point where it suggests addiction? How is your behavior affected by your need to be stimulated and bombarded? Do you keep the radio or TV on all the time, even when you are not watching or listening? Do you read the newspaper for hours just to "kill time"? Do you get angry if it is not delivered in the morning?

3. Be aware of how you use your television. What do you choose to watch? What needs does it satisfy in you? How do you feel afterward? How often do you watch? What is the state of mind that brings you to turn it on in the first place? What is the state of mind that brings you to turn it off?

4. What are the effects of taking in bad news and violent images on your body? On your psyche? Are you ordinarily aware of this domain at all? Notice if you are feeling powerless or depressed in the face of world stress.

5. Try to identify specific issues that you care about that, if you worked on, might help you to feel more engaged and more powerful. Just doing *something,* even if it is a very "little" something, can often help you to feel as if you can have an effect, that your actions count, and that you are connected to the greater world in meaningful ways. You might be able to feel effective if you identified an important health, safety, or environmental issue in your neighborhood or town or city and worked on it, perhaps to raise other people's consciousness of a potential problem or to alleviate one that has already been identified. Since you are a part of the larger whole, it can be inwardly healing to take some responsibility for outward healing in the world. Remember the dictum "Think globally, act locally." It works the other way around too: "Think locally, act globally."

V

THE WAY OF
AWARENESS

33

New Beginnings

$\mathbf{A}$s another cycle of the stress reduction program comes to a close, I look around one last time and marvel at these people who embarked together on this journey of self-observation and healing eight short weeks ago. Their faces look different now. They sit differently. They know how to sit. We started out this morning with a twenty-minute body scan, then went from that into sitting for twenty minutes or so. The stillness was exquisite. It felt as if we could sit forever.

It feels as if they know something very simple now that somehow eluded them before. They are still the same people. Nothing much has changed on a big scale in their lives. Except, in some subtle way that comes out as we review what it has meant for them to come this far on the journey, everything.

They do not want to stop at this point. This happens each time an eight-week cycle comes to an end. It always feels as if we are just getting started. So why stop? Why not keep meeting weekly and continue practicing together?

We stop for many reasons, but the most important one has to do with developing autonomy and independence. Our learning in these eight weeks needs to be tested in the world, when we have nothing to fall back on except our own inner resources. This is part of the learning process, an important part of making the practice one's own.

The practice need not stop just because the course is over. In fact, the whole point is for the practice to keep going. This journey is a lifelong one. It is just beginning. The eight weeks is just to get us launched or to redirect the trajectory we are on. By ending the classes we are simply saying, "All right, you have the basics. Now you are on your own. You know what to do. Do it." We are purposefully taking away the external supports so that people can work at sustaining the momentum of mindfulness on their own and at fashioning their own ways of putting it to work in their lives. If we are to have the strength to face and work with the full catastrophe in our lives, our meditation practice needs a chance to develop on its own, to depend only on our own intentionality and commitment, not on a group, not on a hospital program.

When we started the clinic ten years ago, the thinking was that after eight weeks of training, people would go out on their own. Then, if they wanted to come back after six months or a year or more, we would make this an option by holding graduate programs in which they could take the practice deeper. This model has worked well over the years. The graduate classes are well attended, and clinic graduates also come back regularly to sit with us during our all-day sessions.

But today, because the clinic is approaching its tenth birthday and the staff has been thinking about new ways of doing things, I have come to class with a proposal for a new way to proceed, namely that if there is interest, we might get together now that the classes are over for monthly follow-up sessions over the next half year. In this way people would still have the opportunity to sustain the practice and the momentum they have developed over these eight weeks on their own, but they would receive support periodically along the way. The response to this proposal is unanimously favorable. Everybody is eager to make this new commitment, and so it is arranged.

◆

For you the reader, it is important to remind yourself that classes, groups, follow-up sessions, tapes, and books, can be helpful at certain junctures but they are not essential. What is essential is your vision and your commitment to practice today and then get up tomorrow and practice, too, no matter what else is on your agenda. If you follow the outline of the program our patients follow as described in Chapter 10, eight weeks should be a sufficient time to bring your meditation practice to the point where it begins to feel natural and like a way of life that you might want to continue with. You will certainly have seen before eight weeks is up that the real learning comes from within yourself. Then, by rereading sections of this book, by consulting the books on the reading list in the appendix, and, when possible, by locating other people and groups to meditate with, you can reinforce and support your practice as it grows and deepens.

♦

Looking around the room now, I am struck by the high level of enthusiasm everyone seems to have about what they have accomplished in this brief period of time and by how much they obviously respect and admire each other's strength and determination as well as their own. Their superb attendance reflected that commitment.

Edward didn't miss one day of practice. Since he had started off with the body-scan tape at my suggestion when I first saw him two months before the program began, his effort is even more impressive to me. He feels his life depends on it. He practices every lunchtime at work, either in his office or in his car in the parking lot. Then he does the body-scan tape when he gets home from work, before he does anything else. Only then does he make dinner. He says that practicing this way has lifted his spirits and helps him to feel that he can handle the physical and emotional ups and downs he is going through as a result of having AIDS, the fatigue he often feels, and the numerous tests and protocols to which he is subjected.

Peter feels he has made major changes in his life that will help him to stay healthy and prevent another heart attack. His realization when he caught himself washing his car at night in his driveway was a major eye-opener for him. He, too, continues to practice every day.

Beverly, whose experiences were described in Chapter 25, feels that the program helped her to be calmer and to believe that she can be herself in spite of her bad days. As we saw, she thought to use her meditation training in imaginative ways to maintain control during medical diagnostic procedures that frightened her.

Marge had surgery for removal of a nonmalignant mass in her abdomen right after the program ended, so I didn't get to talk with her until several months later. I had lent her a copy of the hospital stress reduction videotape, *The World of Relaxation*, which she used at home to prepare herself mentally for the surgery and to help her with her recovery in the weeks afterward, in addition to her regular meditation practice. She later told me that she was awake for the one-hour operation with an epidural block and meditated through the whole thing. She heard them talking about dissecting the tumor off the large intestine but remained calm. When she went home, she used the meditation over and over again to speed her recovery process. She said that she had no problems with pain after the anesthesia wore off, as she had had with other surgeries in the past.

She says that before she started in the program, she was wound up like a tight spring. Now she feels much more relaxed and easygoing, even though she still has as much pain in her knees as ever.

Art has fewer headaches now and feels he can prevent them from happening in stressful situations by using his breathing. He feels more relaxed, even though the particular pressures of police work are still there. He is looking forward to retiring from it. He liked the yoga best of all and said he experienced a new level of relaxation on the all-day session, when time fell away completely.

Phil, the French-Canadian truck driver we have met along the way a number of times went through some dramatic experiences with the practice. His way of speaking and his willingness to share what he was going through touched everyone in the class. He now feels he will be better able to concentrate and will not be so ruled by his back pain when he takes the exam for his insurance license. He feels that his pain is more manageable and his ability to appreciate his time with his family has made life richer.

Eight weeks later, Roger remains more or less bewildered about his life situation. He made it through the program, which surprised me, and he says he is more relaxed and less dependent on drugs for pain; but he still does not have much clarity about how to face his domestic situation. He lost his temper on at least one occasion, and his wife had to get a court order to keep him away from the house. He clearly needs some individual attention. However, he has been in therapy before and rejects the suggestion of any more at this time, much as I encourage him to pursue it again.

Eleanor is glowing like a light bulb this morning. She came to the clinic because she was having panic attacks. She hasn't had one since the program started, but she feels that if one comes up, she will know how to handle it now. The all-day session was extremely important for her. She touched areas of inner peace she said she has never known in sixty years.

And Louise, who told us on the first day that her son "made" her take the program by saying to her, 'Mom, it worked for me and now you absolutely *have* to do it," found it started helping right away with her whole attitude toward her life, as well as with her pain from rheumatoid arthritis and the restrictions it was imposing on her ability to live the way she wanted to. She found she was able to get behind her pain in the body scan and then learned to pace herself throughout her day. A few weeks ago, she triumphantly told the class of going in the car to Cooperstown for the weekend, something she would never have thought possible before. Of course she visited the Baseball Hall of Fame with family and friends, and each time that she felt she had had enough of the crowds and the press of people, she went outside, found a place to sit, closed her eyes, and just did her meditation, completely unselfconsciously, in spite of all the people. She knew that that was what she needed to do to stay balanced during this potential ordeal for her. She did it a number of times that day and that weekend and was able to sail through her trip. She exclaimed, "My son was absolutely right. I thought he was crazy, but this has given me another chance at life."

Loretta, who came for hypertension, found her life changed as well. She works as a consultant to corporations and public agencies. She said before the program that she was always afraid to show her clients the reports she had prepared for them. Now she feels much more confident about her work, declaring, "So what if they don't like it? For that matter, so what if they *like* it? Now I see that it's whether *I* feel good about it that is most important. It's made for a lot less anxiety about my work, and a lot better work too."

This insight—"so what if they do like it"—speaks volumes about Loretta's growth in the past eight weeks. She has clearly seen that she can be trapped by the positive, by approval, by acclaim, as much as by criticism and failure. She has seen that she must define her experiences on her own terms for them to hold real meaning for her. The rest is just an elaborate fiction, an illusion, although one it is easy to become stuck in.

And Hector leaves feeling he has learned to control his anger better. Since he was a wrestler and carries his three hundred pounds effortlessly, like a delicate but massive bird, it was great fun to do the pushing exercises with him. He knew how to hold his center physically, and now he knows how to hold it emotionally as well.

◆

All these people and the many others who are completing the program this week have worked hard on themselves. Most changed in one way or another, even though our emphasis was and continues to be on non-striving and self-acceptance. The gains most of them did make did not come out of idleness, nor did they come solely from attending class each week and giving each other support. They came, for the most part, out of the loneliness of the long-distance meditator, out of their willingness to sit and to be, to dwell in silence and stillness and encounter their own minds and bodies;

to practice non-doing, even when their minds and bodies resisted and clamored for something more entertaining and requiring less effort.

Before we close, Phil, who has by this time become the class storyteller, shares the following memory with us, which he says he has been carrying around since he was twelve years old, not knowing exactly why. Suddenly its meaning struck him this week as he was practicing;

"We were going to a Baptist church in Canada. It was a small church, there was maybe about ninety people going to that church, ya know. There was a lot of problems at the church at that time. And my father isn't the type of person to go to a church where there was always a kind of problem. The church is supposed to be united, ya know, and working together. And so he says, 'Let's get away from here for a while.' We knew this small church out in the country, in the middle of nowhere. It's like a four-corner, and there was the church and that was about it. There was all farmers around there. They only had a group of maybe ten, fifteen, twenty people at the most going to the church and, well, we figured we'd go there for support, ya know. They'll increase their people and we'll meet new people and make new friends.

"So we went there and they had no ministers there. Ministers would come in from here and there different Sundays and just kinda do the service. And that Sunday we were there waiting and waiting. No minister. It was way past time, so somebody decided that maybe we should start singing some hymns, ya know. And so we got together and sang a few hymns and still no minister, and it's getting late. So one guy says, well maybe someone would like to read something from the Bible and say something, ya know. Nobody said anything, wanted to do anything. But this guy stood up. He didn't have no education, didn't know how to read or nothing. He was a farmer, very plain, very maybe what some people would call uneducated, which he was, for one thing, but not dumb, ya know, just plain, not having an education. So he could not read the Bible to say something. But he asked if somebody could read the Bible for him, he knew of the passage. It was about giving. And then, being a farmer, he gave this example, he says: 'It's just like the pig and the cow had a conversation one day together. And the pig said to the cow, "How come you get grain, bought grain from the store, ya know, all the best of everything, and I get garbage from the table, garbage to eat?" And the cow says, "Well, I give every day, but you, we have to wait till you're dead to get anything good out of you.' " So he says, 'This is what the Lord wants you to do . . . give to the Lord every day, ya know, give your soul to the Lord, ya know, give praise to the Lord every day and you will be rewarded more ways than one, ya know. And don't be like the pig and wait until you're dead for God to get anything out of you.'

"So that was what the message was all about. And this is what kept on coming to my mind as I'm doing the body scan . . . and finally one day it came to me that it's the same thing with the stress reduction program. You have to give something, you have to really work at it, you have to give thanks to your body, ya know, recognize your eyes. Don't wait until you go blind and say, 'Oh my God, my eyes.' Or your feet, don't wait until you're almost crippled, or anything like this . . . your mind, I mean, they say if you had enough faith, the size of a grain of salt, you could move mountains. The same thing . . . most doctors say we use a very little bit of our brain. The brain is a very powerful thing, just like a battery in a car. It's got all kinds of power, but if you don't have good connections, you're not going to get anything out of it, ya know. You have to practice your brain to put it to work, in other words, so you'll get something out of it, ya know.

"And I says, 'My God, this is more or less what this [the stress clinic] is all about,' ya know, I kinda pictured that together. But this message that farmer gave us in church that day, this spiritual message was very powerful. I got goose bumps when I heard it and I still do. Like I say, it came to me and I just translated it as it's the same for your own body. You have to give to be able to receive. I gave this program a lot of effort and time. Sometimes I didn't feel like driving one hundred miles just for this thing. But I came to every class, never missed a meeting, always on time. But see, it's easy once you start getting something out of it. If you put your mind that you want to try, give it the best there is, all the attention you can, you'll get something out of it, ya know."

◆

It is clear as they leave the room today that most people understand that although the classes may be over, this is only the beginning. The journey really is a lifelong one. If they have found an approach that makes sense to them, it is not because someone sold it to them but because they explored it for themselves and found it of value. This is the simple path of mindfulness, of being awake in one's own life. Sometimes we call it the way of awareness.

Walking the path of awareness requires that you keep up the meditation practice. If you don't, the way tends to get overgrown and obscured. It becomes less accessible even though, at any moment that you choose, you can come back to it again because it is always right here. Even if you have not been practicing for some time, as soon as you are back with your breathing, back in the moment, you are right here again, back on the path.

In fact, once you are cultivating mindfulness systematically in your life, it is virtually impossible to stop. Even *not practicing* is practicing in a way, if you are aware of how you feel compared with when you do practice regularly and how it affects your ability to handle stress and pain.

The way to maintain and nurture mindfulness is to develop a daily momentum in the meditation practice and keep it going. The next two chapters give you some concrete and practical recommendations for keeping up both the formal and the informal mindfulness practice so that the way of awareness can lend ongoing clarity and direction to your life as it continues to unfold.

34
Keeping Up the Formal Practice

The most important part of the work of mindfulness is to keep your practice alive. The way you do that is to do it. It needs to become part of your life, in the same way that eating is or working is. We keep the practice alive by making time for being, for non-doing, no matter how much rearranging it takes. Making a time for formal practice every day is like feeding yourself every day. It is that important.

The techniques that you use are not so important. Whether you use tapes for guidance is not so important. The techniques and tapes are just ways of bringing you to yourself. The important thing is to keep coming back to the moment. The best advice for any kind of question in the meditation practice is to keep practicing, to just keep looking at the problem non-judgmentally. Over time, the practice tends to teach you what you need to know next. If you sit with your questions and your doubts, they tend to dissolve in subsequent weeks. What seemed impenetrable becomes penetrable, what seemed murky becomes clear. It is as if you are really just letting your mind settle. Thich Nhat Hanh, the Vietnamese meditation teacher, poet, and peace activist, uses the image of cloudy apple juice settling in a glass to describe meditation. You just sit . . . the mind settles itself. It *is* like that.

It will be helpful to you to reread Part I, "The Practice of Mindfulness" from time to time as your meditation practice deepens, as well as the chapters on the applications of mindfulness in Part IV that are most relevant to you. Many things that you might have thought were obvious at first become less so as the practice deepens. And some details that might not have been meaningful to you before can become more so as your practice deepens. So rereading the instructions from time to time can be helpful. They are so simple that it is easy to misunderstand them.

Even the instructions on watching the breath can be easily misunderstood. For example, many people hear the instruction to "watch" your breath to mean "think about" your breath. They are not the same. The practice does not require that you think about your breathing. It involves "being with" your breathing, observing it, feeling it. True, when the mind wanders away, thinking about your breath will bring it back into awareness. However, at that point, you go back to simply observing.

The instructions on how to handle thinking are also often misunderstood. We are not suggesting that thinking is bad and that you should suppress your thoughts so that you can concentrate on your breathing or on the body scan or on a yoga posture! The way to handle thinking is to just observe it as thinking, to be aware of thoughts as events in the field of your consciousness. Then, depending on your practice, you can do various things. For example, if you are working at developing calmness and concentration using your breathing, you let go of the thoughts and go back to the breath as soon as there is an awareness that thinking has carried your attention off the breath. Letting go is not a pushing away of your thoughts or a shutting them off, or repressing them or rejecting them. It is more gentle than that. You are allowing the thoughts to do whatever they do as you keep your attention on the breath as best you can, moment by moment.

Another way of working with thinking is to watch *it* instead of your breath. In this practice, which we do for a short while at the end of the sitting tape, you simply bring your attention to the flow of thought itself. In doing this, we are not oriented toward the content of our thoughts even though we are aware of their content. We let them register and work at just seeing them as thoughts, observing them come and go without getting pulled into their content.

In mindfulness practice it is okay to have any thoughts at all. We don't try to censor our thinking nor do we judge it as we observe it. You may find this difficult to do, especially if as a child you were brought up to believe that certain thoughts were "bad" and you were bad for having them. The work of mindfulness practice is very gentle. If a thought or a feeling is here, why not admit it and look at it? Why suppress the content we dislike and favor the content we like when, in the process, we are compromising our chance to see ourselves clearly and know our minds more as they really are?

Here is where the work of acceptance comes in. We need to remember to be gentle and kind with ourselves as we allow ourselves to be receptive not only to the breath but to any moment and what it might bring.

In the practice the pull of the mind is invariably *away* from looking deeply within, *away* from awareness of your internal state of being. The pull of our minds tends toward externals, what we have to do today, what is going on in our lives. But when these thoughts capture our attention and we momentarily become involved in their *content*, our awareness ceases at that moment. So the real practice is not what technique you are using but your commitment to wise attention from moment to moment, your willingness to see and let go, to see and let be, whatever thoughts preoccupy the mind.

Problems in addition to those stemming from misunderstanding the meditation instructions may arise that can also undermine your practice. A big one is thinking that you are getting someplace. As soon as you notice that you are feeling proficient at the meditation or that you are getting into "special states" or good "spaces," you have to be careful and watch what is going on in your mind very closely. While it is only natural to be pleased by signs of progress such as deeper concentration and calmness, liberating insights, feelings of relaxation and self-confidence, and of course changes in your body, it is very important to just let them happen without taking too much credit for them. For one thing, as we have already seen, as soon as the mind comments on an experience, it distances you from it and makes it into something else. Also, it is not really accurate for the mind to claim that "you" are responsible, that you did something. After all, the essence of the practice is *non-doing*.

The mind runs after anything and everything. One minute it might be saying how wonderful the meditation practice is, the next it is convincing you of the opposite. Neither really comes from wisdom. What is important is to recognize this impulse to build up how good your meditation practice is when it comes up and to work with it in awareness as you would work with any other thought, by letting it be and letting it go. Otherwise, practically speaking, you could easily get into talking a great deal about how wonderful meditation and yoga are, how much they have helped you, how everybody else should do them, and bit by bit, become more of an advertising agent for them than a practitioner. The more you talk, the more energy you dissipate that might serve you better if it went into your practice. If you keep an eye out for this common pitfall of meditation, your practice will grow in depth and maturity and your mind will become less ruled by its own little delusions. For this reason, we actually recommend to the people in the stress clinic at the very beginning that they not tell a lot of people that they are meditating, and also that they try not to talk *about* their meditation but just do it. This is the best way to make use of those well-intentioned but often diffuse and confused energies of mind and focus them through the lens of mindfulness.

These are some of the most common misunderstandings about the formal practice. They are all easily corrected by reminding yourself of what I saw on a T-shirt one day. It said, "Meditation, it's not what you think!"

◆

In Chapter 10 we outlined the eight-week schedule that we use in the stress clinic. For convenience it is encapsulated below. We suggest that you follow it for eight weeks and then continue on your own under your own direction. Further suggestions for keeping up your momentum and commitment are given following the eight-week schedule.

EIGHT-WEEK PRACTICE SCHEDULE

WEEKS 1 & 2	Body scan, 6 days per week, 45 minutes a day. Sitting with awareness of breathing, 10 minutes per day.
WEEKS 3 & 4	Alternate body scan with yoga (45 minutes) if possible, 6 days per week. Continue sitting with awareness of breathing, 15–20 minutes per day.
WEEKS 5 & 6	Sit 30–45 minutes per day, alternating with yoga. Begin walking meditation if you haven't already.
WEEK 7	Practice 45 minutes per day using your own choice of methods, either alone or in combination. If you have been using tapes, try not to use them this week.
WEEK 8	Go back to using tapes. Do body scan at least twice this week. Continue the sitting and the yoga.

BEYOND EIGHT WEEKS:

- Sit every day. If you feel the sitting is your major form of practice, sit for *at least* twenty minutes at a time, and preferably thirty to forty-five minutes. If you feel the body scan is your major form of practice, then make sure you sit as well for at least five to ten minutes per day. If you are having a "bad" day and have "absolutely no time," then sit for three minutes or even one minute. Anybody can find three minutes or one minute. But when you do it, let it be a minute of concentrated non-doing, letting go of time for that minute. Keep your focus on the breath for stability and calmness.
- If at all possible, try to sit in the morning. It will have a positive effect on your whole day. Other good times to practice are: (a) right away when you get home from work, before dinner; (b) before lunch, at home or in your office; (c) in the evening or late at night, especially if you are not tired; (d) any time at all . . . every moment is a good time for formal practice, sometimes.
- If you feel the body scan is your major form of practice, then do it every day for *at least* twenty minutes at a time and preferably 30 to 45 minutes.
- Practice the yoga four or more times per week for 30 minutes or more. Make sure you are doing it mindfully, especially with awareness of breathing and bodily sensations and resting between postures.

◆

You may find it helpful to practice together with other people from time to time. I make a point of going to talks or classes or group sittings as much as I can, and I also try to make time for intensive practice, times when I go off on meditation retreats, similar to our all-day sessions but longer. You might try seeking out groups in your area with whom you could sit and practice. For mindfulness sitting groups in your area, you can write to

Insight Meditation Society
Pleasant Street
Barre, Massachusetts 01005-9701

The Insight Meditation Society runs mindfulness meditation retreats led by some of the most effective and experienced meditation teachers in the world. Many of them lead retreats in different parts of the country. You can write to them for their brochure of scheduled programs. In the western part of the country, write to

Insight Meditation West
P.O. Box 909
Woodacre, California 94973

These groups both have a slightly Buddhist orientation but they do not proselytize. They provide excellent supportive environments for deepening one's meditation practice and for meeting other people who are committed to living mindfully.

Another alternative is to contact hospitals in your area that might be offering programs in stress reduction or stress management. However, be aware that most will not be offering mindfulness training. You might also contact holistic education groups of various kinds, such as Interface, in Watertown, Massachusetts; The Open Center, in New York City; and Omega Institute, in Rhinebeck, New York; and peruse their catalogs for meditation programs.

In the Boston area, you might contact

> Cambridge Insight Meditation Center
> 331 Broadway
> Cambridge, Massachusetts 02139

for meditation classes and group meditations. Here the practice is taught from the perspective of the Thai forest tradition. While it too has a Buddhist orientation, the quality of the teaching is excellent and the community it serves is broad and varied.

◆

Reading can also support your practice. Read from the books on the reading list in the appendix as well as rereading pertinent sections of this book from time to time.

◆

Finally, just sit, just breathe, and if you feel like it, allow yourself to smile inwardly.

35

Keeping Up the Informal Practice

"Dear Jon: I could write a book on how my anxieties have become controllable since I have taken the stress reduction program. . . . Moment to moment has been a real key for me, and every day I get more confident in my abilities to cope with stress. Regards, Peter." May 1988

As we have seen, the essence of mindfulness is paying attention on purpose. So keeping up the informal practice means paying attention, being awake, owning your moments. This can be great fun. You can ask yourself at any point, "Am I fully awake?" "Do I know what I am doing right now?" "Am I fully present in the doing of it?" "How does my body feel right now?" "My breathing?" "What is my mind up to?"

We have touched on numerous strategies for bringing mindfulness into daily life. You can tune in to standing, walking, listening, speaking, eating, and working. You can tune in to your thoughts, your mood states and emotions, your motives for doing things or for feeling a certain way, and, of course, the sensations in your body. You can tune in to other people, children and adults—their body language, their tension, their feelings and speech, their actions and the consequences of those actions. You can tune in to the larger environment, the feel of the air on your skin, sounds of nature, light, color, form, movement.

As long as you are awake, you can be mindful. All it takes is wanting to and remembering to bring your attention into the present moment. Once again it is important to emphasize that paying attention does not mean "thinking about." It means directly perceiving what you are attending to. Your thoughts will only be *a part* of your experience. They may or may not be an important part. Awareness means seeing the whole, perceiving the entire content and context of each moment. We can never grasp this entirely through thinking. But we can perceive it in its essence if we get beyond our thinking, to direct seeing, direct hearing, direct feeling. So mindfulness is seeing and knowing that you are seeing, hearing and knowing that you are hearing, touching and knowing that you are touching, going up the stairs and knowing that you are going up the stairs. You might respond, "Of course I know I am going up the stairs when I am going up the stairs," but mindfulness means not just knowing it as an idea, it means *being with* going up the stairs, it means moment-to-moment awareness of the experience. By practicing in this way, we can break loose from the automatic-pilot mode and gradually bring ourselves to live more in the present and know its energies more fully. Then, as we have seen, we can respond more appropriately to change and to potentially stressful situations, because we are aware of the whole and of our relationship to it. You can practice this anytime you are awake.

Chapter 9 explored the topic of mindfulness in daily life in some detail and should be reviewed for ideas for keeping up this aspect of the practice. Chapter 10 suggests a number of informal awareness exercises that we do in the stress clinic along with the formal mindfulness practice. First and foremost is practicing tuning in to our breathing in moments throughout the day. As we have seen, this anchors us in the present. It grounds us in our body and helps us to be centered and awake to the moment.

We also practice being mindful of routine activities, such as waking up in the morning, washing, getting dressed, taking out the garbage, doing errands. The essence of the informal practice is always the same. It involves inquiring of yourself, "Am I here now?" "Am I awake?" The very asking usually brings us more into the present, puts us more in touch with what we are doing.

ADDITIONAL AWARENESS EXERCISES YOU MAY FIND USEFUL

1. Try to be mindful for one minute in every hour.
2. Touch base with your breathing throughout the day wherever you are, as often as you can.

3. For one week, be aware of one pleasant event per day while it is happening. Record these, as well as your thoughts, feelings, and bodily sensations, in a calendar (see Appendix) and look for patterns.

4. During another week do the same for one unpleasant or stressful event per day while it is happening. Again, record your bodily sensations, thoughts, feelings and reactions/responses. Look for underlying patterns.

5. Bring awareness to one difficult communication per day during another week, and record what happened, what you wanted from the communication, what the other person wanted, and what actually transpired in a similar calendar (see Appendix). Look for patterns over the week. Does this exercise tell you anything about your own mental states and their consequences as you communicate with others?

6. Bring awareness to the connections between physical symptoms of distress that you might be having, such as headaches, increased pain, palpitations, rapid breathing, muscle tension, and preceding mental states and their origins. Keep a calendar of these for one full week.

7. Be mindful of your needs for formal meditation, relaxation, exercise, a healthy diet, enough sleep, intimacy and affiliation, and humor, and honor them. These needs are the mainstays of your health. If adequately attended to on a regular basis, they will provide a strong foundation for health, increase your resilience to stress and lend greater satisfaction and coherence to your life.

8. After a particularly stressful day or event, make sure that you take steps to decompress and restore balance that very day if at all possible. In particular, meditation, cardiovascular exercise, sharing time with friends, and getting enough sleep will help in the recovery process.

◆

In summary, every moment of your waking life is a moment to which you might bring greater stillness and awareness. Our suggestions for how to do this will pale next to your own as you cultivate mindfulness in your life.

36

The Way of Awareness

In our culture we are not so familiar with the notion of ways or paths. It is a concept that comes from China, the notion of a universal law of being, called the *Tao*, or simply "the way." The Tao is the world unfolding according to its own laws. Nothing is done or forced, everything just comes about. To live in accord with the Tao is to understand non-doing and non-striving. Your life is already doing itself. The challenge is whether you can see in this way and live in accordance with the way things are, to come into harmony with all things and all moments. This is the path of insight, of wisdom, and of healing. It is the path of acceptance and peace. It is the path of the mind-body looking deeply into itself and knowing itself. It is the art of conscious living, of knowing your inner resources and your outer resources and knowing also that, fundamentally, there is neither inner nor outer.

There is little of this in our education. Our schools do not emphasize being. We are left to sort that one out by ourselves. It is *doing* that is the currency of modern education. Sadly, though, it is a fragmented doing for the most part, divorced as it is from any emphasis on who is doing the doing and from what we might learn in the domain of being. So often the doing is under the pressure of time, as if we were being pushed through our lives by the pace of the world, without the luxury of stopping and taking our bearings, of knowing who is doing the doing. Awareness itself is not highly valued, nor are we taught the richness of it and how to nurture and use it.

It might have helped us considerably to have been shown, perhaps through some simple exercises in elementary school, that we are not our thoughts, that we can watch them come and go and learn not to cling to them or run after them. Even if we didn't understand it at the time, it would have been helpful just to hear it.

Likewise, it would have been helpful to know that the breath is an ally, that it leads to calmness just by watching it. Or that it is okay to just be, that we don't have to run around all the time doing or striving or competing in order to feel that we have an identity.

We may not have gotten these messages as children, but it is not too late. Anytime that you decide that it is time to connect up to the domain of your own wholeness is the right time to start. In the yogic traditions age is measured from when you started practicing, not from when you were born. So, by this point, if you have started practicing, you may now be only a few days or weeks or months old! How nice.

Strange as it may seem, this is the real work that we invite the people who are referred by their doctors to the stress clinic to engage in. It is the exploring of the notion that there is a way of being, a way of living, a way of paying attention that is like starting afresh, that is liberating in and of itself, right now, within all one's suffering and the turmoil of life. But to explore it as an idea or a philosophy would be a dead exercise in thinking, just more ideas to fill our already overcrowded minds.

You are invited, in the same spirit as our patients, to work at making the domain of being an ally in your own life, to walk the path of mindfulness and see for yourself how things change when you change the way you are in your body and in the world. As we saw at the very beginning, it is an invitation to embark on a lifelong journey, an invitation to see life as an adventure in awareness.

This adventure has all the elements of a heroic quest, a search for yourself along the path of life. It may sound farfetched to you but we see our patients as heroes and heroines in the Greek sense, on their own personal odysseys, battered about by fates and the elements and now, in their willingness to embark upon this journey of wholeness, finally treading the path toward home.

As it turns out, we don't have far to look for ourselves on this quest. At any moment we are very close to home, much closer than we think. If we can just realize the fullness of *this* moment, of *this* breath, we can find stillness and peace right here. We can be at home right now, in our body as it is.

When you walk the path of awareness, you are bringing a systematic consciousness to the experience of living that only makes living more full, more real. The fact that no one ever taught you how to do this or told you that it was worth doing is immaterial. When you are ready for this quest, it finds you. It is part of the Way for things to unfold like this. Each moment truly is the first moment of the rest of your life. Now really *is* the only time you have to live.

Mindfulness practice provides an opportunity to walk along the path of your own life with your eyes open, awake instead of half unconscious, responding consciously in the world instead of reacting automatically, mindlessly. The end result is subtly different from the other way of living in that we know that we are walking a path, that we are following a way, that we are awake and aware. No one dictates to you what that path is. No one is telling you to follow "my way." The whole point is that there is only one way, but that way manifests in as many different ways as there are people and customs and beliefs.

Our real job, with a capital J, is to find *our own way*, sailing with the winds of change, the winds of stress and pain and suffering, the winds of joy and love, until we realize that we have also never left port, that we are never far from our real selves.

There is no way to fail in this work if you pursue it with sincerity and constancy. Meditation is not relaxation spelled differently. If you do a relaxation exercise and you aren't relaxed at the end, then you have failed. But if you are practicing mindfulness, then the only thing that is really important is whether you are willing to look and to be with things as they are in any moment, including discomfort and tension and your ideas about success and failure. If you are, then there is no failure.

Similarly, if you are facing the stress in your life mindfully, you cannot fail in your responses to it. Just being aware of it is a powerful response, one that changes everything and opens up new options for growth and for doing.

But sometimes those options don't manifest right away. It may be clear what you don't want to do but not clear yet what you do want to do. These are not times of failure either. They are creative moments, moments of not knowing, moments to be patient, centered in *not knowing*. Even confusion and despair and agitation can be creative. We can work with them if we are willing to be in the present from moment to moment with awareness. This is Zorba's dance in the face of the full catastrophe. It is a movement that carries us beyond success and failure, to a way of being that allows the full spectrum of our life experiences, our hopes and our fears, to play itself out within the field of our own living.

The Way of Awareness has a structure to it. In this book we

have gone into its structure in some detail. We have touched on how it is connected to health and healing, to stress, pain and illness, and to all the ups and downs of the body, the mind, and life itself. It is a path to be traveled, to be cultivated through daily practice. Rather than a philosophy, it is a way of being, a way of living your moments and living them fully. This way only becomes yours as you travel it yourself.

Mindfulness is a lifetime's journey along a path that ultimately leads nowhere, only to who you are. The way of awareness is always here, always accessible to you, in each moment. After all is said and done, perhaps its essence can only be captured in poetry, and in the silence of your own mind and body at peace.

So, having arrived at this point on our journey together, let this moment be cradled in the vision of the poet, Pablo Neruda, in his poem "Keeping Quiet."

Now we will count to twelve
and we will all keep still.

For once on the face of the earth,
let's not speak in any language;
let's stop for one second,
and not move our arms so much.

It would be an exotic moment
without rush, without engines;
we would all be together
in a sudden strangeness.

Fishermen in the cold sea
would not harm whales
and the man gathering salt
would look at his hurt hands.

Those who prepare green wars,
wars with gas, wars with fire,
victories with no survivors,
would put on clean clothes
and walk about with their brothers
in the shade, doing nothing.

What I want should not be confused
with total inactivity.
Life is what it is about;
I want no truck with death.

If we were not so single-minded
about keeping our lives moving,
and for once could do nothing,
perhaps a huge silence
might interrupt this sadness
of never understanding ourselves
and of threatening ourselves with death.
Perhaps the earth can teach us
as when everything seems dead
and later proves to be alive.

Now I'll count up to twelve
and you keep quiet and I will go.

APPENDIX

AWARENESS
CALENDARS

READING LIST

INDEX

TAPE ORDERING
INFORMATION

AWARENESS OF PLEASANT OR UNPLEASANT EVENTS CALENDAR

Instructions: One week, be aware of one pleasant event or occurrence each day *while it is happening*. At a later time, on a calendar such as the one provided here, record in detail what it was and your experience of it. The next week, be aware of one unpleasant or stressful experience each day and record it in a similar way.

	What was the experience?	Were you aware of the pleasant (or unpleasant) feelings *while* the event was happening?	How did your body feel, in detail, during this experience? Describe the sensations you felt.	What moods, feelings, and thoughts accompanied this event at the time?	What thoughts are in your mind now as you write this down?
MONDAY					
TUESDAY					
WEDNESDAY					

THURSDAY			
FRIDAY			
SATURDAY			
SUNDAY			

AWARENESS OF A DIFFICULT OR STRESSFUL COMMUNICATION CALENDAR

Instructions: One week, be aware of one difficult or stressful communication each day *while it is happening*. At a later time, record the details of your experience on a calendar such as the one provided here.

	Describe the communication. With whom? What was the subject?	How did the difficulty come about?	What did you really want from the person or situation? What did you actually get?	What did the other person[s] want? What did they actually get?	How did you feel during and after this time?	Has this issue been resolved yet? How might it be?
MONDAY						
TUESDAY						
WEDNESDAY						

THURSDAY

FRIDAY

SATURDAY

SUNDAY

READING LIST

MINDFULNESS MEDITATION

Beck, C. *Nothing Special*. San Francisco: Harper Collins, 1993.

Goldstein, J. *One Dharma: The Emerging Western Buddhism*. San Francisco: Harper, 2002.

Goldstein, J., and J. Kornfield. *Seeking the Heart of Wisdom: The Path of Insight Meditation*. Boston: Shambhala, 1987.

Gunaratana, H. *Mindfulness in Plain English*. Boston: Wisdom, 1993.

Hahn, T. N. *The Heart of the Buddha's Teachings*. New York: Broadway, 1998.

Hahn, T. N. *The Miracle of Mindfulness*. Boston: Beacon, 1976.

Kabat-Zinn, J. *Coming to Our Senses: Healing Ourselves and the World Through Mindfulness*. New York: Hyperion, 2005.

Kabat-Zinn, J. *Wherever You Go, There You Are: Mindfulness Meditation in Everyday Life*. New York: Hyperion, 1994.

Krishnamurti, J. *This Light in Oneself: True Meditation*. Boston: Shambhala, 1999.

Levine, S. *A Gradual Awakening*. Garden City, NY: Anchor/Doubleday, 1979.

Rosenberg, L. *Breath by Breath*. Boston: Shambhala, 1998.

Rosenberg, L. *Living in the Light of Death*. Boston: Shambhala, 2000.

Salzberg, S. *Lovingkindness*. Boston: Shambhala, 1995.

Santorelli, S. *Heal Thy Self: Lessons on Mindfulness in Medicine*. New York: Bell Tower, 1999.

Sheng-yen, C. *Hoofprints of the Ox*. New York: Oxford University Press, 2001.

Suzuki, S. *Zen Mind, Beginner's Mind*. New York: Weatherhill, 1970.

Thera, N. *The Heart of Buddhist Meditation*. New York: Weiser, 1962.

APPLICATIONS OF MINDFULNESS AND OTHER BOOKS ON MEDITATION

Bennett-Goleman, T. *Emotional Alchemy: How the Mind Can Heal the Heart*. New York: Harmony, 2001.

Brantley, J. *Calming Your Anxious Mind: How Mindfulness and Compassion Can Free You from Anxiety, Fear, and Panic*. Oakland, CA: New Harbinger, 2003.

Epstein, M. *Thoughts Without a Thinker*. New York: Basic Books, 1995.

Goleman, D. *Destructive Emotions: How We Can Heal Them*. New York: Bantam, 2003.

Kabat-Zinn, M., and J. Kabat-Zinn. *Everyday Blessings: The Inner Work of Mindful Parenting*. New York: Hyperion, 1997.

McLeod, K. *Wake Up to Your Life*. San Francisco: Harper, 2001.

McManus, C. A. *Group Wellness Programs for Chronic Pain and Disease Management.* St. Louis, MO: Butterworth-Heinemann, 2003.

McQuaid, J. R., and P. E. Carmona. *Peaceful Mind: Using Mindfulness and Cognitive Behavioral Psychology to Overcome Depression.* Oakland, CA: New Harbinger, 2004.

Segal, Z. V., J.M.G. Williams, and J. D. Teasdale. *Mindfulness-Based Cognitive Therapy for Depression: A New Approach to Preventing Relapse.* New York: Guilford, 2002.

Tolle, E. *The Power of Now.* Novato, CA: New World Library, 1999.

Wallace, B. A. *Tibetan Buddhism from the Ground Up.* Somerville, MA: Wisdom, 1993

Williams, J.M.G., Z. V. Segal, J. D. Teasdale, and J. Kabat-Zinn. *Mindfulness and the Transformation of Emotion.* New York: Guilford, 2005.

YOGA AND STRETCHING

Boccio, F. J. *Mindfulness Yoga.* Boston: Wisdom, 2004.

Christensen, A. and D. Rankin. *Easy Does It Yoga: Yoga for Older People.* New York: Harper and Row, 1979.

Iyengar, B.K.S. *Light on Yoga,* revised edition. New York: Schocken, 1977.

Kraftsow, G. *Yoga for Wellness.* New York: Penguin/Arkana, 1999.

Meyers, E. *Yoga and You.* Toronto: Random House Canada, 1996.

HEALING

Goleman, D. *Healing Emotions: Conversations with the Dalai Lama on Mindfulness, Emotions, and Health.* Boston: Shambhala, 1997.

Halpern, S. *The Etiquette of Illness: What to Say When You Can't Find the Words.* New York: Bloomsbury, 2004.

Lerner, M. *Choices in Healing: Integrating the Best of Conventional and Complementary Approaches to Cancer.* Cambridge, MA: MIT Press, 1994.

Meili, T. *I Am the Central Park Jogger.* New York: Scribner, 2003.

Moyers, B. *Healing and the Mind.* New York: Doubleday, 1993.

Ornish, D. *Love and Survival: The Scientific Basis for the Healing Power of Intimacy.* New York: HarperCollins, 1998.

Remen, R. *Kitchen Table Wisdom: Stories that Heal.* New York: Riverhead, 1997.

Simmons, P. *Learning to Fall: The Blessings of an Imperfect Life.* New York: Bantam, 2002.

Tarrant, J. *The Light Inside the Dark: Zen, Soul, and the Spiritual Life.* New York: HarperCollins, 1998.

Tenzen Gyatso (the 14th Dalai Lama). *The Compassionate Life.* Boston: Wisdom, 2003.

STRESS

LaRoche, L. *Relax—You May Have Only a Few Minutes Left: Using the Power of Humor to Overcome Stress in Your Life and Work.* New York: Villard, 1998.

Rechtschafffen, S. *Time Shifting: Creating More Time to Enjoy Your Life.* New York: Doubleday, 1996.

PAIN

Cohen, D. *Finding a Joyful Life in the Heart of Pain: A Meditative Approach to Living with Physical, Emotional, or Spiritual Suffering.* Boston: Shambhala, 2000.

Dillard, J. N. *The Chronic Pain Solution.* New York: Bantam, 2002.

Sarno, J. E. *Healing Back Pain: The Mind-Body Connection.* New York: Warner, 2001.

POETRY

Eliot, T. S. *Four Quartets.* New York: Harcourt Brace, 1977.

Lao-Tzu. *Tao Te Ching.* (Stephen Mitchell, transl.) New York: HarperCollins, 1988.

Mitchell, S. *The Enlightened Heart.* New York: Harper and Row, 1989.

Whyte, D. *The Heart Aroused: Poetry and the Preservation of the Soul in Corporate America.* New York: Doubleday, 1994.

OTHER BOOKS OF INTEREST, SOME MENTIONED IN THE TEXT

Bohm, D. *Wholeness and the Implicate Order.* London: Routledge and Kegan Paul, 1980.

Karr-Morse, R., and M. S. Wiley. *Ghosts from the Nursery: Tracing the Roots of Violence.* New York: Atlantic Monthly Press, 1997.

Kazanjian, V. H., and P. L. Laurence, (eds). *Education as Transformation.* New York: Peter Lang, 2000.

Lappe, F. M. *Diet for a Small Planet.* New York: Ballantine, 1971.

Luke, H. *Old Age: Journey into Simplicity.* New York: Parabola, 1987.

Miller, A. *For Your Own Good: Hidden Cruelty in Childrearing and the Roots of Violence.* New York: Farrar, Straus and Giroux, 1983.

Montague, A. *Touching: The Human Significance of the Skin.* New York: Harper and Row, 1978.

Ravel, J.F., and M. Ricard. *The Monk and the Philosopher: A Father and Son Discuss the Meaning of Life.* New York: Schocken, 1998.

Schwartz, J. M., and S. Begley. *The Mind and the Brain: Neuroplasticity and the Power of Mental Force.* New York: HarperCollins, 2002.

Varela F. J., E. Thompson, and E. Rosch. *The Embodied Mind: Cognitive Science and Human Experience,* Cambridge: MIT Press, 1991.

SELECTED SCIENTIFIC PAPERS ON MINDFULNESS AND MBSR

Baer, R. A. Mindfulness training as a clinical intervention: A conceptual and clinical review. *Clinical Psychology: Science and Practice* (2003) *10*:123–143.

Carlson, L. E., Z. Ursuliak, E. Goodey, M. Angen, and M. Specca. The effects of a mindfulness meditation–based stress reduction program on mood and symptoms of stress in cancer outpatients: 6-month follow-up. *Supportive Care in Cancer* (2001) *9*:112–123.

Davidson, R. J., J. Kabat-Zinn, J. Schumacher, et al. Alterations in brain and immune function produced by mindfulness meditation. *Psychosom Med* (2003) *65*:564–570.

Epstein, R. M. Mindful Practice. *JAMA* (1999) *282*:833–839.

Kabat-Zinn, J. An out-patient program in Behavioral Medicine for chronic pain patients based on the practice of mindfulness meditation: Theoretical considerations and preliminary results. *Gen Hosp Psychiatry* (1982) *4*:33–47.

Kabat-Zinn, J., L. Lipworth, and R. Burney. The clinical use of mindfulness meditation for the self-regulation of chronic pain. *J Behav Med* (1985) *8*:163–190.

Kabat-Zinn, J., L. Lipworth, R. Burney, and W. Sellers. Four year follow-up of a meditation-based program for the self-regulation of chronic pain: Treatment outcomes and compliance. *Clin J Pain* (1986) *2*:159–173.

Kabat-Zinn, J., and A. Chapman-Waldrop. Compliance with an outpatient stress reduction program: rates and predictors of completion. *J. Behav Med* (1988) *11*:333–352.

Kabat-Zinn, J., A. O. Massion, J. Kristeller, L. G. Peterson, K. Fletcher, L. Pbert, W. Linderking, S. F. Santorelli. Effectiveness of a meditation-based stress reduction program in the treament of anxiety disorders. *Am J Psychiatry* (1992) *149*:936–943.

Kabat-Zinn, J., E. Wheeler, T. Light, A. Skillings, M. Scharf, T. G. Cropley, D. Hosmer, and J. Bernhard. Influence of a mindfulness-based stress reduction intervention on rates of skin clearing in patients with moderate to severe psoriasis undergoing phototherapy (UVB) and photochemotherapy (PUVA). *Psychosom Med* (1998) *60*:625–632.

Kabat-Zinn, J. Participatory Medicine. *J Euro Acad Dermatol Venereol* (2000) *14*:239–240.

Kabat-Zinn, J. Mindfulness: The Heart of Rehabilitation. Foreword to *Complementary and Alternative Medicine in Rehabilitation*, E. Leskowitz (ed.) Churchill Livingstone, 2000, xi–xiv.

Kabat-Zinn, J. Mindfulness-based interventions in context: Past, present, and future. *Clin Psychol Sci Pract*, (2003) *10*:144–156.

Marcus, M. T., M. Fine, and K. Kouzekanani. Mindfulness-based meditation in a therapeutic community. *J Substance Abuse* (2001) *5*:305–311.

Miller, J., K. Fletcher, and J. Kabat-Zinn. Three-year follow-up and clinical implications of a mindfulness-based stress reduction intervention in the treatment of anxiety disorders. *Gen Hosp Psychiatry* (1995) *17*:192–200.

Randolph, P. D., Y. M. Caldera, A. M. Tacone, et al. The long-term combined effects of medical treatment and a mindfulness-based behavioral program for the multidisciplinary management of chronic pain in West Texas. *Pain Digest* (1999) *9*:103–112.

Reibel D. K., J. M. Greeson, G. C. Brainard, and S. Rosenzweig. Mindfulness-based stress reduction and health-related quality of life in a heterogeneous patient population. *Gen Hosp Psychiatry* (2001) *23*:183–192.

Roth, B. Mindfulness-based stress reduction in the inner city. *Advances in Mind-Body Health* (1997) *13*:50–58.

Roth, B., and T. Creaser. Mindfulness meditation–based stress reduction: Experience with a bilingual inner-city program. *The Nurse Practitioner* (1997) *22*:150–176.

Roth, B. and D. Robbins. Mindfulness-based stress reduction and health-related quality of life: Findings from a bilingual inner-city patient population. *Psychsomatic Med* (2004) *66*:113–123.

Saxe, G. A., J. R. Hebert, J. F. Carmody, J. Kabat-Zinn, et al. Can diet, in conjunction with stress reduction, affect the rate of increase in prostate-specific antigen after biochemical recurrence of prostate cancer? *J Urology* (2001) *166*:2202–2207.

Segal, Z. V., J.M.G. Williams, and J. D. Teasdale. *Mindfulness-Based Cognitive Therapy for Depression: A New Approach to Preventing Relapse.* New York: Guilford, 2002.

Shapiro, S. L., and G. E. Schwartz. Mindfulness in medical education: Fostering the health of physicians and medical practice. *Integrative Med* (1998) *1*:93–94.

Shapiro, S. L., G. E. Schwartz, G. Bonner. Effects of mindfulness-based stress reduction on medical and premedical students. *J Behav Med* (1998) *21*:581–599.

Shapiro, S. L., and G. E. Schwartz. Intentional systemic mindfulness: An integrative model for self-regulation and health. *Advances* (2000) *16*:128–134.

Speca, M., L. E. Carlson, E. Goodey, and E. Angen. A randomized wait-list controlled clinical trial: The effects of a mindfulness meditation–based stress reduction program on mood and symptoms of stress in cancer outpatients. *Psychosom Med* (2000) *6*:2613–2622.

Teasdale, J. D., Z. V. Segal, J.M.G. Williams, V. A. Ridgeway, et al. Prevention of relapse/recurrence in major depression by mindfulness-based cognitive therapy. *J Consult Clin Psychol* (2000) *68*:615–623.

Weissbecker, I., P. Salmon, J. L. Stuidts, A. R. Floyd, E. A. Dedert, S. E. Sephton. Mindfulness-based stress reduction and sense of coherence among women with fibromyalgia. *J Clin Psycol Med Settings* (2002) *4*:297–307.

Williams, K. A., M. M. Kolar, B. E. Reger, and J. C. Pearson. Evaluation of a wellness-based mindfulness stress reduction intervention: A controlled trial. *Am J Health Promotion* (2001) *15*:422–432.

WEB SITES

www.umassmed.edu/cfm Website of the Center for Mindfulness, UMass Medical School

www.mindandlife.org Website of the Mind and Life Institute

INDEX

Wise attention, 279–281
Workaholism, 257–258, 383–384
Work stress, 211, 386–395
    automatic-pilot and, 388
    change and, 387–388
    control and, 386
    example of reduction of, 390–392
    hints and suggestions for reduction
      of, 393–395
    wholeness concept and, 387–389
World Health Organization, 412
World of Relaxation, The (TV program),
    180–182
World stress, 410–420
    future, 417–418
    hints and suggestions for dealing
      with, 419–420
    information, 414–415
    movies, 415–416
    nuclear weapons and waste, 413–414
    pollution, 410–413
    television, 415–417
Wounds, psychological, 226

Xanax, 277, 363

Yoga, 94–113
    being mode and, 96–97
    benefits of, 100
    body awareness and, 97–98
    breathing in, 103–105
    concept of, 101
    healing and, 168, 171
    importance of, 98–100
    postures in, 102–113
    practice schedule for, 142, 144, 145,
      434, 435
    procedures, 103–105
    rejuvenating effect of, 100
    sleep stress and, 363, 364
    trust and, 36

Zantac, 277
Zone purification, 87–88
Zorba the Greek (film), 5

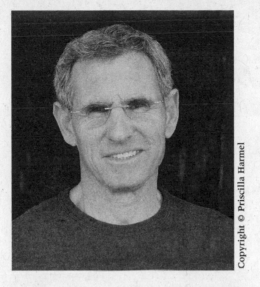

Copyright © Priscilla Harmel

JON KABAT-ZINN, Ph.D., is a scientist, writer, and meditation teacher engaged in bringing mindfulness into the mainstream of medicine and society. He is Professor of Medicine emeritus at the University of Massachusetts Medical School, where he was founding executive director of the Center for Mindfulness in Medicine, Health Care, and Society, and founder and former director of its world-renowned Stress Reduction Clinic. He is the author of *Wherever You Go, There You Are: Mindfulness Meditation in Everyday Life, Coming to Our Senses: Healing Ourselves and the World Through Mindfulness,* and coauthor, with his wife Myla, of *Everyday Blessings: The Inner Work of Mindful Parenting.* He is also Senior Advisor to the Consortium of Academic Health Centers on Integrative Medicine, and a board member of the Mind and Life Institute, a group that organizes dialogues between the Dalai Lama and Western scientists. He lectures and leads retreats on mindfulness-based stress reduction for health professionals worldwide.

Mindfulness Meditation Practice CDs
with Jon Kabat-Zinn

There are three sets of Mindfulness Meditation Practice CDs.

They can be ordered directly from the web site:
www.mindfulnesstapes.com

Series 1 (4 CDs) contains the guided meditations [the body scan and sitting meditation] and guided mindful yoga practices used by people who enrolled in Dr. Kabat-Zinn's classes in the Stress Reduction Clinic at the University of Massachusetts Medical Center. These practices are described in detail in this book. Each CD is 45 minutes in length.

◆

Series 2 (4 CDs) is designed for people who want a range of shorter guided meditations to help them develop and/or expand a personal meditation practice based on mindfulness. The series includes the mountain and lake meditations (each 20 minutes) as well as a range of other 10 minute, 20 minute, and 30 minute sitting and lying down practices. This series was originally developed to accompany *Wherever You Go, There You Are.*

◆

Series 3 (4 CDs) is designed to accompany Dr. Kabat-Zinn's latest book, *Coming to Our Senses.* Program include mindfulness of breath and body sensations; mindfulness of sounds and hearing; mindfulness of thoughts and feelings; the practice of choiceless awareness; and lovingkindness meditation. All programs are 20–30 mintes in length.

For more information, as well as to order,
see *www.mindfulnesstapes.com*

Note: **Series 1** and **Series 2** are also available as audiocassette programs.

Mindfulness Meditation Practice Tapes
with Jon Kabat-Zinn

Name _____

Address _____

_____

City / State / Zip _____

Country* _____

Telephone (____) _____

Please note: Telephone orders cannot be accepted.

Send orders to:

STRESS REDUCTION TAPES

P.O. BOX 547

LEXINGTON, MA 02420

SERIES I	# of sets		Total $
Set of 2 tapes	_____	$20.00 per set	_____
	add $2.00 *per set* for postage & handling		_____
	Massachusetts residents add 5% ($1.00) sales tax *per set*		_____
		TOTAL SERIES I ORDER	_____

All order shipped First Class.

*For orders outside North America, please *add an* ADDITIONAL *postage
charge of $3.00 per set.*

SEE NEXT PAGE FOR METHOD OF PAYMENT

METHOD OF PAYMENT

Check ❑   Amount Enclosed $ _____

Visa ❑   MasterCard ❑   DiscoverCard ❑   American Express ❑

ACCOUNT NUMBER

| | | | | | | | | | | | | | | | |

MO / YR

_____ / _____

Expiration Date

_____

Signature of Authorized Buyer

Make checks payable to: STRESS REDUCTION TAPES

For tape orders from outside the U.S. please use credit card,
or check drawn on a U.S. bank in U.S. dollars, or an International
Postal Money Order in U.S. dollars

For more information on these and other mindfulness meditation
practice tapes by Dr. Kabat-Zinn, or to place a secure order online via the
internet, please visit the Stress Reduction Tapes website at
www.mindfulnesstapes.com